THE PSYCHOLOGICAL CONSTRUCTION OF EMOTION

Also Available

Emotion and Consciousness
Edited by Lisa Feldman Barrett, Paula M. Niedenthal,
and Piotr Winkielman

Handbook of Emotions, Third Edition
Edited by Michael Lewis, Jeannette M. Haviland-Jones,
and Lisa Feldman Barrett

The Mind in Context
Edited by Batja Mesquita, Lisa Feldman Barrett,
and Eliot R. Smith

The Wisdom in Feeling:
Psychological Processes in Emotional Intelligence
Edited by Lisa Feldman Barrett and Peter Salovey

THE PSYCHOLOGICAL CONSTRUCTION OF EMOTION

Edited by

Lisa Feldman Barrett
James A. Russell

THE GUILFORD PRESS
New York   London

Library of Congress Cataloging-in-Publication Data

The psychological construction of emotion / edited by Lisa Feldman Barrett,
James A. Russell.
    pages cm
  Includes bibliographical references and index.
  ISBN 978-1-4625-1697-1 (hardback)
  1. Emotions.   I. Barrett, Lisa Feldman.   II. Russell, James A.
(James Albert), 1947–
  BF531.P776 2014
  152.4—dc23

                                     2014025248

About the Editors

Lisa Feldman Barrett, PhD, is University Distinguished Professor of Psychology and Director of the Interdisciplinary Affective Science Laboratory at Northeastern University, with research appointments at Harvard Medical School and Massachusetts General Hospital. Dr. Barrett's research focuses on the nature of emotion from both psychological and neuroscience perspectives, and incorporates insights from anthropology, philosophy, linguistics, and the history of psychology. She is the recipient of a Pioneer Award from the National Institutes of Health, among numerous other awards, and is a Fellow of the Royal Society of Canada, the American Association for the Advancement of Science, and the Association for Psychological Science. She was a founding Editor-in-Chief of the journal *Emotion Review* and cofounder of the Society for Affective Science. Dr. Barrett has published more than 160 papers and book chapters.

James A. Russell, PhD, is Professor of Psychology and Director of the Emotion Development Lab at Boston College. His research centers on human emotion, with interests in how large-scale environments influence emotion, the nature of emotion, how emotions can be described and assessed, a circumplex model of core affect, cultural similarities and differences in emotion concepts, and the perception of emotion from facial expressions. Dr. Russell is an Editor-in-Chief of *Emotion Review* and a Fellow of the American Psychological Association and the Association for Psychological Science. He has published more than 100 articles in scientific journals.

Contributors

Lisa Feldman Barrett, PhD, Department of Psychology, Northeastern University, Boston, Massachusetts

Lawrence W. Barsalou, PhD, Department of Psychology, Emory University, Atlanta, Georgia

William Bechtel, PhD, Department of Philosophy and Interdisciplinary Program in Cognitive Science, University of California, San Diego, La Jolla, California

Kent C. Berridge, PhD, Department of Psychology, University of Michigan, Ann Arbor, Michigan

Michael Boiger, PhD, Center for Social and Cultural Psychology, University of Leuven, Leuven, Belgium

Gerald Clore, PhD, Department of Psychology, University of Virginia, Charlottesville, Virginia

James A. Coan, PhD, Department of Psychology, University of Virginia, Charlottesville, Virginia

Mercè Correa, PhD, Division of Behavioral Neuroscience, Department of Psychology, University of Connecticut, Storrs, Connecticut

William A. Cunningham, PhD, Department of Psychology and Marketing, University of Toronto, Toronto, Ontario, Canada

Kristen Dunfield, PhD, Department of Psychology, Concordia University, Montreal, Quebec, Canada

Jennifer M. B. Fugate, PhD, Department of Psychology, University of Massachusetts Dartmouth, Dartmouth, Massachusetts

Marlen Z. Gonzalez, MA, Department of Psychology, University of Virginia, Charlottesville, Virginia

Mitchell Herschbach, PhD, Department of Philosophy, California State University, Northridge, Northridge, California

Ian R. Kleckner, PhD, Department of Psychology, Northeastern University, Boston, Massachusetts

Morten L. Kringelbach, DPhil, Department of Psychiatry, Warneford Hospital, University of Oxford, Oxford, United Kingdom, and Centre for Functionally Integrative Neuroscience, University of Aarhus, Aarhus, Denmark

Joseph LeDoux, PhD, Center for Neural Science, New York University, New York, New York

Kristen A. Lindquist, PhD, Department of Psychology, University of North Carolina at Chapel Hill, Chapel Hill, North Carolina

Batja Mesquita, PhD, Center for Social and Cultural Psychology, University of Leuven, Leuven, Belgium

Eric J. Nunes, PhD, Division of Behavioral Neuroscience, Department of Psychology, University of Connecticut, Storrs, Connecticut

Suzanne Oosterwijk, PhD, Department of Psychology, University of Amsterdam, Amsterdam, The Netherlands

Andrew Ortony, PhD, Department of Psychology, Northwestern University, Evanston, Illinois

Karen S. Quigley, PhD, Department of Psychology, Northeastern University, Boston, Massachusetts, and Edith Nourse Rogers Memorial VA Hospital, Bedford, Massachusetts

Patrick A. Randall, PhD, Division of Behavioral Neuroscience, Department of Psychology, University of Connecticut, Storrs, Connecticut

James A. Russell, PhD, Department of Psychology, Boston College, Chestnut Hill, Massachusetts

John D. Salamone, PhD, Division of Behavioral Neuroscience,
Department of Psychology, University of Connecticut, Storrs, Connecticut

Andrea Scarantino, PhD, Department of Philosophy and Neuroscience Institute,
Georgia State University, Atlanta, Georgia

Tobias Schröder, PhD, Institute for Urban Futures, Potsdam University
of Applied Sciences, Potsdam, Germany

Paul E. Stillman, MA, Department of Psychology, The Ohio State University,
Columbus, Ohio

Paul Thagard, PhD, Department of Philosophy, University of Waterloo,
Waterloo, Ontario, Canada

Alexandra Touroutoglou, PhD, Department of Neurology,
Harvard Medical School, Charlestown, Massachusetts

Christine D. Wilson-Mendenhall, PhD, Department of Psychology,
Northeastern University, Boston, Massachusetts

Acknowledgments

Preparation of this volume was supported by a National Institutes of Health Director's Pioneer Award (DP1OD003312), by U.S. Army Research Institute for the Behavioral and Social Sciences contracts (W5J9CQ-11-C-0046 and W5J9CQ-11-C-0049), and by grants R01 AG030311, R01 MH093394, and R21MH099605 awarded to Lisa Feldman Barrett. The views, opinion, and/or findings contained in this volume are solely those of the authors and should not be construed as an official Department of the Army or Department of Defense position, policy, or decision.

Contents

PART III. CORE AFFECT

PART IV. COMMENTARY AND CONSILIENCE

PART V. INTEGRATION AND REFLECTION

THE PSYCHOLOGICAL CONSTRUCTION OF EMOTION

CHAPTER 1

An Introduction to Psychological Construction

LISA FELDMAN BARRETT
JAMES A. RUSSELL

Two Intuitive Theories of the Human Mind

Throughout the ages, the human mind has been understood using two intuitive theories within the Western philosophical and scientific tradition. In the first theoretical approach, the mind is understood as a collection of separate and independent abilities, or *faculties*, that reflect separate *processes*, each with its own *distinct physical properties* that are innate (neurons in a brain region, a modular brain circuit, or bodily correlate). This is known as *faculty psychology*. In the second approach, the mind is understood as an ongoing stream of mental activity, or sequences of *mental states*, that are caused by a set of *common or domain-general processes* (with physical properties typically left unspecified). This second theoretical approach has been called by many different names, but these have recently been united and collectively are referred to as *psychological construction* or just *construction* (cf. Gendron & Barrett, 2009; Lindquist & Barrett, 2012). The last several thousand years of Western scholarly inquiry into the nature of the mind can be understood as an ongoing debate between these two intuitive theories of how the mind is structured.

The faculty psychology approach is the de facto "common-sense" approach, in which the mind is presumed to comprise a number of independent psychological abilities. Faculties are often conceived of as functionally encapsulated "mental organs" akin to the organs of the body (e.g., Chomsky, 1980; de Gelder & Vandenbulcke, 2012; Fodor, 1983; Wolff, as discussed in Klein, 1970). Although the assumptions of faculty psychology

1

date back as early as the Greek philosophers (see Klein, 1970, and Uttal, 2001, for reviews), Christian Wolff (1679–1754) is credited as the first faculty psychologist, because he clearly argued that the mind contains as many faculties as there are words to describe them. Wolff believed that the categories humans name with words have a deep metaphysical essence that makes them what they are (that is, he engaged in what modern-day psychologists refer to as "psychological essentialism"; Medin & Ortony, 1989). Some faculty psychologists went further by suggesting that each mental faculty has a specific and distinct physical cause in the brain (e.g., Broca, 1865, cited in Berker, Berker & Smith, 1986; Gall, 1835; Spurzheim, 1832). For much of its history, neuroscience has used faculty psychology assumptions to understand the functional architecture of the human brain (cf. Uttal, 2001). Faculty psychology is implicit in folk psychology, has often been referred to as the "common-sense" approach to psychology, and has had tremendous gravitational pull as an explanatory framework within scientific psychology.

Because psychological construction approaches have not really been unified as a philosophical or scientific tradition until recently, there is still work to be done in tracing the exact history of these ideas in philosophy of mind and neuroscience. Still, there are some easily recognizable clues. For example, empiricist philosophers (who believed that mental life is built from sensation) criticized the faculty psychology idea that innate mental powers structure the human mind. Also, the associationist philosophers argued against faculty psychology by claiming that mental states are complex events assembled from simpler, constituting elements, and a science of the mind should discover these elements. Even behaviorism can be thought of as a type of constructionist approach (in which all behavior results from a common set of learning principles). And there are also examples, within neuroscience, that were early arguments against the strong localizationist ideas of Broca (another faculty psychologist) that have a constructionist flavor (for a discussion, see Harrington, 1987).

As mental philosophy transformed into the science of psychology in the mid 1800s, this debate on the structure of the mind was clearly in evidence. Both James (1884, 1890/1950) and Wundt (1897/1998) were highly critical of faculty psychology as a basis for the scientific study of the mind. They believed that faculties were nothing but subjective categories, and that such categories could not support scientific induction. For example, James (1890/1950, p. 195) argued:

> The cardinal passions of our life, anger, love, fear, hate, hope, and the most comprehensive divisions of our intellectual activity, to remember, expect, think, know, dream, with the broadest genera of aesthetic feeling, joy, sorrow, pleasure, pain, are the only facts of a subjective order which this vocabulary deigns to note by special words.

In a similar vein, Wundt (1897/1998, p. 2) argued that even internal versus external sensations were not different in kind, "but different points of view from which we start in the consideration and scientific treatment of a unitary experience."

As an alternative to faculty psychology, James and Wundt both assumed that mental states are constituted from more basic, domain-general ingredients. For example, when writing about emotion, James described his proposed ingredients in physiological and motor terms, arguing that emotions can be reduced to the perception of afferent information from the body. Wundt, on the other hand, described his ingredients in psychological terms, arguing that subjective feelings of the body as pleasant or unpleasant, highly arousing or quiescent (i.e., "affect"), form the core of all mental life. According to Wundt, representations of prior experiences (i.e., "ideas") help make that affect meaningful as an emotion or thought. Unlike James, who treated the ingredients (physical changes) and the resultant (mental states such as emotions) as separate phenomena, Wundt assumed that emotions *emerge from* the elements. Unfortunately for James and Wundt, it was difficult to identify the basic elements of the mind in the 19th century. They had to rely on either introspection or the limited experimental methods available at the time, and solid scientific evidence was not particularly forthcoming using either approach. Both men were dismissed for a time for various reasons (Wundt was mistakenly accused of relying on introspection (Danziger, 1980), and James was dismissed for his unsophisticated understanding of the relation between the peripheral and central nervous systems (e.g., Cannon, 1927). During this same period, however, faculty psychology did not fare well in the laboratory, and psychology turned to functionalism, then ultimately to behaviorism as a solution. In the process, the mind was abandoned as a viable topic of scientific study. When psychology finally returned to the study of the mind during the cognitive revolution, a more sophisticated version of faculty psychology emerged from the ashes to dominate psychological science for decades.

Since then, history has been repeating itself. Whether explicitly labeled or not, constructionist theories have emerged in many domains of psychology and neuroscience applying to memory, perception, concept development, person perception, social categories, psychopathology, and the functional architecture of the brain (e.g., Barrett & Satpute, 2013; Bechtel, 2008; Bruner, 1990; Mareschal et al., 2007; Hassabis & Macguire, 2009; Jablonski, 2012; Lindquist & Barrett, 2012; Menon, 2011; Neisser, 1976; D. L. Schacter, 2012; D. L. Schacter & Addis, 2007; Spunt & Lieberman, 2012; Xu & Kushnir, 2013). Furthermore, without explicitly labeling their work "constructionist," a handful of psychologists beginning in the early 20th century wrote about emotional phenomena as events that emerge from more basic processes (in chronological order: Harlow & Stagner, 1932, 1933; Duffy, 1934a, b; 1941; Hunt, 1941; S. Schachter & Singer, 1962;

Mandler, 1975, 1990). Recently, these views were collected together and their shared assumptions were articulated as "constructionist" approaches (Gendron & Barrett, 2009; Gross & Barrett, 2011). This volume celebrates psychological construction as a growing family of accounts with its own history and an exciting future.

Psychological Construction as an Approach to Study the Nature of Emotion

Psychological construction can be viewed as a research program in same sense as that meant by Lakatos (1978). Family members share related (although not always identical) assumptions, methods, hypotheses, and historical models. The core assumption of this program is that each emotional episode is constructed rather than triggered. The program denies the common intuition that all instances of what we English speakers call "fear," for example, are highly similar because they are all caused by a hidden common agent unique to fear (e.g., an "affect program" or a neural circuit); that is, the psychological construction research program explicitly eschews essentialism (cf. Barrett, 2013).

For the past half-century, most emotion researchers have typically followed their intuitions, with the result that their research is guided by some version of faculty psychology. This can been seen in the questions that have guided (and baffled) the field. If each class of emotion is assumed to be a homogeneous set of recurring preorganized components, then certain questions naturally arise. What are the different classes of emotion? How many are there? How can we define emotion? And what is an emotion anyway? After decades of research, these questions remained largely unanswered. It is tempting to hope that these questions will be resolved with better-designed experiments, more precise measurements, and more sophisticated analytic strategies, but another possibility is that they will never be properly settled because they are based on underlying assumptions that are faulty. Indeed, Lakoff (2013) recently called emotion an *essentially contested concept*: everyone agrees that emotions exist, but no one can agree on their definition; there are a variety of meanings employed for emotion, but scientific inquiry seems unable to settle the matter. The reason for this conundrum can be found in what these unanswered questions (What are the classes of emotion? How many? Definition? What is it?) have in common: an assumption that the components (nonverbal expressions, physiological changes, etc.) in an emotional episode are caused by and therefore explained by a common agent behind them, the essence of each emotion. The different emotions, in turn, are fixed psychic and physical entities, primitive kinds of psychological and biological events that are countable, classifiable, and definable. Indeed, William James (1890/1950, p. 449) wrote: "The trouble with the emotions in psychology is that they are regarded too much as . . . psychic entities, like the old immutable species in natural history."

Because intuition tells us that emotions are predetermined response patterns generated by a common mechanism, psychological construction often implies the counterintuitive approach of revealing why these questions are ill-posed. What are the different classes of emotion? James (1890/1950) observed that "any classification of the emotions is seen to be as true and as 'natural' as any other" (p. 454). How many emotions are there? James again: "There is no limit to the number of possible different emotions" (p. 454). How can we define emotion? Mandler (1984) observed "that there is no commonly, even superficially, acceptable definition of what a psychology of emotion is about" (p. 279), a point confirmed more recently by Izard (2010).

Consistent with the psychological construction program, James denied that emotion is an agent that causes its "expressions"—that is, the facial movements, bodily changes, and instrumental acts commonly thought to be triggered by the emotion. Although reversing the common-sense order of events (we run and then feel afraid rather than vice versa) is the most famous aspect of James's theory, this reversal flows from a more fundamental idea: a rejection of the common-sense presupposition that each emotion word names a physical category, with a physical essence, and a power specifically and mechanistically to cause certain predetermined changes in behavior. According to Deigh (2014, p. 9), James characterized emotional feelings not as "isolable, recurring units of consciousness whose nature and composition is the subject of scientific study. They are, rather, like rapids and eddies in a river, to be understood as disturbances and agitations in an unbroken stream of thought, which one studies by examining the forces and conditions that produce such changes in the flow."

This Volume

Our goal in organizing *The Psychological Construction of Emotion* is to introduce readers to the assumptions, hypotheses, and scientific approaches that embody this research program's approach to studying the nature of emotion. In the past, psychological construction ideas on the nature of emotion were nascent, embedded in critiques of faculty psychology approaches. More recently, a new generation of psychological construction theories has emerged, articulating a more detailed and nuanced scientific agenda for the study of emotion. Moreover, several of the chapters in this volume propose biological hypotheses for how construction is accomplished within the brain and body, providing an opportunity to bridge psychological construction to other levels of analysis (and countering the mistaken assumption that any biological evidence on the nature of emotion is support for a faculty psychology view). The volume, while not comprehensive, is a sampling of the different approaches within the emerging family of psychological construction theories. Several other theories that implicitly rely on psychological construction assumptions, but that were not included in this volume, are worth reading for a more complete picture of the modern constructionist research program on emotion (e.g., Lane & Schwartz, 1987; LeDoux, 2012, 2014; Olsson & Ochsner, 2008; Roy, Shohamy, & Wager, 2012; Seth, 2013; Uddin, Kinnison, Pessoa, & Anderson, 2014).

As an attempt to draw out the themes and assumptions that unify the psychological construction approach, contributing authors (where appropriate) were asked explicitly to consider and respond to four questions:

1. If emotions are psychological events constructed from more basic ingredients, then what are the key ingredients from which emotions are constructed? Are they specific to emotion or are they general ingredients of the mind? Which, if any, are specific to humans?
2. What brings these ingredients together in the construction of an emotion? Which combinations are emotions and which are not (and how do we know)?
3. How important is variability (across instances within an emotion category, and in the categories that exist across cultures)? Is this variance epiphenomenal or a thing to be explained? To the extent that it makes sense, it would be desirable to address issues such as universality and evolution.
4. What constitutes strong evidence to support a psychological construction to emotion? Point to or summarize empirical evidence that supports your model or outline what a key experiment would look like. What would falsify your model?

Part I: Foundations

The volume's first section comprises two chapters that set the philosophical stage for the rest of the chapters. In Chapter 2, Herschbach and Bechtel discuss how psychological construction approaches are consistent with the new, dynamic mechanistic philosophy of science. They observe that the psychological construction research program is not critical of a mechanistic approach to emotion in general; rather, it criticizes a particular (somewhat impoverished) mechanistic view that is often found in faculty psychology approaches to emotion, characterized as a "machine metaphor" (Barrett, Chapter 3). In this view, the mind is understood primarily as a sequential stimulus → response enterprise in which different emotions (and cognitions and perceptions) arise from distinct mechanisms that can be studied like bits and parts of a machine. In its place, Herschbach and Bechtel offer a more sophisticated mechanistic account that dissolves old fault lines (e.g., reductionism and holism) and provides a useful foundation for constructionist approaches.

Along the way, Herschbach and Bechtel make several intriguing points that are helpful to keep in mind while reading the rest of the volume's chapters. First, they discuss how two aspects of science—the characterization of a phenomenon and the discovery of its mechanism—are not independent of one another; together, both characterizations make an ongoing, transactive process. Conventionally, scientists are supposed to delineate a phenomenon, then search for the mechanisms that cause the phenomenon, in that order. But a phenomenon and its mechanism are not separable. Scientists might start out with an a priori stipulation about what counts as the same phenomenon (and what to distinguish as different phenomena), but the search for mechanisms can sometimes cause a revision in what counts as the phenomenon of interest. This transactional process is an example of categorization in action. The initial delineation of psychological phenomena often goes unexamined by the scientists themselves, usually because they are using the intuitive folk psychological concepts of faculty psychology (cf. Danziger, 1997). In fact, constructionist approaches have tended to emerge in psychology precisely when the process of searching for a mechanism reveals that instances grouped together as the same phenomenon do not share sufficient organizational coherence to be explained by a common mechanism (e.g., recognition of meaningful variation within instances referred to as the phenomenon of anger), or more recently, that instances designated as different phenomena (e.g., "stress," "emotion," and "memory") turn out not to have categorically different mechanisms, revealing shared regularities across these instances that have thus far been ignored (i.e., recognizing similarities across categories).

Herschbach and Bechtel make a second important point—that a mechanism need not be unitary, and it can be decomposed into different operations. Various types of decomposition are possible (structural, functional, and phenomenal). Herschbach and Bechtel note that some psychological construction approaches have relied on phenomenal deconstruction, using phenomenological distinctions to identify component operations, and they caution us to be mindful of the approach's limitations for developing a dynamic, mechanistic account of emotion. This relates to the question, for example, of whether core affect (a construct discussed in several chapters; e.g., Barrett et al., Chapter 4; Russell, Chapter 8; Kringelbach & Berridge, Chapter 10; Kleckner & Quigley, Chapter 12) is a component operation that is part of the mechanism for emotion, or whether it is a property or feature of the emotion that is constructed (a way of describing a property of the product that itself is more than the sum of its parts). Or put another way, is core affect an ingredient, or is core affect itself constructed? Herschbach and Bechtel's point about decomposition also points out the virtues of a brain-based epistemology for psychological construction, several of which are proposed in this volume (e.g., Barrett et al., Chapter 4; Ooster-wijk, Touroutoglou, & Lindquist, Chapter 5; Thagard & Schröder, Chapter 6; Cunningham, Dunfield, & Stillman, Chapter 7; Kringelbach & Berridge, Chapter 10; Salmone, Correa, Randall, & Nunes, Chapter 11).

Finally, Herschbach and Bechtel introduce the concept of reconstitution in mechanistic explanations—the idea that the search for domain-general psychological ingredients potentially leads scientists to revise their phenomenon of interest without defining emotions out of existence. This point is important because it deals with one of the lingering misunderstandings of psychological construction—that the goal is to deny emotions any biological reality or to define them out of existence. Herschbach and Bechtel's analysis highlights the fact that emotions can be constructed from more basic operations without being illusions of the mind (see also Barrett, Chapter 3).

In Chapter 3, Barrett discusses 10 common misconceptions of the psychological construction approach to emotion that result from its failure to adhere to the common narrative structure typically found in faculty psychology explanations (which serves as the metanarrative structure of psychological theories). Barrett suggests that psychological construction seems unintuitive, because these theories actively eschew the machine metaphor's stimulus → response enterprise. Furthermore, psychological construction seems needlessly complex, because it tends to dissolve much cherished, simplifying distinctions in psychological theory, such as automatic versus controlled processing, social versus biological, linear cause versus effect, and nature versus nurture. Psychological construction also actively works against the idea that psychological categories have biological essences, without denying that each emotional episode has a biological cause. Scientific ideas that actively deny essentialism are often difficult for people to understand (Gelman & Rhodes, 2012).

Barrett cautions readers explicitly to replace a faculty psychology mindset with a constructionist mindset as they read through the rest of the volume (see also Barrett, 2012). Instead of asking "What is an emotion?" the psychological construction research program asks "How is an emotional episode made?" Instead of asking "Are emotions real?" we ask "How do emotions become real?" because the hypothesis is that the reality of emotions is conditional, based on a set of a processes and contexts. From a constructionist mindset, the questions "How many emotions are there?" and "Which ones are basic?" become nonquestions. Instead of asking "Are emotions hardwired?" the psychological construction research program asks "How does the brain's functional architecture construct emotional episodes?" A question about dedicated biological modules—"Is there a brain network or region with neurons that are dedicated to a type of emotion?"—becomes "Is it possible to identify a distributed pattern of brain activity to diagnose the instances of a category of emotion?" The rephrasing of this question acknowledges that diagnosis is not explanation, because even abstract, conceptual categories can be associated with reliable patterns of brain activity without being natural kinds. Instead of asking "How did emotions evolve as adaptations," we ask "Which evolved mechanisms that construct an emotional episode are species-general and which are species- or even person-specific?" The rephrasing of this question acknowledges that the "nature versus nurture" dichotomy is false, because life experiences and learning have the capacity to change the wiring of the brain. And instead of asking "What is the affect program or neural circuit dedicated to each emotion?" the psychological construction research program asks "Why do people stereotype emotions and look for biological essences, in the same way they essentialize other perceiver-dependent categories, such as race?"

Part II: Psychological Construction Theories

The volume's second section comprises six chapters that introduce various psychological construction theories of emotion. These theories share the assumption that emotions are not just physiological changes, or perceptions of those changes, or social constructions, but are unified events or episodes that have physiological, cognitive/perceptual, and social elements. These theories explain emotional episodes using domain-general approaches, because they share the view that the basic operations governing emotion construction are no different from those governing cognition, perception, and social interaction, all of which have implications for regulating homeostasis. For example, in Chapter 4, Barrett et al. propose that emotions are categorized physical states and offer specific hypotheses for how emotional episodes arise within the brain's functional architecture for creating situated conceptualizations of sensations from the body and the world. As discussed by Oosterwijk et al. in Chapter 5, this architecture involves domain-general functional networks that interact in unique ways to create the variety of mental events that are experienced as emotions and are named with emotion words. Thagard and Schröder propose in Chapter 6 that instances of emotion (i.e., emotional episodes) are *semantic pointers*, which they define as a patterns of large, widely distributed neural populations that fire with varying dynamics and can be organized into functional networks. Their computational model proposes a different way in which situated conceptualizations (discussed by Barrett et al. in Chapter 4) might be implemented within the widely distributed neural populations of the human brain, and represents a more computational way of understanding the network dynamics proposed by Oosterwijk et al. Similar to Thagard and Schröder's proposal, Cunningham et al., in their iterative reprocessing model, propose in Chapter 7 that an emotional episode is a "macrostate" constructed from a variety of different patterns of neural activity (what they refer to as "microstates") that result from hierarchically organized brain systems that interact through time. While the two theories are similar in their goals, they are distinct in their implementation: Cunningham et al. employ a dynamical systems framework as a heuristic for understanding how the emotional episodes are constructed, whereas Thagard and Schröder use a semantic pointer architecture. All of the theories detailed in Chapters 4 to 7 represent the new wave of psychological construction theories that cross levels of analysis to propose the neural operations by which construction takes place. In this regard, the theories agree that emotional episodes are represented as distributed, dynamic patterns of neural activity, and augment more classic psychological construction models in which constituent elements of emotional episodes are specified mainly at the psychological level of analysis.

In Chapter 8, Russell moves the reader from the neurophysiological level to the psychological level. He reviews his earlier arguments that psychological construction is counterintuitive and explicitly challenges our intuitions in a number of ways. Russell then reminds us of the empirical research that gradually chipped away at the standard faculty psychology textbook account, leading to a rejection of the classical view of emotion concepts and challenges to the alleged universality of emotion signaling via facial expression. He then focuses on his psychological construction account of subjective affective experience, emphasizing the heterogeneity of the events included in this category. He replaces the oversimplified concept of "emotional experience" with a set of distinct concepts (e.g., core affect, meta-experience, attributed affect, and perceptions of affective quality).

Next we move from a substantive level to a more methodological one. All psychological construction theories propose that emotional episodes emerge dynamically from their constituent components, an idea that is nicely captured and discussed in Chapter 9 by Coan and Gonzalez. Synthesizing prior discussions about how a statistical approach reflects a philosophical stance, even if implicitly (Barrett, 2006, 2011; Coan, 2010), Coan and Gonzalez offer an alternative measurement model to the standard latent variable model, which at a deep level captures the faculty psychology approach. Their alternative is meant to be more consistent with a constructionist approach.

Part III: Core Affect

The psychological construction research program contains a core hypothesis that internal sensory or affective states are understood as meaningfully related to or caused by the external surroundings via the involvement of additional processes or operations. The specifics of what internal source undergoes a meaning analysis vary considerably across theories. For example, James (1884, 1890/1950) emphasized the importance of raw sensory processing of somatic, visceral, vascular, and motor cues from the body as the basic building block of the mind. Wundt (1897/1998) focused on the mental counterpart of those internal cues, which he called "affect." Duffy (1957) emphasized arousal. More recent psychological construction theories tend not to separate the physical from the mental, as can be found in the concept of core affect.

Core affect is a concept that figures prominently in several psychological construction theories of emotion. It deliberately discards the commonsense mind–body distinction and is stipulatively defined as a neurophysiological state that is potentially accessible to consciousness as a primitive affective feeling. Core affect is a concept that also illustrates the assumption in psychological construction that processes underlying emotional episodes are not unique to emotional episodes. Comprised of the feelings that correspond to the body's ever-changing physiological state, core affect is a general feature of consciousness and is therefore not unique to emotion (Barrett & Bliss-Moreau, 2009; Duncan & Barrett, 2007). Psychological treatments of core affect have been well-explored (e.g., Russell, 2003; Russell & Barrett, 1999). From a phenomenological perspective, core affect is experienced as a single feeling that, when named, may be called feelings of excitement or stress, calm or depression, and so on. From a psychometric perspective, a circumplex provides a mathematical model of core affect (Yik, Russell, & Steiger, 2011). There are also stable individual differences in core affective responding (summarized in Barrett & Bliss-Moreau, 2009). To round out the existing psychological focus on core affect, the third part of our volume contains three chapters that provide a more biological account of core affect.

Chapters 10 and 11, by Kringelbach and Berridge, and Salamone et al., respectively, both discuss the brain systems involved in core affect. Both focus on the mesolimbic dopamine system in the brain. Kringelbach and Berridge discuss research that has identified distinctive *liking* and *wanting* systems that they believe roughly correspond to the valence and arousal dimensions of human core affective feelings (see the circumplex model of affect discussed by Russell in Chapter 8). Salamone et al. review research that points to limitations of the hedonic hypothesis of dopamine function, indicating that dopamine should not be thought of as the neurotransmitter of reward or pleasure. Rather, they argue that dopamine is engaged whenever an effortful response is required, whether appetitive or aversive. In fact, there is emerging evidence that both pleasure and displeasure have common substrates in opioid and dopamine transmission (e.g., Leknes & Tracey, 2008).

Kleckner and Quigley frame Chapter 12 with what is perhaps the most basic goal of psychological science—to find the physical basis of subjective experience. With this as their starting point, they discuss the peripheral nervous system contributions to affective feelings using concepts and principles from psychophysiology. They also discuss the dynamic interactions between the central and peripheral nervous systems that play a role in creating affective feelings, drawing heavily on neuroscience evidence from the anatomist Bud Craig. Kleckner and Quigley provide a general overview of how prior studies have attempted to map measures of physiological change to measures of mental features that characterize core affect, and offer specific suggestions for how the psychological construction research program provides additional hypotheses for exploration.

Part IV: Commentary and Consilience

The volume's fourth part contains four chapters that discuss common ground and points of disagreement between the psychological construction research program and other research programs for emotion. In Chapter 13, Ortony and Clore discuss the theoretical ways in which psychological construction is consistent with their brand of appraisal theory. The appraisal research program is quite heterogeneous (Barrett, Mesquita, Ochsner, & Gross, 2007); Gross & Barrett, 2011; Moors, 2009). One class of appraisal theories defines *appraisals* as cognitive mechanisms that evaluate the situation and cause the emotional episode. This class shares the assumptions of faculty psychology. In contrast, Ortony and Clore characterize appraisals as descriptions of how the world is experienced during an emotional episode. In their view, emotions are situated affective states that are embodied representations of situations. In this way, Ortony and Clore's theory is the counterpart to psychological construction. Their theory focuses mainly on describing the emergent product (what an emotion feels like), whereas psychological construction concentrates more on understanding how interacting elements or operations produce the emergent emotional episode.

One function of alternative theories in science is to create a dialogue that encourages each side in the debate to revise in light of the advances of the other. This can be seen in Chapter 14 by Scarantino, who discusses his proposed revision to the basic emotion research program through the lens of psychological construction, with the goal of fashioning a new and improved basic emotion theory that is immune to constructionist critiques. In the process, Scarantino casts a critical eye on key assumptions within the family of psychological construction theories, offering nuanced reflections of how various constructionist accounts differ from one another. His chapter provides the next installment of the ongoing, centuries-long dialogue between faculty psychology and constructionist theories of emotion. His discussion represents a serious attempt to assimilate some of the key observations from a psychological constructionist approach into a "new and improved" version of basic emotion theory. To advance the dialogue, Russell critiques Scarantino's theory in Chapter 8.

In Chapter 15, Boiger and Mesquita discuss the similarities and differences between psychological and social varieties of construction. Their discussion is particularly important in the evolution of constructionist accounts, because scientists often confuse the two perspectives, or fail to see their difference. In fact, psychological and social constructionist theories offer complementary accounts on the nature of emotion. The psychological construction research program tends to focus its scientific lens on the *within-person* operations involved in constructing emotional episodes, whereas the social constructionist research program tends to focus on the *between-person* operations. But this is a matter of emphasis. Psychological constructionist accounts do *not* deny the importance of the social interaction as a dynamically unfolding process that shapes the construction of an emotional episode, but they leave such influences unspecified. Without denying the importance of within-person processes during emotion construction, Boiger and Mesquita focus their discussion on how social dynamics is part of the system through which emotions emerge, and they discuss how three scales of social context—moment-to-moment interactions, ongoing interpersonal relationships, and the broader cultural context—provide the social matrix within which emotional episodes are constructed. The psychological construction research program seriously considers the role of context in emerging emotional episodes, and Boiger and Mesquita's ideas offer concrete scientific options for how to operationalize context. Moreover, they suggest the unintuitive but intriguing possibility that an emotional episode might not occur within a single individual, but its fuller specification requires some quantification of the transactions that occur within a specific context.

In Chapter 16, the final chapter of this section, Fugate offers insights on the evolutionary continuity of emotion from a psychological construction standpoint. If emotional episodes are not natural kinds, but are perceiver-dependent products of a human mind (Barrett, 2006, 2012), then the question of whether nonhuman animals have emotions takes center stage. Fugate's answer is that it depends on the kind of animal mind one is talking about. Specifically, she considers the role of language and abstract conceptual reasoning for the emotion construction process, and placing cognition on a continuum, speculates as to which animal species have the kind of mind that is equipped for experiencing emotion (vs. core affective feelings).

Part V: Integration and Reflection

To conclude the volume, we offer our thoughts on how psychological construction presents an opportunity for more a integrated research program, incorporating a number of theoretical and methodological perspectives. Chapter 17 by Russell introduces a new project—termed the Greater

Constructionist Project—that uses the basic assumptions of constructionist approaches to psychology to provide an integrated theoretical approach for the science of emotion, helping, perhaps, to transform *emotion* from an essentially contested concept into a scientifically viable one. In Chapter 18, Barrett summarizes her earlier observations on points of contact between psychological construction and other emotion research programs, then offers additional insights into the potential for psychological construction to integrate the science of emotion across levels of analysis. Her chapter includes a suggestion that psychological construction has value as a research program well beyond science of emotion. Specifically, she proposes that a psychological construction approach has value for conceptualizating the functional architecture of the human brain, for uniting the major psychological categories (cognitions, perception, emotion, and action) into one unified theoretical framework. Finally, the volume concludes with an Afterword by Joseph LeDoux, who in recent years has developed his research on the brain's basic threat circuitry into a theoretical account of emotional experience that shared many features with other psychological constructionist accounts.

ACKNOWLEDGMENTS

Preparation of this chapter was supported by a National Institutes of Health Director's Pioneer Award (No. DP1OD003312); by grants from the National Institute on Aging (No. R01AG030311), the National Institute of Mental Health (No. R21MH099605), and the National Science Foundation (No. BCS-1052790); and by contracts from the U.S. Army Research Institute for the Behavioral and Social Sciences (Contract Nos. W5J9CQ-11-C-0046 and W5J9CQ-12-C-0049) to Lisa Feldman Barrett. The views, opinions, and/or findings contained in this chapter are solely those of the authors and should not be construed as an official Department of the Army or Department of Defense position, policy, or decision.

REFERENCES

Barrett, L. F. (2006). Emotions as natural kinds? *Perspectives on Psychological Science, 1*, 28–58.

Barrett, L. F. (2011). Bridging token identity theory and supervenience theory through psychological construction. *Psychological Inquiry, 22*, 115–127.

Barrett, L. F. (2012). Emotions are real. *Emotion, 12*, 413–429.

Barrett, L. F. (2013). Psychological construction: A Darwinian approach to the science of emotion. *Emotion Review, 5*, 379–389.

Barrett, L. F., & Bliss-Moreau, E. (2009). Affect as a psychological primitive. *Advances in Experimental Social Psychology, 41*, 167–218.

Barrett, L. F., Mesquita, B., Ochsner, K. N., & Gross, J. J. (2007). The experience of emotion. *Annual Review of Psychology, 58*, 373–403.

Barrett, L. F., & Satpute, A. B. (2013). Large-scale brain networks in affective and social neuroscience: Towards an integrative architecture of the human brain. *Current Opinion in Neurobiology, 23*, 361–372.

Bechtel, W. (2008). *Mental mechanisms: Philosophical perspectives on cognitive neuroscience.* London: Routledge.

Berker, E. A., Berker, A. H., & Smith, A. (1986). Translation of Broca's 1865 report: Localization of speech in the third left convolution. *Archives of Neurology, 43*, 1065–1072.

Bruner, J. (1990). *Acts of meaning.* Boston: Harvard University Press.

Cannon, W. B. (1927). The James–Lange theory of emotions: A critical examination and alternative theory. *American Journal of Psychology, 39*, 106–124.

Chomsky, N. (1980). Rules and representations. *Behavioral and Brain Sciences, 3*, 1–61.

Coan, J. A. (2010). Emergent ghosts of the emotion machine. *Emotion Review, 2*, 274–285.

Danziger, K. (1980). The history of introspection reconsidered. *Journal of the History of the Behavioral Sciences, 16*, 241–262.

Danziger, K. (1997). *Naming the mind: How psychology found its language.* London: Sage.

de Gelder, B., & Vandenbulcke, M. (2012). Emotions as mind organs. *Behavioral and Brain Sciences, 35*, 147–148.

Deigh, J. (2014). Willliam James and the rise of the scientific study of emotion. *Emotion Review, 6*, 4–12.

Duffy, E. (1934a). Is emotion a mere term of convenience? *Psychological Review, 41*, 103–104.

Duffy, E. (1934b). Emotion: An example of the need for reorientation in psychology. *Psychological Review, 41*, 184–198.

Duffy, E. (1941). An explanation of "emotional" phenomena without use of the concept "emotion." *General Journal of Psychology, 25*, 283–293.

Duffy, E. (1957). The psychological significance of the concept of "arousal" or "activation." *Psychological Review, 64*, 265–275.

Duncan, S., & Barrett, L. F. (2007). Affect is a form of cognition: A neurobiological analysis. *Cognition and Emotion, 21*, 1184–1211.

Fodor, J. A. (1983). *The modularity of mind: An essay on faculty psychology.* Cambridge, MA: MIT Press

Gall, F. J. (1835). *On the origin of moral qualities and intellectual faculties of man* (W. Lewis, Trans.). Boston: Marsh, Capen & Lyon.

Gelman, S. A., & Rhodes, M. (2012). "Two-thousand years of stasis": How psychological essentialism impedes evolutionary understanding. In K. S. Rosengren, S. Brem, E. M. Evans, & G. Sinatra (Eds.), *Evolution challenges: Integrating research and practice in teaching and learning about evolution* (pp. 3–21). New York: Oxford University Press.

Gendron, M., & Barrett, L. F. (2009). Reconstructing the past: A century of ideas about emotion in psychology. *Emotion Review, 1*, 316–339.

Gross, J. J., & Barrett, L. F. (2011). Emotion generation and emotion regulation: One or two depends on your point of view. *Emotion Review, 3*, 8–16.

Harlow, H. F., & Stagner, R. (1932). Psychology of feelings and emotions: I. Theory of feelings. *Psychological Review, 39*, 570–589.

Harlow, H. F., & Stagner, R. (1933). Psychology of feelings and emotions: II. Theory of emotions. *Psychological Review, 40*, 184–195.

Harrington, A. (1987). *Medicine, mind and the double brain: A study in 19th century thought.* Princeton, NJ: Princeton University Press.

Hassabis, D., & Macguire, E. A. (2009). The constructive system of the brain. *Philosophical Transactions of the Royal Society B, 364*, 1263–1271.

Hunt, W. A. (1941). Recent developments in the field of emotion. *Psychological Bulletin, 38*, 249–276.

Izard, C. E. (2010). The many meanings/aspects of emotion: Definitions, functions, activation and regulation. *Emotion Review, 2*, 363–370.

Jablonski, N. G. (2012). *Living color: The biological and social meaning of skin color.* Berkeley: University of California Press.

James, W. (1884). What is an emotion? *Mind, 9*, 188–205.

James. W. (1950). *The principles of psychology* (Vol. 2). New York: Dover. (Original work published 1890)

Klein, D. B. (1970). *A history of scientific psychology: Its origin and philosophical backgrounds.* New York: Basic Books.

Lakoff, G. (2013, August 3). Invited address. International Society for Research on Emotion, Berkeley, CA.

Lakatos, I. (1978). Philosophical papers (Vol. 1). In J. Worrall & G. Currie (Eds.), *The methodology of scientific research programmes.* Cambridge, UK: Cambridge University Press.

Lane, R., & Schwartz, G. E. (1987). Levels of emotional awareness: A cognitive-developmental theory and its application to psychopathology. *American Journal of Psychiatry, 144*, 133–143.

LeDoux, J. (2012). Rethinking the emotional brain. *Neuron, 73*, 653–676.

LeDoux, J. (2014). Coming to terms with fear. *Proceedings of the National Academy of Sciences.* Available at *www.pnas.org/content/early/2014/02/04/1400335111.full.pdf+html.*

Leknes, S., & Tracey, I. (2008). A common neurobiology for pain and pleasure. *Nature Reviews Neuroscience, 9*, 314–320.

Lindquist, K., A., & Barrett, L. F. (2012). A functional architecture of the human brain: Insights from the science of emotion. *Trends in Cognitive Sciences, 16*, 533–540.

Mandler, G. (1975). *Mind and emotion.* New York: Wiley.

Mandler, G. (1984). *Mind and body: Psychology of emotion and stress.* New York: Norton

Mandler, G. (1990). William James and the construction of emotion. *Psychological Science, 1*, 179–180.

Mareschal, D., Johnson, M., Sirois, S., Spatling, M., Thomas, M., & Weatermann, G. (2007). *Neuroconstructivism—I: How the brain constructs cognition.* New York: Oxford University Press.

Medin, D., & Ortony, A. (1989). Psychological essentialism. In S. Vosniadou & A. Ortony (Eds.), *Similarity and analogical reasoning* (pp. 179–195). New York: Cambridge University Press.

Menon, V. (2011). Large-scale brain networks and psychopathology: A unifying triple network model. *Trends in Cognitive Sciences, 15*, 483–506.

Moors, A. (2009) Theories of emotion causation: A review. *Cognition and Emotion, 23*(4), 625–662.

Neisser, U. (1967). *Cognitive psychology.* New York: Appleton-Century-Crofts.

Olsson, A., & Ochsner, K. N. (2008). The role of social cognition in emotion. *Trends in Cognitive Sciences, 12,* 65–71.

Roy, M., Shohamy, D., & Wager, T. D. (2012). Ventromedial prefrontal-subcortical systems and the generation of affective meaning. *Trends in Cognitive Sciences, 16*(3), 147–156.

Russell, J. A. (2003). Core affect and the psychological construction of emotion. *Psychological Review, 110,* 145–172.

Russell, J. A., & Barrett, L. F. (1999). Core affect, prototypical emotional episodes, and other things called emotion: Dissecting the elephant. *Journal of Personality and Social Psychology, 76,* 805–819.

Schacter, D. L. (2012). Adaptive constructive memory processes and the future of memory. *American Psychologist, 67,* 603–613.

Schacter, D. L., & Addis, D. R. (2007). The cognitive neuroscience of constructive memory: Remembering the past and imagining the future. *Philosophical Transactions of the Royal Society B, 362,* 773–786.

Schachter, S., & Singer, J. (1962). Cognitive, social, and physiological determinantsof an emotional state. *Psychological Review, 69,* 379–399.

Seth, A. K. (2013). Interoceptive inference, emotion, and the embodied self. *Trends in Cognitive Sciences, 17,* 565–573.

Spunt, R. P., & Lieberman, M. D. (2012). An integrative model of the neural systems supporting the comprehension of observed emotional behavior. *NeuroImage, 59*(3), 3050–3059.

Spurzheim, J. G. (1832). *Outlines of phrenology.* Boston: Marsh, Capen & Lyon.

Uddin, L., Kinnison, J., Pessoa, L., & Anderson, M. (2014). Beyond the tripartite cognitive–emotion–interoception model of the human insular cortex. *Journal of Cognitive Neuroscience, 26*(1), 16–27.

Uttal, W. R. (2001). *The new phrenology: The limits of localizing cognitive processes in the brain.* Cambridge, MA: MIT Press.

Wundt, W. (1998). *Outlines of psychology* (C. H. Judd & W. Engelmann, Trans.). New York: Williams & Norgate. (Original work published 1897)

Xu, F., & Kushnir, T. (2013). Infants are rational constructivist learners. *Current Directions in Psychological Science, 21,* 28–32.

Yik, M., Russell, J. A., & Steiger, J. H. (2011). A 12-point circumplex structure of core affect. *Emotion, 11,* 705–731.

PART I

FOUNDATIONS

CHAPTER 2

Mental Mechanisms and Psychological Construction

MITCHELL HERSCHBACH
WILLIAM BECHTEL

Psychological construction represents an important new approach to psychological phenomena, one that has the promise to help us reconceptualize the mind as both a behavioral and a biological system. It has so far been developed in the greatest detail for emotion, but it has important implications for how researchers approach other mental phenomena such as reasoning, memory, and language use. Its key contention is that phenomena characterized in (folk) psychological vocabulary are not themselves basic features of the mind, but are constructed from more basic psychological operations. The framework of mechanistic explanation, currently under development in philosophy of science, can provide a useful perspective on the psychological constructionist approach. A central insight of the mechanistic account of explanation is that biological and psychological phenomena result from mechanisms in which component parts and operations do not individually exhibit the phenomena of interest but function together in an orchestrated and sometimes complex, dynamical manner to generate it.

While at times acknowledging the compatibility of the mechanist approach with the constructionist approach (Lindquist, Wager, Kober, Bliss-Moreau, & Barrett, 2012), proponents of the constructionist approach have at other times pitched their approach as antimechanist. For example, Barrett (2009) claims that the psychological constructionist approach rejects machines as the primary metaphor for understanding the mind, instead favoring a recipe metaphor; constructionism also purportedly rejects the "mechanistic" picture of causation, which it portrays as linear

21

1. *If emotions are psychological events constructed from more basic ingredients, then what are the key ingredients from which emotions are constructed? Are they specific to emotion or are they general ingredients of the mind? Which, if any, are specific to humans?*

The mechanistic approach to philosophy of science we describe is not itself a theory of psychological phenomena such as emotions. Rather, it offers a framework for how discovery and explanation operate in sciences such as biology and psychology. Therefore, such a framework is not itself committed to the psychological constructionist hypothesis that emotions are constructions from more basic ingredients. But what philosophers have noticed about the processes of discovery and explanation for other biological phenomena do point in favor of psychological constructionism about psychological phenomena. It is common for scientists initially to identify a single entity as the mechanism responsible for a phenomenon, and they describe this part using the vocabulary originally reserved for the phenomenon of interest. Subsequent research, however, often reveals that this simple, direct localization of the phenomenon is false; they then find the mechanism comprises a host of interacting parts, each of which performs activities that are distinct from the phenomenon to be explained. This general pattern of finding complex, multipart mechanisms is at a minimum consistent with, and can be seen to provide indirect support for, the psychological constructionist approach. In the case of psychological phenomena, mechanists agree with constructionists that psychologists need to work to discover the more basic operations of the mind that are realized in regions and networks of the brain. Which, if any, of these basic psychological operations are unique to humans, and whether human-specific psychological phenomena involve the unique combination of psychological operations present in some nonhuman animals, are questions that cannot be answered a priori simply by adopting a mechanistic approach.

2. *What brings these ingredients together in the construction of an emotion? Which combinations are emotions and which are not (and how do we know)?*

The mechanistic approach is agnostic about how scientists should conceptualize emotions, and what particular parts, operations, and organization should be identified in a mechanistic explanation of emotional phenomena. As in many other scientific inquiries, everyday categories are a starting point for delineating mental phenomena, and if neural mechanisms do not respect these folk categories, conceptual revision of the type proposed by psychological constructionism may be necessary. A host of neuroscientific research does support the constructionists' view that the brain does not respect the traditional division between "mental faculties" such as cognition and emotion. But researchers are only at the stage of proposing initial hypotheses about the basic psychological operations that will go into mechanistic accounts of mental

(continued)

phenomena such as emotion, so it is not yet clear how drastically we may need to revise our folk psychological categories. We do, however, believe a mechanistic approach offers some lessons about how this inquiry should proceed. First, we emphasize the importance of looking to neuroscience to guide such hypotheses, even if neuroscientific research at times is at too low a level to immediately impact our mechanistic understanding of agents' psychological phenomena. Second, we should expect our emotion mechanisms' parts and operations to be endogenously active and organized in a complex, nonlinear fashion.

3. *How important is variability (across instances within an emotion category, and in the categories that exist across cultures)? Is this variance epiphenomenal or a thing to be explained? To the extent that it makes sense, it would be desirable to address issues such as universality and evolution.*

Mechanistic accounts treat regularities as the phenomena to be explained in terms of underlying mechanisms. This is not inconsistent with recognizing that each instance of a phenomenon differs on a variety of dimensions, but it does require finding regularity even in variable instances. Too much variability across instances of a proposed category of phenomena, or great regularity across instances of different categories, points toward a need to redescribe or reconstitute the phenomena to the explained—possibly dissolving boundaries between phenomena considered distinct, or even more radically recategorizing the phenomena to be explained. Discovering that phenomena have overlapping mechanisms is one major reason for uniting phenomena previously considered distinct, and being able to identify distinct mechanisms is a reason to continue to differentiate phenomena, even if those phenomena are always in fact interconnected.

4. *What constitutes strong evidence to support a psychological construction to emotion. Point to or summarize empirical evidence that supports your model or outline what a key experiment would look like. What would falsify your model?*

Evidence that specific emotion categories are not grounded in discrete, localized neural mechanisms would speak in favor of the psychological constructionist's general approach of finding more basic psychological operations from which emotional episodes are constituted. This would follow the general pattern of researchers finding that biological phenomena often are explained by dynamical mechanisms that consist of many parts organized in complex ways. Furthermore, evidence indicating that regularities at the level of the actions and physiological responses of whole agents do not track folk emotion categories would suggest revising these categories and the relation between emotion and other mental phenomena. Mechanistic research often involves such reconstitution of the phenomena to be explained.

or sequential in nature (see also Barrett, Wilson-Mendenhall, & Barsalou, 2014). While some mechanistic accounts do fit this description, we will see that the mechanisms generating phenomena can be complex and dynamic, producing phenomena far less stereotypical and more adaptive than people often associate with machines. Our goal, however, is not just to render constructionism and mechanism compatible. Philosophers of science have been examining the nature of mechanistic explanation in biology, with the goal of gaining new insights into the operation of science. We will identify some of the places where the mechanistic account can shed new light on the constructionist project.

The constructionist account of emotion is presented as an alternative to what Barrett (2006) calls the "natural kind" approach, which segregates emotion from other psychological kinds (e.g., perception, memory), differentiates and treats different kinds of emotion (fear, anger, happiness, sadness, etc.) as psychologically primitive, and treats these as causal processes in the mind that are ultimately to be localized in the brain either in distinct brain regions (e.g., fear in the amygdala) or in discrete neural networks. The categories emotion, perception, memory, etc., and the subdivision of emotion into fear, anger, etc., are parts of our folk accounts through which we describe our own and other agents' mental states and activities. In this context they have an important role to play—they enable us to assess the individuals with whom we interact and coordinate our activities appropriately. They become problematic, for the constructionist and for us, when they are viewed, as in the natural kind approach, as identifying basic activities performed in the mind. These mental activities are constructed from operations that are different in character and therefore require a different vocabulary to be described. In our view, it is the orchestrated functioning of a mechanism operating in a particular physical and social environment (and shaped by its history in that environment) that exhibits these mental activities.

The points of difference between the natural kind and constructionist approaches map onto fundamental issues highlighted in accounts of mechanism. In the mechanist approach, mechanisms are characterized in terms of the phenomena for which they are responsible. This makes the project of delineating the phenomenon critical, since different types of phenomena require different explanations. The constructionist's contention is that when we appreciate that emotions are constructed, we are attuned to such things as the wide variability found in the facial expressions, behaviors, and physiology associated, for example, with fear. We concur with this, but emphasize in another section (pages 27–30) the need nonetheless to develop an account of phenomena that identifies regularities, for it is such regularities that become the touchstones of explanatory endeavors. On pages 30–35, we focus on what is the key element in mechanistic science—the appeal to component parts and operations of a mechanism. This requires decomposing the mechanism. It is out of the component parts and operations that the mechanist and constructionist both view mental phenomena such as emotions as arising; but here the mechanist can give some perspective on both why it is so difficult to identify component parts and operations of a mechanism, and on the historical process by which they have been identified in mechanistic sciences that are further along than psychology at present. As a result of the emphasis on decomposition in mechanistic science, mechanistic accounts are often viewed as reductionistic. But, as we develop in that section on pages 35–38, accounts of mechanism also require attention to how the whole mechanism is organized and situated in its environment—a mechanistic account requires both a reductionist and a holist perspective. This becomes particularly important when the organization of the mechanism is nonsequential and the operations are nonlinear, because these conditions can give rise to complex dynamics. On pages 38–41, we turn to one of the intriguing consequences of mechanistic research—it sometimes leads to a reconception, or what we call a *reconstitution*, of the initial phenomenon for which an explanation is sought. We consider whether psychological phenomena themselves need to be reconceptualized in light of our understanding of the mechanisms that generate them. Before turning to these issues, however, we begin with a brief primer on the new mechanistic philosophy of science.

A Primer on the New Mechanistic Philosophy of Science

If one consults traditional accounts of explanation in philosophy of science, one learns that explanation requires showing how the phenomenon to be explained follows from one or more laws, together with some initial conditions (Hempel, 1965, 1966). While this nomological account of explanation may fit some cases in physics, it fares poorly in psychology, in which there are few examples of laws, and the laws that may be found serve not to explain but to characterize phenomena in need of explanation (see Cummins, 2000, who notes that such laws in psychology are often called "effects"). It also fares poorly in biology (including neuroscience). When scientists advance explanations in both biology and psychology, they often speak of identifying the mechanism responsible for a given phenomenon. Responding to this, a number of philosophers of science have offered accounts of what counts as a mechanism in these disciplines. While the accounts differ in vocabulary and in some of their claims, they agree that a mechanism comprises an organized set of parts performing different operations whose orchestrated functioning results in the phenomenon of interest[1] (Bechtel & Richardson, 1993/2010; Bechtel & Abrahamsen, 2005; Craver, 2007; Darden, 2006; Machamer, Darden, & Craver, 2000). A mechanistic explanation both describes the mechanism and shows how it gives rise to the phenomenon. For example, beginning with William Harvey in the 17th century, explaining the phenomenon of the circulation of blood in animals involved identifying the heart as the responsible mechanism, then showing how the periodic contraction and relaxation of the muscles in the various chambers and the opening and closing of the valves (operations involving specific parts) resulted in the phenomenon. Over time the phenomenon was more fully characterized, capturing, for example, the precise timing of the muscle contraction, and new components such as neurons were included in the account. Although eventually researchers found it useful to characterize the phenomenon and the operations involved mathematically, the parts and operations are central to the account. Researchers do not simply construct the law of heart behavior and derive the behavior of a heart given initial conditions from such a law.

We have introduced the mechanistic account by contrasting it with more traditional accounts of explanation that present explanation as deriving a statement of the phenomenon from laws and initial conditions. The mechanistic approach also recasts a number of important issues in philosophy of science, such as the format in which explanations may be represented and how scientists reason about mechanisms. Whereas it is natural to represent laws in propositions or equations, the challenge in understanding a mechanism is to grasp the types of parts and operations it employs, and how these are organized. A diagram is often most effective in conveying this information. Logical deduction provides a way of showing that an instance (e.g., the movement of a given pendulum) follows from a law. But to see how a variety of operations generate a phenomenon, one must simulate the operation of the mechanism, either in a physical model, in one's head, or in a computational simulation.[2] Two issues on which mechanistic philosophy of science offers a different perspective than more traditional nomological ones are of particular concern here.

One involves reduction. In one sense that is familiar to scientists, mechanistic research is inherently reductionistic insofar as it appeals to entities and events at a lower level of organization—parts and operations—to explain the behavior of the whole mechanism. But in another sense, it is inherently holistic in that mechanisms must be organized and appropriately situated in their environment in order to function. Accordingly, mechanistic accounts are multilevel and do not privilege the lowest level.

The second issue involves discovery. Advocates of the traditional nomological accounts of science generally eschewed discovery, focusing instead on justification. The reason was that although there was reason to hope that one could articulate processes of logical inference through which theories were justified (or at least could be falsified), there seemed to be little prospect of a logical specification of how one discovers laws (but see Langley, Simon, Bradshaw, & Zytkow, 1987; Thagard, 1988). Philosophers focused on mechanistic explanation have, however, identified some important aspects of how mechanisms are discovered. Of special relevance to us is how reasoning can progress from initial proposals for localizing operations in the parts of a mechanism, to much richer accounts involving many parts that are organized in complex ways.

The Challenge of Delineating Emotional Phenomena

In referring to what is to be explained as a *phenomenon*, and considering examples such as biological respiration or encoding of long-term memories, it may seem as though phenomena are immediately apparent and obvious to anyone who looks for them. But, in fact, a great deal of scientific, often experimental, work is typically required to delineate phenomena in a manner that renders them appropriate as the target of explanation. Even something that we take to be basic to the life of mammals, circulation of blood, was not apparent even to physicians prior to the work of Harvey. Until then, physicians held that there were two distinct types of blood, arterial and venous, both of which flowed out from the heart to the peripheral tissues. Although Harvey himself was not able to show how the circuit from the arteries to the veins was completed, since capillaries were too small to be identified with the tools he had available, he presented what now seems like overwhelming evidence that the blood must circulate. First, he showed that the valves where the veins connect to the heart are oriented in the wrong direction for blood to flow out through the veins. Second, he calculated that the amount of blood that would have to be created from food on a regular basis, if it were not recirculated, vastly exceeded dietary intake. Finally, he showed that if veins were restricted in a limb, the limb would soon bloat from the amount of arterial blood reaching it. But none of this was compelling to many of his contemporaries, who insisted on the traditional account of the phenomenon in terms of two types of blood, both traversing outward from the heart.

It is not just obstinacy that renders phenomena challenging to identify. Rather, the activities that get characterized as phenomena and then explained typically depend on relations between entities that have to be identified. For example, Darwin had to notice how traits of organisms (e.g., the beaks of the finches he observed in the Galapagos) made them fit for the conditions in their environment. Previous theorists, such as Paley, whom Darwin much admired, focused on the complexity of the characteristics of organisms, but only once Darwin identified traits as adaptive did it make sense to seek an explanation in a process such as natural selection. Moreover, sometimes quantification is required to delineate phenomena. It was widely known by anyone who thought about it that objects left unsupported near the surface of the earth drop. Yet it took Galileo to show that objects near the surface of the earth always fall 32 feet/sec^2, a phenomenon that would later be explained by Newton's law of universal gravitation.

With this as background, let us turn to the phenomena we expect psychology to explain. Here several challenges arise. First, the English word *emotion*, like many other words in our mental vocabulary, likely refers to a host of different psychological phenomena that may share a family resemblance but also exhibit great variability. This extends not only to our folk talk of emotions but also to the use of the term *emotion* by scientists. One finds emotions presented as conscious feelings, cognitive states (e.g., appraisals), peripheral physiological responses (e.g., heart rate, respiration), and behavioral tendencies or overt behavior (e.g., facial, bodily, verbal); sometimes they are treated as collections of these mental and bodily phenomena (see reviews, e.g., Gendron & Barrett, 2009; Gross & Barrett, 2011; Prinz, 2004, Chapter 1). Such differences are of fundamental importance from the perspective of mechanistic explanation, since a mechanism is identified according to the phenomenon it explains.

The challenge is apparent if one considers the question of where the mechanism responsible for emotion is located. For mechanists, a phenomenon and its mechanism are not separate entities, with the mechanism *causing* the phenomenon. Rather, the activity of the mechanism is said to *constitute* or *realize* the phenomenon of interest. So if bodily events are literal parts of emotions, then clearly the mechanisms of emotion cannot be purely in the brain. But if emotions are disembodied mental states that can have bodily effects (which are not themselves literal parts of the emotions), and if the mechanisms of the mind are indeed to be found in the brain, then mechanisms of emotion will be neural mechanisms.

Second, as the constructivists emphasize (e.g., Barrett, 2006), emotional phenomena are highly variable. Episodes of fear, even when elicited in the same person by the same stimulus, show considerable variability in behavioral responses, autonomic activity, and subjective experience. The goal of a mechanistic account is not to construct a separate mechanism for each episode but to identify a mechanism that accounts for regular patterns. The concept of a phenomenon, as presented by Bogen and Woodward (1988), as the appropriate target of explanation involves regularities that can be exhibited repeatedly. This is not inconsistent with recognizing that each instance differs on a variety of dimensions, but it does require finding regularity even in variable instances.

The relation between phenomenon, regularity, and mechanism is more complex than these remarks suggest. Not every well-established quantitative regularity constitutes a phenomenon to be explained by a separate mechanism. Rather, there is often a reciprocal relation between identifying a phenomenon and identifying a mechanism—as an account of the mechanism develops, it may enable us to account for a variety of regularities, which may then be grouped together as aspects of the same phenomenon. It is at this point that the constructionist contention that emotion is constructed from many of the same operations that figure in other cognitive activities becomes a serious issue for scientists.

If the connections between components lead scientists to treat them as components of one mechanism, and we view all the activities to which this mechanism gives rise as aspects of the same phenomenon, then we have a recipe for an extremely problematic holism, at least across biology and psychology.[3] One of the consequences of identifying the molecular basis of many biological activities has been the discovery that many are shared, and that there are important pathways by which the activities affect one another. For example, there is increasingly compelling evidence that nicotinamide adenine dinucleotide (NAD), a central component of metabolic activities, affects circadian rhythms, which have traditionally been assigned to different mechanisms. The consequence would seem to be that we should identify one phenomenon involving basic metabolism and circadian timekeeping. This same line of reasoning quickly leads us to identify only one biological phenomenon and one mechanism (the whole organism, plus perhaps its environment).

If the goal is explanation, we must resist such thorough-going holism. In practice, mechanistic scientists differentiate phenomena and avoid holism, while acknowledging points of interaction between the responsible mechanisms. Thus, they differentiate circadian timekeeping from myriad related phenomena to which it and the mechanisms responsible for it are linked. Scientists in part make the decision as to what to count as one phenomenon and hence one mechanism pragmatically in terms of what they think they can productively integrate into one account. But if decisions as to how to delineate phenomena are to generate scientific understanding, they must also aspire to track actual distinctions in nature. The mechanisms identified with different phenomena will not be totally separable from each other, but each must have sufficient organizational coherence to make it appropriate to treat it as one mechanism responsible for one phenomenon (see the discussion of clusters in small-world networks on pages 37–38; different clusters may constitute mechanisms for specific phenomena, but their behavior may be modified in real time through the long-range connections to other clusters).

Adopting the mechanistic perspective does not simply resolve the challenge this poses to delineating psychological phenomena and mechanisms, but it does give some guidance. The question of whether emotional phenomena and cognitive phenomena should be distinguished, or whether some other differentiation is needed, in part depends on how successful researchers are at developing mechanistic accounts that distinguish them. It may be that one can maintain a productive distinction between emotion and some other mental phenomena and identify mechanisms that can be distinguished even if they are always interconnected. Likewise, it may be possible to distinguish particular emotion types from each other in the same manner.

Here we do not take a stand on whether the constructionists are right in challenging the traditional distinction between emotion and other mental phenomena, or between different emotions as distinct phenomena; rather, we have only tried to show some of what is at stake from a mechanistic perspective. One thing we hope we have made clear, though, is that the question is not whether there are totally distinct or totally integrated phenomena/mechanisms, but whether the phenomena and the mechanisms responsible for them are sufficiently differentiable that they can be treated separately. On pages 38–41, we return to the question of delineating the phenomena and whether the constructionists' description of psychological phenomena so transforms traditional conceptions that they *reconstitute* the phenomena themselves.

Decomposition and Localization

Central to the mechanistic approach to explanation is the idea that components parts perform different operations than the mechanism as a whole, and are organized and orchestrated to produce the phenomenon of interest. Thus, once one has delineated a phenomenon and linked it with an appropriate mechanism, a key task is to decompose that mechanism. Two types of decomposition are relevant to mechanistic explanation: decomposition into structural parts (*structural decomposition*) and into functional operations (*functional decomposition*). Decomposing in either way can be an extremely challenging endeavor—the appropriate ways of dividing a mechanism into parts or component operations are not obvious to all those who look. It requires developing both the appropriate conceptual framework and adequate experimental tools. On the conceptual side, researchers must develop the concepts for particular sorts of parts or operations and the vocabulary for identifying them.[4] For example, in distinguishing regions of the brain, Brodmann (1908) had to construct the concept of brain areas distinguished by their cytoarchitecture. Likewise, in decomposing fermentation into component operations, biochemists needed concepts for the relevant different types of chemical reactions (oxidation, phosphorylation, etc.). In addition, researchers needed the requisite experimental tools to determine when these concepts are satisfied. Moreover, a given group of researchers may only have the tools for one type of decomposition; indeed, at a given time, only one set of tools may be available in the scientific community. Brodmann aspired to distinguish brain regions that would perform distinct mental operations, but he had no tools for picking out such operations; biochemists in the 1930s sought to link reactions with specific enzymes, but they could not determine the chemical constitution of enzymes (or even determine whether they were macromolecules or colloids). The ultimate goal, though, is to localize component operations in component parts of the mechanism, but the understanding of how to do so may only develop at the end of a sustained inquiry.

The process of decomposing a mechanism takes place over time. The importance of functional decomposition is often ignored in the early stages of a mechanistic research project, where it is common to attempt to localize a whole phenomenon in a single part of the mechanism. For example, Broca (1861) localized the faculty of articulate speech in the left prefrontal region that bears his name, and Buchner (1897) localized fermentation in a single enzyme he named *zymase*. Bechtel and Richardson (1993/2010) refer to this as "direct" or "simple" localization. Sometimes such localization is correct, but even when it is, it simply relocates the mechanism in a component of what was taken to be the mechanism. As such it does not directly constitute any explanatory advance, for it offers no account of how the phenomenon is produced. Yet it can play an important heuristic role in opening a line of empirical inquiry.

One can view what Barrett (2006) calls "natural kind" approaches to emotion as engaged in the project of directly localizing individual emotions in brain regions. She identifies not only basic emotion theories but also some appraisal theories as exemplars of the approach. What distinguishes these approaches is that (1) emotions are a discrete, basic category of psychological phenomena distinct from perception, memory, reason, etc.; (2) fear, anger, happiness, sadness, etc., are discrete types of emotions, irreducible to more basic psychological phenomena; and (3) the discrete emotion types are localized in distinct areas of the brain, whether these are single brain regions or discrete networks. Lindquist et al. (2012) call this the "locationist approach." What is characteristic of this approach is that the decompositions proposed in steps (1) and (2) are in terms of phenomena, not the operations realizing them. The reliance on such *phenomenal decompositions* (Bechtel, 2008) is extremely common in psychology. It was the strategy of the faculty psychologists, and it provided the basis for Gall's program of phrenology. Although faculty psychology and phrenology are widely denigrated today, their approach to decomposing psychological processes is evident in the division of psychological processes into categories such as memory, perception, and language, of memory into long-term versus short-term memory, and of long-term memory itself into episodic and semantic memory. With the advent of functional magnetic resonance imaging (fMRI), these categories have often provided the psychological activities to be localized in the brain.

The constructionists' contention is that the delineation of natural kinds of emotion "has outlived its scientific value and now presents a major obstacle to understanding what emotions are and how they work" (Barrett, 2006, p. 29). We agree that this approach needs to be supplanted by one that engages in decomposition of emotional phenomena into their operative parts and operations, and that these will not be properly characterized in the language of emotion, memory, or perception, but in more basic vocabulary that identifies the general operations that constitute the mind. But an important question is how to move forward to the "promised land." Here it is important to recognize that even when it turns out to be incorrect, direct localization can be heuristically productive in the development of a science. One way that it does so is by promoting the discovery of evidence that the part in which the phenomenon was localized is not the only part involved. Then researchers start to ask what the various parts are doing, and this prompts finally decomposition into the contributions of the different parts. It can also bring the realization that different phenomena rely on the same part, prompting the question of what operation might be involved in these various phenomena. Lindquist et al.'s (2012) meta-analysis of the neuro-imaging literature on human emotion is one recent example of this kind of research framed in opposition to direct localization accounts of emotion (see also Oosterwijk, Touroutoglou, & Lindquist, Chapter 5, this volume).

While it is easy to identify examples where psychologists and cognitive neuroscientists have settled for simple localizations, neuroimaging (as well as the other main tool of cognitive neuroscience, analysis of lesions) has itself provided evidence of the need to decompose psychological phenomena and not just localize them in the brain. In one of the first positron emission tomographic (PET) studies of cognitive processes, Petersen, Fox, Posner, Mintun, and Raichle (1988) found that the verb-generation task elicited increased blood flow in left dorsolateral prefrontal cortex, the anterior cingulate, and the cerebellum. Although much of the interest focused on the left dorsolateral prefrontal cortex, the researchers themselves were puzzled by the activity in the anterior cingulate, and interested in what it and the cerebellum contributed. Moreover, the fact that nearly the same region of left dorsolateral prefrontal cortex showed increased activation in a semantic memory task led Gabrieli, Poldrack, and Desmond (1998) to conclude that "operations may be the same whether they are considered in the context of language, working memory, episodic memory, or implicit memory. The left prefrontal cortex thus serves as a crossroads between meaning in language and memory" (p. 912). The current generation of neuroimaging studies that focuses on networks of brain regions that exhibit synchronized behavior in the resting state and are then recruited in specific cognitive tasks (Mantini, Perrucci, Del Gratta, Romani, & Corbetta, 2007; Fox & Raichle, 2007; van den Heuvel, Mandl, Kahn, & Pol, 2009; Sporns, 2010; Moussa, Steen, Laurienti, & Hayasaka, 2012) is the outgrowth of the earlier attempts to localize cognitive activities in single brain regions. Barrett and Satpute (2013) describe this transition in neuroscientific research on emotion and social cognition (see also Lindquist & Barrett, 2012).

Attempts to directly localize phenomena in single components of an organism have often revealed the limitations of such an approach. In anticipating this, the vitalists (a diverse group of 17th- through the 19th-century biologists who rejected mechanist approaches to the activities of living organisms and often appealed to a vital force to explain these phenomena) were often correct in their objections to early proposals of mechanistic biologists. But whereas the vitalists lacked a positive research program of their own, an important virtue of the mechanist project was that it generated hypotheses for which falsifying evidence (e.g., that other parts were involved) could emerge, forcing researchers to address the question of what operations they performed and to develop a functional decomposition of the phenomenon into multiple operations.

As difficult as it often is to identify the parts of a mechanism, identifying operations can be even more challenging. The problem is that when the mechanism is functioning, the component operations interact smoothly, so that the result of one operation feeds directly into others. Barrett (2009) captures this point when she comments, "The contents of a psychological state reveal nothing about the processes that realize it, in much the same way that a loaf of bread does not reveal the ingredients that constitute it" (p. 330; however, we would prefer a better analogy, since a loaf of bread is not an active mechanism). Often the clues as to the component operations must come from sources other than direct interventions on the mechanism, such as lesioning or stimulating its parts. In biochemistry, for example, they were provided by organic chemists, who discovered that organic compounds comprise groups, such as hydroxyl or phosphate groups, and that operations might involve adding or removing whole groups or modifying them in predicable ways. With these operations in mind, researchers could attempt to organize the different potential intermediates they identified when the reaction was interrupted at various points into comprehensible sequences of chemical reactions.

Only in a few areas has it been possible to propose psychological operations out of which mechanisms responsible for psychological phenomena can be constructed. In the case of sensory systems, it has been possible in some cases to identify the types of stimuli to which particular neurons are responsive—center–surround contrasts in the retina and lateral geniculate nucleus (LGN), oriented and moving edges in V1 (primary visual cortex), illusory contours in V2, shapes in V4—and then to ask what sorts of information-processing operations would enable the downstream region to identify a feature such as an illusory contour from representations of edges. Likewise, the discovery of different cells that respond to information relevant to navigation in the medial temporal lobe (place cells, head-direction cells, grid cells, boundary-vector cells) has provided researchers a basis on which to hypothesize about the information-processing operations that enable navigation by path integration. In many regions, such as the hippocampus and surrounding areas, the neural architecture provides both clues and evidence for hypotheses about the operations being performed.

It is noteworthy that the examples in the previous paragraph appeal to neuroscience to identify the information-processing operations underlying the cognitive activities of whole agents (e.g., seeing or navigating). In contrast, constructionists often focus on *psychological* primitives and appeal to examples such as categorizing and core affect as the basic operations (Barrett, 2009; Russell, 2003). There are, however, virtues in appealing to neuroscience in identifying operations. The first is that the operations to which constructionists appeal are often surprisingly close to the phenomena to be explained. Categorizing is an activity that agents (even single-celled organisms such as bacteria) perform. Moreover, it is an activity that may be performed in different ways, relying on different operations. We worry that despite constructionists' concern to supplant folk psychological operations with ones from which they are generated, they may have stayed too close to the folk level. This is not surprising, since, short of insight from outside, theorists have few places to go to identify the component activities. However, we are sympathetic to the view that appealing directly to the operations of the brain is to look to too low a level of organization to develop explanations of psychological phenomena. Contrary to some philosophical reductionists (Bickle, 2003), the goal in explanation is not to descend to the lowest possible level, but to the level at which one finds operations out of which a mechanism can generate the phenomenon of interest. For many higher cognitive phenomena we need more complex operations than those that might be performed by single neurons. The virtue, though, of operations specified in terms of the neural architecture is that they are independently grounded and not just the projections of phenomena onto the mechanism that is to explain them. Even if, for many purposes, they are operations at too low a level of organization to figure directly in the explanation of cognitive phenomena, they do afford the prospect of identifying higher-level structures whose operations may be appropriate to the phenomena of interest. These might include neural columns or brain regions. Barrett (2009) is critical of the suggestion of appealing to columns on the grounds that they have many projections beyond themselves. This, however, is not a reason to reject them as the structures whose operations support cognition, since we expect the parts of a mechanism to interact with each other to generate phenomena.

A second concern is with the prospect of differentiating psychological and neural operations. Barrett's (2009) proposal of psychological primitives seems to impose an unnecessary and unhelpful boundary between psychology and neuroscience. In mechanistic research there is always a level of decomposition beyond which particular researchers, with the tools and techniques available to them, typically do not go. Often this presents no problem—to explain the phenomenon they seek to explain, it is enough to show the parts and operations out of which it is constructed. They or someone else may then become interested in the components themselves, treat them as phenomena, and seek to explain them mechanistically. This does not mean denying the higher-level construction! In going further down, these researchers are asking different questions and appealing to different types of parts and operations to explain the component mechanism. For purposes of explanation, one may establish a level of parts and operations one takes as primitive, but there is nothing magical or necessarily psychological about the operations in terms of which one decomposes a phenomenon—especially given the lack of consensus over the nature of the "mental" or "psychological." Researchers trained in and employing techniques of psychology may in fact identify and invoke the same parts and operations as someone trained in and employing the tools of neuroscience. One of the goals of inquiry in neuroscience is to identify the operations (information-processing activities) that various brain regions perform. As these are characterized, they may equally be employed by psychologists as the operations they invoke in psychological explanations.

Identifying the parts and operations into which to decompose psychological phenomena remains a major challenge for psychology. It is, however, a challenge that all mechanistic sciences face. Moreover, even if the early attempts have stuck too close to folk categories and have not identified the parts and operations required to explain psychological phenomena, there is no reason for despair. In particular, collaboration with neuroscience may help to generate higher-level psychological operations in terms of which the desired explanations can be developed. In recent work, Barrett (Barrett & Satpute, 2013; Lindquist & Barrett, 2012) appears to be taking these lessons to heart, by exploring intrinsic functional neural networks as the "core systems" realizing higher-level, domain-general psychological operations out of which emotions and other agent-level psychological phenomena are constructed. In addition to using neuroscience as a guide to discovering higher-level psychological operations, Barrett's newer terminology of "core systems" better suggests that these domain-general psychological ingredients are not essentially "primitive" and can themselves be structurally and functionally decomposed into parts and operations.

Decomposition and Recomposition

As we have stressed, the goal of decomposition is to identify parts and operations that contribute to the phenomenon but do not individually exhibit the phenomenon. The gain in explanation comes from understanding how components that do not themselves exhibit the phenomenon can nonetheless exhibit it when working collaboratively. The challenge is to understand how such collaboration can yield the phenomenon. Again, in pressing this point, we concur with Barrett (2009, p. 332) that "there must be an explicit accounting (i.e., a mapping) of how categories at each level relate to one another." To emphasize how this endeavor complements decomposition, we refer to it as *recomposition*. Even though, just as in the case of decomposition, researchers may not literally put the parts back together, they must at least do so conceptually.

Recomposition, however, turns out to be considerably harder than decomposition, because we have only begun to understand the consequences of different modes of organization. When humans think about combining operations, they tend to do so sequentially, as in an assembly line. The same holds true for scientists trying to recompose mechanisms. When operations are envisaged as sequentially ordered, researchers can recompose them in their minds, imagining the results of executing the first operation, then imagining the second applied to it, and so forth. Thus, one can imagine DNA being transcribed into various RNAs, them being transported to the cytoplasm, where transfer RNA (tRNA) binds with an amino acid and then with a locus on a messenger RNA (mRNA), the amino acid forming a bond with the last amino acid to have been added to the polypeptide sequence, and so forth. Likewise, one can imagine visual perception resulting from processing first by center–surround cells in the retina and LGN, then by edge detection cells in V1, and so forth.

This sequential conception of a mechanism has been enshrined in Machamer et al.'s (2000, p. 3) characterization of a mechanism as operating "from start or set-up to finish or termination conditions." It, moreover, is a factor behind the frequent view that mechanisms are impoverished in what they can accomplish and are not up to the challenges of producing cognition. For example, Barrett and colleagues' (2014; Barrett, 2009) critique of the "machine" metaphor for the mind often targets this linear organization as one its main inadequacies.

This sequential conception of mechanism is, however, both inadequate for most biological mechanisms and vastly underestimates what can be accomplished when mechanisms are organized in a more complex manner. But the failure to look beyond sequentially organized mechanisms is not surprising, because it turns out to be very difficult for humans to understand how systems organized in a nonsequential manner will behave. One of the simplest departures from sequential order is negative feedback, in which a later process in an imagined sequence affects the execution of an earlier one. Its first known use in human design was a water clock by Ktesibios in the third century B.C., but it had to be continually reinvented over the next 2,000 years when designers sought to maintain a system at a target level. In the early 20th century it became more widely used and was then heralded by the cyberneticists as a fundamental principle found in both biological and social systems.

Negative feedback is sufficiently simple that most people can grasp how it works in their imagination: As a furnace heats the air, it causes metal to expand, opening a switch, causing the furnace to stop. When the temperature drops sufficiently, the metal contracts, the switch is closed, and the furnace again generates heat. But while this use of negative feedback to control a mechanism so as to maintain or approach a target state can be intuitively understood, another important effect of negative feedback—that it can generate sustained oscillations—is even today not widely recognized except by engineers who view it as a nuisance they seek to minimize. The reason is that by mentally simulating a system with negative feedback, one cannot ascertain whether it will continue to oscillate or it will dampen. Whether it will do so depends on whether the operations are appropriately nonlinear, a feature we cannot capture in our mental rehearsal. Confronted with nonsequential mechanisms with nonlinear operations, researchers adopt a different strategy to recompose the mechanism: They mathematically or computationally model it by representing the operations in terms of differential equations and employing them in a computational model to simulate the functioning of the mechanism.

The nonsequential, nonlinear nature of biological mechanisms not only serves to make them more challenging for scientists to understand, but it also provides them the resources to behave in a manner very different from the way machines they have designed typically behave. Moreover, these behaviors are crucial to the ability of living organisms to maintain themselves as distinct entities, recruiting matter and energy from their environment and continually building and repairing themselves. Biological organisms are in this sense *autonomous* (Ruiz-Mirazo, Peretó, & Moreno, 2004). Autonomous systems are not just reactive systems; they are endogenously active. Endogenous activity is already manifested in the simplest life forms—single-celled organisms without neurons or brains, including prokaryotes that lack differentiated organelles. Even such "simple" organisms carry out complex processing of information about their environment and use it to modulate their endogenous activity, including motor behavior, a task for which animals employ a nervous system. This endogenously active feature of organisms carries over to brains—a signature of this endogenous activity is the oscillatory behavior that can be identified at a wide range of frequencies and shows up in the synchronized activity across networks in the brain (Abrahamsen & Bechtel, 2011).

In rejecting the machine model for the mind, Barrett (2009) opts instead for the recipe model: Mental phenomena are constructions in accord with recipes (see also Barrett et al., 2014). But the entries in a recipe book are static entities, and only when utilized by a skilled chef do they figure in the generation of the rich variety of foods that we associate with them. It is the chef, not the recipes, that is critical to this process, and he or she does so as an endogenously active system engaged in ongoing, variable interactions with an environment. We suggest that it is more appropriate to maintain the mechanistic perspective but recognize that the mechanisms involved in the brain involve nonlinear operations organized in complex ways that we are only beginning to identify and understand.[5] One feature of brain organization that researchers are beginning to understand is that at different levels of organization, it exhibits a small-world architecture in which units (neurons, columns, brain regions) are primarily connected to their neighbors, but with a few long-range connections (Watts & Strogratz, 1998). The high clustering of local units allows clusters to specialize in specific types of information processing, while the short path length enables these clusters to coordinate their activities as appropriate. The local clusters in such an organization can be viewed as specialized information-processing mechanisms whose operations cognitive science and neuroscience are trying to identify. The mental activities and behaviors of cognitive agents result from the coordinated operation of many of these clusters as a person, as a whole, engages his or her environment. This is the conception of the functioning of the brain that the metaphor of construction is advanced to capture, and we suggest that when the complex dynamic behavior that is possible in mechanisms is recognized, their account is best served by the framework of mechanistic explanation. Cunningham, Dunfield, and Stillman (Chapter 7, this volume) and Thagard and Schröder (Chapter 6, this volume) offer examples of mechanistic accounts of emotion emphasizing a complex, dynamic organization of neural parts and operations.

Reconstituting the Phenomena

Mechanistic research is directed at explaining phenomena that have already been delineated. But as we have already noted, delineating phenomena is an ongoing activity, and it goes on even as explanations are being developed. Researchers might devote considerable effort to explaining a phenomenon only to realize that it has quite a different character than initially assumed. In one particularly dramatic example, biologists spent over a century trying to explain the phenomenon of animal heat. For much of that time, heat was presumed to be an energy resource. In the process of trying to explain animal heat, researchers came to understand many of the important operations that go into basic metabolism. But, eventually, heat came to be recognized as a waste product—once free energy was turned into heat, it was no longer available to do useful work in living organisms. Only the energy that was captured in chemical bonds, such as those of adenosine triphosphate (ATP), is available for work. Bechtel and Richardson (1993/2010) refer to such revisions in the characterization of the phenomenon as *reconstituting the phenomenon*.

Does the fact that the operations performed in the brain are not themselves appropriately characterized in terms of the folk categories of emotion, thought, memory, self-knowledge, etc., entail that mental phenomena themselves should be reconstituted? Eliminativists in the philosophy of mind have long contended that these and other categories of folk psychology should be eliminated from science when they are found to be incapable of being reduced to the best available theory of how the brain works (Churchland, 1981). But the assumption that these categories track internal operations in the mind or brain may misrepresent their role in a fundamental way. Whole persons use folk psychological concepts to characterize themselves and other people, and these characterizations can have significant psychological and behavioral consequences. For example, if we can conceptualize what our goals are, we may be better able to identify and avoid acting on desires that are incompatible with them. And when we attribute beliefs and desires to others, we may be able to anticipate their behavior and better coordinate our own actions with theirs. These uses of folk idioms have consequences for behavior and so make them an appropriate focus of psychological research even if they do not track the basic operations of our mental mechanisms.

Barrett (2012; Barrett, Wilson-Mendenhall, & Barsalou, Chapter 4, this volume) and other psychological constructionists take a position along these lines about the psychological phenomena identified by folk categories. They treat emotion, cognition, etc., as genuine psychological phenomena rather than endorsing their complete elimination from the science of psychology. But they endorse an alternative characterization of these psychological phenomena. Rather than being primitive categories of the mind, these phenomena are constructed from more basic psychological ingredients, many of which are shared across psychological phenomena the folk distinguish as emotional or cognitive. In the case of the different emotion categories, constructionists deny that they are distinguished by unique psychological ingredients (and the mechanisms that realize them). Rather, emotional episodes of anger, fear, etc., are ones in which core affect and other interoceptive and exteroceptive sensory information are conceptualized by the agent as instantiating an emotion category. According to psychological constructionists, the psychological and behavioral components of emotional episodes do not exhibit the tight correlations assumed by natural kind theories of emotion. These psychological ingredients are involved in many phenomena that the folk distinguish as emotional and non-emotional. Emotional episodes in ourselves and others occur, for constructionists, when sets of these loosely correlated ingredients are conceptualized by an observer as an instance of an emotion category. This categorization process is a real phenomenon that can have psychological, behavioral, and social consequences, which are to be studied by psychologists. It is just that these emotional phenomena do not exist independent of agents' conceptualization process. Accordingly, Barrett (2012, 2009) describes emotions as "observer-dependent" phenomena, distinct from "observer-independent" phenomena, whose existence does not depend on being recognized or conceptualized by minded beings.

We accept this metaphysical distinction between entities that depend on minded beings for their existence and those that do not, but we question its being given any special status. Many metaphysical categories, especially ones in biology, may be in this way relational (i.e., the metaphysical nature of the entities depend on their relations with other entities), without depending on the existence of *minds*. Niches are defined with respect to the traits of the organisms that inhabit them, and chemical attractants for bacteria are defined with respect to the organism's chemical receptors. Furthermore, we reject that the distinction between ontologically dependent and independent entities entails a sharp *epistemological* divide between folk and scientific concepts, or between psychological and neuroscientific concepts. Concepts across both divides are heavily dependent on the theories and interests of human cognizers, and may not carve reality (whether it is mind-dependent or independent) at its joints.[6] As humans, we have as much scientific interest in developing categories that facilitate understanding of ourselves and directing our actions as we do in those that characterize the physical, chemical, and biological processes that constitute us.

Making these points, however, does not call into question the psychological constructionist view that some psychological phenomena are constructions rather than psychological primitives, and dependent upon the psychological concepts of the people under study. We agree that "psychology must explain the existence of cognition and emotion because they are part of the world that we (in the Western hemisphere) live in" (Barrett, 2009, p. 330). This makes the study of emotion part of the larger interdisciplinary research program examining people's folk psychological or "mind-reading" abilities. It is a debated issue in the literature whether attributing mental states to oneself involves a distinctive sort of introspective access to one's own mental states, or engages the same nonintrospective methods one uses to attribute mental states to others (e.g., Carruthers, 2009). The latter position can easily be accommodated by constructivists, since, on this view, the process of attributing mental states to others and oneself can be seen as a construction based on a variety of available forms of evidence. But so can a version of the introspectionist account, if the objects of introspection are restricted to the sensory states that constructionists include in their accounts of emotion categorization. While much of the mind-reading literature assumes that Western folk psychological concepts do reflect the actual architecture of the mind, some emphasize that the importance of mind reading depends on its usefulness in mediating social interaction and regulating one's own behavior, rather than on its accurately describing our inner workings (e.g., Godfrey-Smith, 2004, 2005; Zawidzki, 2013). Such accounts have clear affinities toward psychological constructionism.

We do not here take a stand on whether psychological constructionism is correct in its call to reconstitute psychological phenomena. From the perspective of mechanistic explanation, we emphasize that such revision in how the phenomena are described can be the result of research at the level of the whole—such as when constructionists call into question the proposed correlations between the various behavioral measures of emotion—or the indirect result of research at lower levels investigating the mechanisms responsible for these phenomena. In the latter case, for example, the finding that basic emotion categories fail to be localized in distinct brain regions can motivate inquiry into whether these categories should or should not be retained at the level of characterizing persons. In the case of psychological constructionism, its central contention is that psychology has been restricted by its adherence to Western folk psychological concepts, especially in the case of emotion. While many folk concepts have been eliminated as science has progressed, folk psychological concepts have the unique status of being used by us humans to characterize ourselves, and thus partially constitute and influence our own minds. Therefore, folk concepts of emotion have an important place in psychological research, whether or not they accurately reflect the nature of our mental mechanisms.

Conclusion

In this chapter we have highlighted several ways that the new mechanistic philosophy of science can shed light on psychological constructionism. The mechanistic approach offers a multilevel framework for conducting research and explaining psychological phenomena in terms of more basic components. Research into the psychological construction of mental phenomena can benefit from the mechanistic approach's emphasis on both decomposition of a mechanism into its basic parts and operations, and recomposing those parts into an organized whole that is environmentally situated. In this context, we can understand the move from natural kind theories of psychological phenomena to the psychological construction approach as the transition from simple localization to more complex and dynamic accounts of the neural mechanisms responsible for these psychological phenomena, and potentially to a reconceptualization or reconstitution of mental phenomena themselves.

NOTES

1. The relationship between phenomena and mechanisms allows for multiple perspectives. Typically, mechanistic philosophers of science have emphasized the delineation of the phenomenon as the reference point and construed the mechanism as consisting of whatever parts and operations are responsible for it. The same parts and operations may, on this view, be constituents of multiple mechanisms depending on what phenomenon one is explaining. However, sometimes researchers focus on the parts and operations constituting a mechanism, then identify additional phenomena for which they are responsible. While there are contexts in which scientists operate in the latter manner, one reason to prefer the former approach is that mechanisms often do not come well delineated in nature (as is more likely in a human-made machine). Especially in biological systems, different components can be recruited into a functioning system when one activity is required, and into another functioning system on another occasion. A similar problem arises with

phenomena (biological phenomena are often integrated with each other), but in the context of a given research endeavor, the approach of the investigators provides a basis for characterizing the phenomenon for which explanation is sought.

2. Recognizing that scientists sometimes model mechanisms via computational simulations is compatible with, but does not entail that the modeled activities of the mechanism and/or their parts are themselves computational processes. A mechanistic approach in psychology is therefore compatible with, but not necessarily committed to, a computational theory of mind that metaphysically characterizes psychological processes as computational or information-processing activities.

3. Russell (2009) seems to support the idea that psychological constructionism involves a holism across psychology: "The traditional assumption is that a 'theory of emotion' will differ from a theory of cognition, or behaviour, or conation. My claim, in contrast, is that any theory that explains all cases called emotion will be close to the whole of psychology, a theory that of course will not be limited to emotion but will extend to all psychological processes" (p. 1268).

4. Mechanists agree with Barrett (2009) that "the categories at each level of the scientific ontology capture something different from what their component parts capture, and each must be described in its own terms and with its own vocabulary" (p. 332).

5. Barrett et al. (2014) introduce two other supposedly "more apt" nonmachine-based models for the relation between the mind and brain: "molecules that are constructed of atoms" and "chamber music emerging from the interplay of instruments." Unfortunately neither quite captures both the nonlinear organization and endogenous activity we emphasize in the dynamic mechanistic perspective.

6. Although it may seem strange to say a metaphysical category that is constructed via the conceptualization of minded beings is not accurately conceptualized, this is not contradictory. It is possible for agents to use one set of concepts in unreflectively constructing the category, but use another set in their reflective thought about that metaphysical domain (see also Barrett, 2012, p. 422).

REFERENCES

Abrahamsen, A., & Bechtel, W. (2011). From reactive to endogenously active dynamical conceptions of the brain. In K. Plaisance & T. Reydon (Eds.), *Philosophy of behavioral biology* (pp. 329–366). New York: Springer.

Barrett, L. F. (2006). Are emotions natural kinds? *Perspectives on Psychological Science, 1,* 28–58.

Barrett, L. F. (2009). The future of psychology: Connecting mind to brain. *Perspectives on Psychological Science, 4,* 326–339.

Barrett, L. F. (2012). Emotions are real. *Emotion, 12,* 413–429.

Barrett, L. F., & Satpute, A. B. (2013). Large-scale brain networks in affective and social neuroscience: Towards an integrative functional architecture of the brain. *Current Opinion in Neurobiology, 23*(3), 361–372.

Barrett, L. F., Wilson-Mendenhall, C. D., & Barsalou, L. W. (2014). A psychological construction account of emotion regulation and dysregulation: The role of situated conceptualizations. In J. J. Gross (Ed.), *The handbook of emotion regulation* (2nd ed., pp. 447–465). New York: Guilford Press.

Bechtel, W. (2008). *Mental mechanisms*. London: Routledge.

Bechtel, W., & Abrahamsen, A. (2005). Explanation: A mechanist alternative. *Studies in History and Philosophy of Biological and Biomedical Sciences, 36,* 421–441.

Bechtel, W., & Richardson, R. C. (2010). *Discovering complexity: Decomposition and localization as strategies in scientific research.* Cambridge, MA: MIT Press. (Original 1993 edition published by Princeton University Press)

Bickle, J. (2003). *Philosophy and neuroscience: A ruthlessly reductive account.* Dordrecht, The Netherlands: Kluwer.

Bogen, J., & Woodward, J. (1988). Saving the phenomena. *Philosophical Review, 97,* 303–352.

Broca, P. (1861). Remarques sur le siége de la faculté du langage articulé, suivies d'une observation d'aphemie (perte de la parole) [Remarks on the seat of the faculty of articulated language, following an observation of aphemia (loss of speech)]. *Bulletin de la Société Anatomique, 6,* 343–357.

Brodmann, K. (1908). Beiträge zur histologischen Lokalisation der Grosshirnrinde. VI. Mitteilung: Dei Cortexgliederung des Menschen [Contributions to a histological localization of the cerebral cortex. VI. Communication: The division of the human cortex]. *Journal für Psychologie und Neurologie, 10,* 231–246.

Buchner, E. (1897). Alkoholische Gärung ohne Hefezellen (Vorläufige Mittheilung) [Alcoholic fermentation without yeast cells]. *Berichte der Deutschen Chemischen Gesellschaft, 30,* 117–124.

Carruthers, P. (2009). How we know our own minds: The relationship between mindreading and metacognition. *Behavioral and Brain Sciences, 32,* 121–138.

Churchland, P. M. (1981). Eliminative materialism and propositional attitudes. *Journal of Philosophy, 78,* 67–90.

Craver, C. F. (2007). *Explaining the brain: What a science of the mind-brain could be.* New York: Oxford University Press.

Cummins, R. (2000). "How does it work?" versus "What are the laws?": Two conceptions of psychological explanation. In F. Keil & R. Wilson (Eds.), *Explanation and cognition* (pp. 117–144). Cambridge, MA: MIT Press.

Darden, L. (2006). *Reasoning in biological discoveries: Essays on mechanisms, interfield relations, and anomaly resolution.* Cambridge, UK: Cambridge University Press.

Fox, M. D., & Raichle, M. E. (2007). Spontaneous fluctuations in brain activity observed with functional magnetic resonance imaging. *Nature Reviews Neuroscience, 8,* 700–711.

Gabrieli, J. D. E., Poldrack, R. A., & Desmond, J. E. (1998). The role of left prefrontal cortex in language and memory. *Proceedings of the National Academy of Sciences USA, 95,* 906–913.

Gendron, M., & Barrett, L. F. (2009). Reconstructing the past: A century of ideas about emotion in psychology. *Emotion Review, 1,* 316–339.

Godfrey-Smith, P. (2004). On folk psychology and mental representation. In H. Clapin, P. Staines, & P. Slezak (Eds.), *Representation in mind: New approaches to mental representation* (pp. 147–162). Amsterdam: Elsevier.

Godfrey-Smith, P. (2005). Folk psychology as a model. *Philosopher's Imprint, 5,* 1–16.

Gross, J. J., & Barrett, L. F. (2011). Emotion generation and emotion regulation: One or two depends on your point of view. *Emotion Review, 3,* 8–16.

Hempel, C. G. (1965). Aspects of scientific explanation. In C. G. Hempel (Ed.), *Aspects of scientific explanation and other essays in the philosophy of science* (pp. 331–496). New York: Macmillan.

Hempel, C. G. (1966). *Philosophy of natural science.* Englewood Cliffs, NJ: Prentice-Hall.

Langley, P., Simon, H. A., Bradshaw, G. L., & Zytkow, J. M. (1987). *Scientific discovery: Computational explorations of the creative process.* Cambridge, MA: MIT Press.

Lindquist, K. A., & Barrett, L. F. (2012). A functional architecture of the human brain: Emerging insights from the science of emotion. *Trends in Cognitive Sciences, 16,* 533–540.

Lindquist, K. A., Wager, T. D., Kober, H., Bliss-Moreau, E., & Barrett, L. F. (2012). The brain basis of emotion: A meta-analytic review. *Behavioral and Brain Sciences, 35,* 121–143.

Machamer, P., Darden, L., & Craver, C. F. (2000). Thinking about mechanisms. *Philosophy of Science, 67,* 1–25.

Mantini, D., Perrucci, M. G., Del Gratta, C., Romani, G. L., & Corbetta, M. (2007). Electrophysiological signatures of resting state networks in the human brain. *Proceedings of the National Academy of Sciences, 104,* 13170–13175.

Moussa, M. N., Steen, M. R., Laurienti, P. J., & Hayasaka, S. (2012). Consistency of network modules in resting-state fMRI connectome data. *PLoS ONE, 7,* e44428.

Petersen, S. E., Fox, P. T., Posner, M. I., Mintun, M., & Raichle, M. E. (1988). Positron emission tomographic studies of the cortical anatomy of single-word processing. *Nature, 331,* 585–588.

Prinz, J. J. (2004). *Gut reactions: A perceptual theory of emotion.* New York: Oxford University Press.

Ruiz-Mirazo, K., Peretó, J., & Moreno, A. (2004). A universal definition of life: Autonomy and open-ended evolution. *Origins of Life and Evolution of the Biosphere, 34,* 323–346.

Russell, J. A. (2003). Core affect and the psychological construction of emotion. *Psychological Review, 110,* 145–172.

Russell, J. A. (2009). Emotion, core affect, and psychological construction. *Cognition and Emotion, 23,* 1259–1283.

Sporns, O. (2010). *Networks of the brain.* Cambridge, MA: MIT Press.

Thagard, P. (1988). *Computational philosophy of science.* Cambridge, MA: MIT Press/Bradford Books.

van den Heuvel, M. P., Mandl, R. C. W., Kahn, R. S., & Pol, H. E. H. (2009). Functionally linked resting-state networks reflect the underlying structural connectivity architecture of the human brain. *Human Brain Mapping, 30,* 3127–3141.

Watts, D., & Strogratz, S. (1998). Collective dynamics of small worlds. *Nature, 393,* 440–442.

Zawidzki, T. D. (2013). *Mindshaping: A new framework for understanding human social cognition.* Cambridge, MA: MIT Press.

CHAPTER 3

Ten Common Misconceptions about Psychological Construction Theories of Emotion

LISA FELDMAN BARRETT

Humans communicate through stories—in fictional novels and movies, in memoirs and autobiographies, and even in science. Scientists run experiments and use their data to tell stories about how the world works. Every story belongs to a family that shares foundational beliefs and assumptions. These beliefs and assumptions belong to the *metanarrative structure* of a story. For example, in Western storytelling, narratives usually have a beginning, a middle, and an end. Stories with a hero must also have a villain. There can be no redemption without a temptation or at least a conflict. And so on. Even though we might not be explicitly aware of these metanarrative elements, writers and readers use them in tacit agreement. Writers automatically rely on them to make their stories comprehensible, and listeners automatically employ them to predict where an author is going and to understand what he or she is saying. In science, a family of stories sharing a metanarrative structure can be thought of as a "scientific paradigm" (in the tradition of Thomas Kuhn) with a conventionally agreed-upon explanatory framework. Scientific revolutions (to the extent that they actually occur) might be described as one metanarrative story structure replacing another. When a story violates the expected metanarrative structure (e.g., a listener from one culture is parsing a story with a different metanarrative structure from another culture, or a scientist from a scientific paradigm is reading the work of another scientist who fundamentally challenges the assumptions of that paradigm), confusions and misunderstandings usually ensue.

The story will not be easily understood, because the listener is employing a different set of assumptions than is the storyteller. As a result, the story will seem unintuitive and needlessly complex.

As a scientific approach, psychological construction violates several elements of psychology's dominant metanarrative structure for theories about minds and brains, making it vulnerable to misconceptions and misunderstandings. The purpose of this chapter is to consider explicitly some of the misconceptions in light of the metanarrative elements that cause them. The elements considered here are, of course, broad generalizations. No one is claiming that every theory of mind or brain contains every element, or that exceptions to these generalizations can never be found. The main observation is that certain metanarrative elements within psychology make it challenging to communicate psychological construction as a testable scientific approach to emotion, because the theory itself is often misunderstood.

MISCONCEPTION 1. Emotions are creations of the human mind and therefore they are illusions. They not real, and they have no utility or function.

Two metanarrative elements contribute to the mistaken claim that psychological construction considers emotions to be functionless illusions.

Metanarrative Element: Essentialism

Modern psychology theories tend to conceive of the mind as a system of categories, each one representing an organ of computation (mental module or psychological faculty) as an individual and separable process. Each process is presumed, more or less, to be a physical type that can be localized to a specific and distinct set of physical measurements (e.g., distinct and specific brain tissue, autonomic correlates, or behaviors).[1] The physical correlates are usually treated as its essence. This essentialist view of the mind has been labeled "the greatest historical contribution to the development of theoretical psychology" (Marshall, 1984, p. 216). Progress in science typically involves the use of more fine-grained mental categories, more sophisticated measurement and computational methods, and localization of function to networks or individual neurons instead of to gross anatomical brain regions, patterns of peripheral nervous system activation, or overt behaviors. In this view, an emotion category, for example, *fear*, is assumed to be a physical type (Barrett, 2006a, 2012, 2013; Lindquist & Barrett, 2012). Subtypes of *fear* might exist (e.g., Gross & Canteras, 2012; Kreibig, 2010), becoming the mental faculties of interest and replacing *fear* because it is too broad a category.

Why Psychological Construction Is Misunderstood

Psychological construction theorists hypothesize that each emotion category is populated with a variety of instances that do not share an essence. This hypothesis, which denies the metanarrative element of essentialism, is mistakenly understood as a claim that emotion categories are arbitrary groupings of instances, or in the extreme, that emotion words do not name anything real. To my knowledge, no scientist has actually claimed that emotions are random, illusory phenomena, perhaps other than Knight Dunlap and Elizabeth Duffy. In 1932, Dunlap wrote, "The search for 'primary emotions' is as much an anachronism in psychology today as is the search for the soul; and it is a search of the same sort. We must face the fact that the 'emotions' are names to which correspond no concrete realities" (p. 573). Duffy, in 1941, wrote, " 'Emotion' as a scientific concept is worse than useless" (p. 283). Dunlap and Duffy, along with many of their contemporaries (reviewed in Gendron & Barrett, 2009), were addressing the issue that physiological and behavioral studies had, up to that point, failed to find consistent and specific physical correlates to distinguish one emotion category from another (i.e., they had failed to find what scientists of the time had presumed to be each category's biological essence). Since that time, a number of reviews have made similar empirical observations (e.g., Barrett, 2006a; Cacioppo, Berntson, Larsen, Poehlmann, & Ito, 2000; Mandler, 1975; Ortony & Turner, 1990). Although these scientists often come to the conclusion that emotional faculties or modules are not real as physical (or perhaps even as universal psychological) types, this is not a claim that emotions are not real. Emotions can be real without being essentialized types.

Correction

A more modern hypothesis, typical of the psychological construction program of research, is that an emotion word such as "fear" corresponds to a conceptual category. An emotion category is not a physical type, with a physical essence, but a collection of instances that vary in their physical manifestations. These instances are not random but are functionally linked to the immediate situation or environment in which they emerge. This implies that an emotion word names a set of diverse events (or instances) that emerge from multiple causes, and not a single process that produces a set of similar instances or events. This observation also calls into question whether the traditional categories for emotion, such as *fear*, are too broad to allow for the accumulation of knowledge supporting induction and scientific generalization. This point was first made by William James (1884), and it has been echoed by several modern psychological constructionist writers (e.g., Barrett, 2006a; Russell, 2003). The point is not that instances of fear are random, but that *fear*, an emotion category, is too heterogeneous to be a scientifically useful way to explain why people act or feel the way that they do (because across instances of fear, they feel and act in a variety of ways). As a consequence, to understand fear properly, it is necessary to (1) map the heterogeneity and (2) understand the causal processes responsible for producing this heterogeneity. The claim is that instances of fear are highly functional in a situated way, even if the category *fear* does not, itself, represent a single function. This does not mean that fear serves no functions at all; instead, it means that fear can serve several functions (see Barrett, 2012; Barrett, Wilson-Mendenhall, & Barsalou, Chapter 4, this volume). The fact that emotions do not name brain networks or circuits or body systems does not necessarily mean that emotions have no explanatory value in the economy of behavior (e.g., see work by David DeSteno). An emotion does not have to be hardwired into the mammalian nervous system to be functional.

It is interesting to note that essentialism, as a metanarrative element, routinely causes misunderstandings in science. Essentialist beliefs keep people from accepting the reality of evolution, or cause people who believe in evolution to misunderstand the concept of natural selection (cf. Gelman & Rhodes, 2012; Lewontin, 2000). In particular, essentialism prevents people from understanding the kind of population-based thinking that Darwin used when he reformulated the concept of a *species* (as a conceptual category of unique individuals rather than as a physical type; Mayr, 1988). Similarly, essentialism has kept people from understanding population thinking about emotion, and population thinking is a key feature of some psychological construction theories of emotion (e.g., Barrett, 2013; also see Barrett et al., Chapter 4, this volume).

The bottom line is that by denying essentialism, psychological construction is claiming that an instance of emotion is not exclusively realized in the body of the emoter, or in the brain regions that regulate the body. The very existence of an emotional episode (either the self, in emotional experience, or another person, in emotion perception) also requires participation from other parts of the brain that are involved in storing prior experience and knowledge within a perceiver. To those who rely on essentialist assumptions, however, this is sometimes understood as claiming that an emotion is entirely in the mind of a perceiver. This kind of either-or thinking (if emotion is not in your body, then it is all in your head) relates to the second metanarrative element at play here.

Metanarrative Element: Top-Down (Perceiver-Based) Influences Always Cause Illusions

Modern psychological theories (other than those explicitly about perception) still assume that top-down (perceiver-based) contributions to perception are largely *modulatory* on veridical bottom-up readouts of the world and that when top-down influences *drive* perception this causes false impressions or misapprehensions (i.e., illusions). Psychology often delights in revealing how perceivers are mistaken, and are therefore naive, in their experiences of themselves and the world.

Why Psychological Construction Is Misunderstood

The standard view of emotions is that, as natural kind categories, emotions are *recognized* in the outputs of one's own body or in another person's actions. Psychological construction, in contrast, hypothesizes that a perceiver creates an emotion out of those mere physical changes by adding information from past experience about the psychological meaning and utility of those changes. From this perspective, then, an emotion is not recognized by a human mind in the outputs of the body or another's actions but is *constructed* by a human mind using those changes. Thus, psychological construction proposes that top-down (perception-based) contributions are necessary drivers of emotion. If one assumes that top-down influences create illusions, then it is easy to mistakenly assume that psychological construction theorists must be claiming that emotions are illusions. Of course, the construction process does not imply that the resulting perception is an illusion—the hypothesis is that perceiver-based contributions to perception occur as a normal consequence of how the human brain works.

Correction

A perceiver creates an instance of emotion without it being an illusion in the colloquial sense. In certain domains of psychology and increasingly in neuroscience, the hypothesis that perceivers actively contribute to their own perceptions and cognitions is a well-accepted story line. Within neuroscience there is increasing acceptance of the idea that the brain is a predictive organ that creates mental life by a process called "predictive coding," in which it continually generates hypotheses based on past experience in a top-down fashion and tests them against incoming data; in this view, top-down influences drive perception, they do not merely modulate it (e.g., Adams, Shipp, & Friston, 2013; Bastos et al., 2012; Clark, 2013; Friston, 2002; Hohwy, 2013; Shipp, Adams, & Friston, 2013). Predictive coding is the way that a normally functioning brain works. The brain's wiring is even set up this way. For example, it is well-established fact that top-down (perceiver-based) processing characterizes the normal functioning of every human brain. For every neural connection that brings sensory inputs from the thalamus to the cortex, there are 10 feedback connections from the cortex to the thalamus (Golshani, Liu, & Jones, 2001). The number of connections from visual cortex to the subcortical lateral geniculate nucleus far exceeds the number of connections from the lateral geniculate nucleus to the visual cortex (Sillito & Jones, 2002).

This driving "top-down" narrative element is not yet accepted in theories of emotion, however. Appraisal theories hypothesize top-down processes in emotion generation, but these are usually thought to react to and modulate in coming, bottom-up stimulation. The conceptual act theory of emotion, by contrast, implicitly uses ideas that are similar to the logic of predictive coding in its hypotheses about how the brain creates situated conceptualizations (which are the content of emotional episodes). As part of constructing a situated conceptualization, the brain makes predictions about what incoming interoceptive sensory input is expected (based on past experience with the rest of the immediate sensory array). This was once referred to as an "affective" prediction (Barrett & Bar, 2009) but more recently it has been called "interoceptive" prediction (Seth, 2013). Through a series of iterations, the brain compares the incoming sensory input to the prediction and corrects any prediction error, either by changing the prediction based on the exteroceptive input, or changing the sampling of sensory information (by moving the body, or by attentional shifts) to match the prediction. As a consequence, an instance of an emotion is a series of brain states that includes representations of the body and/or actions *and* the additional information that is necessary to create the new functions that make emotions real—that is, the parts that are crucial for creating the situated conceptualizations that are responsible for emotional gestalts (Barrett, 2012; Barrett et al., Chapter 4, this volume).

Some scientists, like myself and my co-authors (Barrett, 2012; Barrett, Wilson-Mendenhall, & Barsalou, 2014; Chapter 4, this volume) and Russell (2003), are partly responsible for the misunderstanding that emotions are illusions, because we employ visual illusions (or related phenomena) as analogies to make a point about the top-down influences in emotion construction. A visual illusion, by its nature, nicely reveals the presence of top-down influences, because the perception includes information that the perceiver supplies and that is not present in the exteroceptive stimulus. It therefore makes a good analogy for how an instance of emotion cannot exist without a perceiver. The goal, to illuminate the role of the perceiver in creating a perception, is not meant to imply that emotions are literally fictions. What a visual illusion demonstrates, such as the Müller–Lyer illusion, is that a perception is the joint product of sensory input from the world (two lines of equal length, one bounded by the inward facing arrowheads and the other bounded by outward pointing arrowheads), as well as knowledge from the perceiver (i.e., his or her prior experience with rectilinear objects and environments). No perception is solely determined by the sensory input (e.g., the lines) alone, and visual illusions are useful for demonstrating this. (Although analogies are often helpful to make a point in science, they are almost always limited in some way.)

Psychological construction theorists make the same point about emotions: They hypothesizes that emotions are not determined solely by sensory changes in a body. Emotions are perceptions that, in part, are a function of the perceiver's prior knowledge and experience. They further hypothesize that construction processes are not unique to emotions (or to visual illusions): The processes are at play in memories, in language comprehension, in moral reasoning, and so on. To claim that emotions are illusions would be to claim that every perception occurring in every moment of waking life is an illusion.

MISCONCEPTION 2: There is no synchrony in the physiology, behaviors, or experiences during emotions. The components of an emotion fluctuate randomly.

Metanarrative Element: Essentialism

It is traditional to assume that an emotion word such as "anger" corresponds to a consistent, coordinated packet of nervous system responses, behaviors (facial actions, action tendencies) and experiences. Many papers on emotion claim this as a scientific fact. Thus, "anger," "sadness," "fear," and some other emotion words are each assumed to refer to a physical type that is observable in nature. Because this pattern is the type's essence, it is assumed that the pattern will occur during each instance of anger. In the science of emotion, essentialism is often labeled as a "straw man" argument. It is often said that no one is really expecting the pattern for a given emotion to occur each and every time in an obligatory way. There will be some degree of variation, either because of stochastic, probabilistic influences, or because other non-emotional processes (e.g., display rules or regulatory strategies) come into play. But essentialism does appear to be implied here, even though it is less overt. Although some variation around each emotion type is to be expected, a modal physical pattern for each category (i.e., a prototype) is still expected (e.g., Tracy & Randles, 2011; Roseman, 2011), and it is still assumed that each emotion can be identified by its specific pattern.

Why Psychological Construction Is Misunderstood

Psychological constructionist theorists assume that an emotion category contains a population of heterogeneous instances. It is therefore assumed that the heterogeneity is real and meaningful as an intrinsic part of what emotions are and how they work. Therefore, this heterogeneity deserves to be understood as part of the nature of emotion in scientific terms, and should not be treated as error, or as reflecting some non-emotional process such as a display rule. Some theories, like the approach of Ortony and Clore (Chapter 13, this volume), assume that the heterogeneity is primarily in the physical manifestations of instances but hypothesize that an emotion category is a cognitive type; a variety of physical instances have the same psychological meaning. Other theories, such as my conceptual act theory, hypothesizes that heterogeneity exists even at the conceptual level within a category (e.g., Barrett, 2006b). These approaches stand in contrast, however, to what are called "basic" or traditional "appraisal" emotion theories, in which the pattern for each emotion category should either be obligatory (e.g., Ekman, 1992) or occur probabilistically (e.g., Roseman, 2011) across instances; a limited amount of variation in the observed pattern from the platonic form is acceptable, but significant deviation is treated as error, or as caused by processes outside the boundaries of the emotional response itself (e.g., display rules or regulatory mechanisms). With such assumptions, it makes sense to attempt a Linnaean-type classification of emotions. To deny the biological reality of this typology, as psychological construction does, is often considered to be synonomous with an argument for randomness, or a claim that emotions have no relationships whatsoever to facial actions or other bodily changes.

Correction

Psychological construction theorists do not deny that there are links between the body and behavior during emotions. Instead, they propose that these relationships are learned, probabilistic, produced by associative processes, and, most importantly, that there is not necessarily a single pattern of relations for each emotion category. This is another way of emphasizing that an emotion word such as "anger" refers to a conceptual category of variable instances.

In psychological construction, heterogeneity across instances within a category can manifest itself in two ways. First, it might not be possible to distinguish the instances of one category from the instances of every other category by consistent patterns of measurable changes (in the peripheral nervous system, the brain, the facial movements, or in other behaviors). That is, a given pattern (in a given experiment) might be *sufficient* to distinguish one emotion instance from another emotion instance, *but not necessary* (the pattern might not hold every time): A given instance of anger might be distinguishable from an instance of fear, but these patterns might not replicate across all instances of anger and fear. In fact, pattern classifiers that distinguish emotion categories with peripheral physiology measurements do not replicate across studies, even when exactly the same stimuli and methods are used (e.g., Kragel & LaBar, 2013; Stephens, Christie, & Friedman, 2010). This is because pattern classifiers should be understood as a disjunction of sufficient conditions. A second possibility is that an observed pattern might *be necessary but not sufficient*: A pattern might represent features that are repeatable across all instances of an emotion, and is therefore diagnostic for the category but insufficient for representing all that is meaningful and functional about each instance within the category. Put another way, diagnosis is not explanation. While both of these possibilities are distinct from a typological approach to emotion, neither proposes that emotional instances are random, or that the changes that occur during an emotional instance are random. Both of these possibilities are examples of how population-based thinking can be applied to understanding the structure of emotion categories, and as such are made more difficult to grasp by essentialistic thinking; in biology, population-based thinking was the last of Darwin's concepts to be understood, in part because of essentialist assumptions (Mayr, 1988).

At the very least, psychological construction offers an antidote for the emotion paradox (Barrett, 2006b): People routinely experience and perceive emotions, yet for over 100 years scientists have been trying unsuccessfully to find the unique biological substrates for each emotion. We have failed, despite having more sophisticated methods and improved experimental control at our disposal. So rather than assume that the biological signatures are there but we cannot find them, perhaps our starting position should be more neutral: Perhaps we should assume that our goal is to map the heterogeneity. Naturalistic observation and comparison is an important part of the scientific paradigm in biology (cf. Mayr, 1988) but it has largely been underutilized in psychology because it is expensive, impractical, and computationally difficult. But new methods and technologies make such observations possible. And who knows? We might just discover those illusive biological substrates for each emotion. One very real possibility is that we might discover idiographic regularities for each emotion category (i.e., a given person might have a repertoire of repeatable instances for *anger*, or *sadness*, or any emotion category).

The issue of whether there are *consistent* patterns of response that are sufficiently repeatable to distinguish all instances of one emotion category from all instances of another is a completely different issue than whether the various changes during a given instance of emotion are *synchronous* with one another (e.g., whether the autonomic nervous system, the brain activations, behaviors, etc., are coordinated with each other to produce a functional response in a given instance). Confusing coherence across instances of a category with synchrony within a given instance, again, reveals the metanarrative element of essentialism. Psychological construction approaches typically assume that various responses are synchronous during an individual emotional episode, because such coordination is part and parcel of healthy functioning. Every moment of life requires such synchronization—emotional episodes are not special in this regard. For example, psychological construction views are completely consistent with Obrist's hypothesis that autonomic nervous system activity is mobilized in response to the metabolic demands associated with an actual behavior (cardiosomatic coupling; Obrist, Wedd, Sutterer, & Howard, 1970) or an expected behavior (suprametabolic coupling; Obrist, 1981; cf. Barrett, 2006a, 2006b). Since limbic tissue in the brain is largely responsible for coordinating visceral and motor responses, thereby regulating the autonomic nervous system, hormonal, and metabolic functions in a way that meets immediate or predicted energy needs, it is reasonable to predict that brain activation patterns might also be situation or behavior specific.

Because psychological construction approaches emphasize that individual instances of an emotion category can vary in the ways that bodies, faces, and brain activation typically vary, some critics claim that psychological constructionists believe that there are no hardwired processes in the body and brain whatsoever. This is an error. Psychological constructionist views acknowledge that certain behavioral adaptations (freezing, fleeing, fighting, etc.) have been identified across a variety of mammalian species, including humans, and are caused by specific neural circuits (e.g., Barrett, 2012, 2013; Barrett et al., Chapter 4, this volume). But these adaptations do not have a one-to-one correspondence to a given emotion category, and they cannot be named with an emotion word, meaning that the circuit for freezing is not the circuit for fear, and the circuit for defensive aggression is not the circuit for anger.[2]

Similarly, because psychological construction emphasizes variability in the measureable outcomes during an emotion, is sometimes claimed that these theories are nonfalsifiable. This is also a mistake. Rather, psychological construction theories are not falsifiable by the standards of traditional emotion theories. Standard emotion theories that propose reliable and specific patterns of measured physiology, facial actions, and brain activations will be supported if they such patterns are found or falsified if they are not found. Psychological construction theories make no claims about specific patterns for each emotion category, so their validity does not rise or fall based on finding them. Psychological construction theories provide an alternative explanation to basic emotion and appraisal theories in the event that such patterns are found (which would have to be ruled out for those theories to be correct), but psychological construction also can explain why such patterns rarely, if ever, materialize. The validity of a psychological construction theory depends on the proposed mechanisms or processes that cause physical changes to be perceived as emotions. Different psychological construction theories propose different mechanisms or processes. If these processes cannot be verified empirically, then the theory is falsified.

MISCONCEPTION 3. True emotions are conflated with emotion schemas. An emotion, as the object of perception, should not be confused with the concept for an emotion.

Metanarrative Element: Essentialism

This is yet another misconception rooted in the metanarrative element of essentialism. Each emotion word is supposed to correspond to a specific pattern of physical (biological or behavioral) response that is observable in an objective (perceiver-independent) way.

Why Psychological Construction Is Misunderstood

From the traditional perspective, a concept for an emotion such as anger is separate from the thing itself (i.e., the perceiver-independent anger response), in the same way that a tree or a plant exists in the real world separately from our concepts of them. As a result, it seems to be a grave error to confuse the two.

Correction

Psychological construction proposes that emotions are not perceiver-independent objects in the physical world like trees and plants. Instead, emotion categories are more like conceptual categories for *flowers* and *weeds*. There is nothing in the physical world that indicates whether a plant is serving as a flower or a weed in a given instance. A plant's status as one or the other is determined by the perceiver's categorization. Flowers and weeds are *perceiver-dependent categories*, because they depend on human perceivers for their existence. Perceiver-dependent categories are not imaginary; they are very real. For example, flowers and weeds *prescribe actions* that mere plants cannot: Flowers are to be cultivated, and weeds are to be pulled from the ground. Flowers and weeds allow people to *communicate* with one another in a relational way: Receiving a dandelion from one's gardener, ragged with its root system attached, communicates an entirely different meaning than when receiving it from one's 5-year-old child. Flowers and weeds are also a form of *social influence*, in that they are a bid to control the mental state and actions of another person in a way that a mere plant cannot achieve.

According to the philosopher John Searle (1995, 2010), humans create ontologically subjective things as part of social reality by imposing functions on physical objects and events that are not based solely on the nature of their physical properties. Searle states this as a general rule: An object or instance (X) counts as having a certain status (Y) in a particular context (C). This status allows X to perform a particular function (or functions) not inherent to its physical structure. Plants (X) become flowers or weeds

(Y) when they are categorized as such by a human mind (C) that exists in consensus with other human minds that also possess categories for flowers and weeds, and agree on the categories' functions (i.e., perceiver-based categories depend on *collective intentionality* for their reality). Of course, flowers and weeds (or any subjectively real objects or events) are not absent from the physical world. A flower or a weed cannot be brought into existence without a plant. A flower or a weed is not a mirage. Rather, the point is that, in a given instance, the physical nature of a flower or a weed (Y) goes beyond just the plant (X) itself—it also involves the top-down, conceptual machinery responsible for human perception available inside the brain of the perceiver (which, for our purposes, can be thought of as C). Understanding how the human brain (in certain instances, C) creates a flower or a weed (Y) from a mere plant (X) is really the question of how flowers and weeds come into existence (because without the perceiver, there is only a plant).

Psychological construction approaches ask the same questions about emotions. Understanding how the human brain (in certain instances, C) creates an emotion (Y) from mere physical changes in the body (X) is really the question of how emotions come into existence (because without the perceiver, there are only changes in heart rate, breathing, actions, etc.). The hypothesis is that the status of these physical changes as instances of anger, sadness, or fear (or even as instances of some other psychological category such as a cognition or a perception) is created in the same way that a plant becomes a flower or a weed: with a human mind making meaning of physical events. Via this meaning, physical changes acquire the ability to perform functions that they do not have on their own (creating social meaning, prescribing actions, allowing communication, and aiding social influence). A body state or an action has a certain physical function (e.g., changes in respiration might regulate autonomic reactivity or widened eyes increase the size of the visual field), but these events do not intrinsically have certain functions *as an emotion*; events are assigned those functions in the act of categorizing them as emotion during categorization. Physical changes (X) *becomes* anger (Y) by *representing* it as anger. From this perspective, then, emotion categories may be folk psychology categories, but they are more than mere "explanatory fictions" (to use Skinner's words; Skinner, 1971, p. 199).

So from the psychological construction standpoint, it does not make sense to claim that concepts for emotion are separable from emotions "themselves." The hypothesis is that emotion concepts play a role in creating perceptions of bodily states as emotions in the moment. They are necessary to the phenomenon of emotion. Furthermore, some psychological construction theories hypothesize that instances of emotion contribute to constituting emotion concepts (discussed in Barrett et al., Chapter 4, this volume). As a consequence, the psychological construction hypothesis does not conflate emotion and emotion concepts —it explicitly hypothesizes that one (the psychological events to which people refer with emotion words) cannot exist as we typically conceive of it without the other (conceptual knowledge for emotion). For another analogy (color), see Barrett, Mesquita, Ochsner, & Gross, 2007).

MISCONCEPTION 4. Psychological construction theories have just recycled Schachter and Singer (1962), who hypothesized that emotions are ambiguous changes in arousal that are subsequently labeled using emotion words. This interpretation process is conscious and deliberate.

Few ideas in science are completely new. Many ideas linked to psychological construction existed before now in some form or another, particularly as critiques of faculty psychology/mental module approaches to emotion. For example, starting as early as the 19th century and continuing into the mid-20th century, literature reviews or commentaries highlighted the fact that physical measurements of the body and behavior do not respect emotion categories as primitive, natural, or modular types (see Gendron & Barrett, 2009). The roots of psychological construction can also be found in the criticism of faculty psychology within the mental philosophy of the 17th century. In fact, criticisms of mental typologies stretch back to pre-Socratic times. Almost all of these proposals suggest what might be considered the unifying assumption of psychological construction approaches to emotions: that anger, sadness, fear, etc. are not the basic building blocks of the mind (i.e., they are not psychological primitives), but instead are emergent products within the mind's system of more basic processes. Unlike earlier psychological construction approaches, which mainly described the gist of psychological construction principles (e.g., see Gendron & Barrett, 2009), the contributors to this volume offer more detailed and nuanced accounts of the psychological construction of emotion, and in certain cases provide specific computational and/or brain-based hypotheses about the mechanisms that allow for psychological construction. The main point is that psychological construction is not one theory—it is a family of theories that share common assumptions (see Barrett & Russell, Chapter 1, this volume) and not all of them are reducible to Schachter and Singer.

If psychological construction ideas have been around for a long time, why is Schachter and Singer (1962) often considered the standard against which all newer theories are evaluated for their novelty and incremental validity? The answer is that the Schachter and Singer's theory employs metanarrative elements that are common in mainstream psychology. This not only makes the Schachter and Singer's version of psychological construction easy to understand, but it also makes other psychological construction theories ripe for misunderstanding when they violate these metanarrative elements.

Metanarrative Element: The Mind Is "Perturbed" by a Stimulus and Issues a "Response"

Perturbation models of the mind are very common in psychology. They usually go something like this: A stimulus (usually defined by the experimenter and exogenous to the person) triggers a hypothetical psychological process within the participant (or the organism) that in turn produces a measurable response in behavior, all in a linear sequence over time. The $S \rightarrow O \rightarrow R$ structure is a description of how a single experimental trial is organized, but it is more than that: It is also the dominant story for how the mind and brain work in many theories in psychology (and particularly in the science of emotion). The roots of this narrative element can be found in the physiology experiments of the 19th century that motivated the first psychology experiments. Just like a muscle cell, the mind is assumed to lie dormant until stimulated, and upon stimulation, a response is assumed to issue reflexively and automatically. The descriptions of psychological events in terms of the stimuli that that provoke them and the effects they produce are so pervasive and deeply rooted in the narrative structure of psychological theories that they invisibly influence how we actually do science (Danziger, 1997, p. 54). For example, trials are assumed to be independent and can therefore be aggregated across conditions of an experiment (because the state of the mind before the stimulus is thought to be irrelevant); when variance across trials is estimated, it is usually modeled as error (rather than part of the phenomenon itself). Chains of these $S \rightarrow O \rightarrow R$ sequences might be linked together to imply that a phenomenon is recursive (see, e.g., Dewey, 1896; Scherer, 2009), but the general structure of causation remains the same. Schachter and Singer (1962) assumed that a stimulus produces a change in arousal that is inherently ambiguous to the experiencer, who then makes an effort to understand it; the experiencer then uses whatever available information is handy to make the ambiguous arousal meaningful, thereby creating an emotional experience.

Why Psychological Construction Is Misunderstood

Using an experimental paradigm that was common at the time, Schachter and Singer (1962) injected participants with epinephrine to create an increase in sympathetic nervous system arousal. Some participants were aware that they were receiving epinephrine and others were not. Schachter and Singer then demonstrated that those participants who experienced ambiguous and unexplained arousal used information from other people (what Schachter [1959] referred to as "social affiliation") to transform their feelings of arousal into an experience of emotion (either euphoria or anger depending on the verbal and nonverbal cues that were being depicted by confederates in the experiment). Although this experiment subsequently failed to replicate, its heuristic value for the science of emotion has been remarkable: It crystalized the hypothesis that an emotion is produced as unexplained arousal erupts, then is subsequently interpreted via a meaning analysis involving the context and emotion words. The typical assumption is that if Schachter and Singer (1962) is a psychological construction theory, and it uses an S → O → R metanarrative structure, then other theories with the same label (i.e., other psychological construction theories) must also use this structure. This assumption is in error.

Correction

Not all psychological construction theories rely on this S → O → R meta-narrative element. While some theories do propose a linear causal sequence, where affective changes come first, followed by meaning making (e.g., Russell, 2003, Chapter 8, this volume; Wundt, 1897), others do not (see, in this volume, Barrett et al., Chapter 4; Thagard & Schröder, Chapter 6; Cunningham, Dunfield, & Stillman, Chapter 7; Coan & Gonzalez, Chapter 9). For example, the conceptual act theory is more consistent with concept of predictive coding (e.g., Adams et al., 2013; Bastos et al., 2012; Clark, 2013; Friston, 2002; Hohwy, 2013; Shipp et al., 2013) to hypothesize how emotions are constructed as situated conceptualizations within the brain's functional architecture (for a similar view, see Seth, 2013; Seth, Suzuki, & Critchley, 2012). As a consequence, most psychological construction views cannot be depicted with a sequence of boxes joined by arrows (i.e., the favorite way for psychologists to depict a psychological process). Even more complex "box and arrow" diagrams with recursive elements do not capture the dynamics of emotion as proposed in many psychological construction theories (see also Misconception 6). The point, in fact, is that a bottom-up, stimulus-driven model of the mind is incorrect (possibly a holdover from the dawn of psychology, when psychological experiments used laboratory methods fashioned after those used in physiology laboratories of the time, where an S → R model might more appropriate; see Danziger, 1997).

Not only is it an error to assume that all psychological construction models hypothesize that affective changes initiate an emotional sequence, but it is an error to assume that the affective changes themselves must have similarly linear and punctate discrete causes (i.e., that affective changes must be driven by conventionally defined stimuli). In S → O → R models of the mind, an embedded assumption is that the relevant process within the mind or brain is "off" until stimulated and then switches to "off" again until the next stimulus appears. When put in such stark terms, this statement might evoke a "straw man" criticism, but it is this mechanistic assumption that allows scientists to treat trials as independent of one another, to aggregate responses across trials, and to assume dependencies across trials or that intertrial variation should be modeled as error. This S → O → R logic leads scientists to ask what causes affect to "turn on." This question reveals a clear misunderstanding of the concept of affective changes within a psychological construction framework. Many psychological construction theories consider affect to be continually changing feelings that are a property of consciousness resulting from the ongoing changes in homeostasis. A body is always "on," requiring energy and sending sensory input to the brain (except during sleep, when this sensory input is somewhat diminished). Any "perturbation" that influences homeostasis (changes in blood glucose levels, hormones, physical activity, etc.) or that the brain *predicts* will change homeostasis, could conceivably produce changes in affect that are meaningfully constructed as emotions.

It is also worth noting that a quick survey of the chapters in this volume, as well as the published literature on psychological construction, reveals that the psychological ingredients of emotion are not always identical to what Schachter and Singer (1962) proposed. Some theories, like that of Schachter and Singer, focus on autonomic arousal as the key bodily component that is interpreted and labeled as emotion (e.g., Duffy, 1957; Mandler, 1975). Others propose raw somatic, visceral, vascular and motor cues (Duffy, 1941; James, 1884) or the mental counterpart of those internal cues as affective feelings characterized by valence and arousal (Harlow & Stagner, 1932, 1933; Hunt, 1941; Wundt, 1897).

Metanarrative Element: Automatic versus Controlled Processes

Many modern psychological theories still rely on a dual-process logic, in which some processes are considered to be automatic and others are controlled and deliberate. Automatic processes are assumed to be more stimulus driven (or bottom-up), whereas controlled processes are assumed to be perceiver driven (or top-down). One guiding assumption has been that the subjective experience of having control over thoughts and actions is the best way of indicating that controlled processing is under way. This idea began with James (1950/1890), and it was elaborated on by Helmholtz (1910/1925), and later by Bargh (1994). Controlled processing is typically defined by the subjective experience of awareness (one is able to self-reflect on one's processing attempts), agency (one experiences oneself as the agent of one's own behavior), effort (one experiences processing as effortful), and control (one is aware that automatic processes may be occurring and motivated and able to counteract them). Varieties of automatic process, in contrast, are defined by the absence of any feeling of awareness, intention, effort, or control. Dual-process theories are alive and well in psychology (cf. Barrett, Tugade, & Engle, 2004). Indeed, some of the most popular psychological theories employ this metanarrative element (e.g., Greene, 2013; Kahneman, 2011). Even the law and economics employ dual-process logic. This is because dual-processes theories embody one of the most cherished metanarrative elements in the Western philosophy of mind: the planful, cognitive, uniquely human aspects of the mind are separate from (and often triumph over) its more reflexive, emotional, and animalistic aspects.

Why Psychological Construction Is Misunderstood

If affective changes occur first, followed by meaningful interpretation of those changes (as proposed by Schachter & Singer, 1962), then a reasonable assumption might be that those meaning-based changes are deliberate and willful. This assumption makes even more sense when Schachter and Singer's experimental method is considered: Injected participants were exposed to a confederate who was explicitly providing them with an interpretive frame for their arousal. Participants were likely searching for an explanation and were aware of the framing provided to them. A related observation is that psychological theories of the mind still tend to reify emotion, cognition, and perception as separate processes in the mind, and as separable networks in the brain. For example, the idea that cognition and emotion interact to produce behavior is still one of the most cherished narratives within a Western philosophy of mind.

Correction

For the most part, psychological construction theories eschew the idea that some processes are automatic and others are controlled. For example, as previously discussed, perceiver-based, top-down influences are not always deliberate or willful. Psychological construction assumes that, typically, all processes involved in creating emotions are automatic and often obligatory, but can be controlled depending on goals, effort, and resources. For example, in the conceptual act theory, categorization is not deliberate or effortful—it occurs as part of the normal functioning of the brain's efforts to make meaning from the changing sensory array (where sensory information is coming both from within the body and from the outside world). Executive control is a necessary ingredient to the construction of emotion, but executive control is not synonymous with deliberate and willful processing (Barrett et al., 2004).

MISCONCEPTION 5. Psychological constructionism has nothing to add above and beyond appraisal theory.

Metanarrative Element: The "Perturbation" Model of the Mind

Most theories in psychology are information-processing theories inspired by or modified from the cognitive revolution and employing the $S \rightarrow O \rightarrow R$ metanarrative element. Top-down (perceiver-based) influences, to the extent that they occur, are prompted by bottom-up stimulus driven influences, and merely modulate those influences.

Why Psychological Construction Is Misunderstood

Appraisal theories use this metanarrative element: A stimulus (S) is interpreted by a perceiver using a certain sequence of evaluations (O) that in turn triggers an emotional response or components of that response (R) (e.g., Scherer, 2009). Schachter and Singer (1962) use a similar approach: Ambiguous arousal (S) is interpreted by the perceiver (O), who in turn creates an emotional response (R). Because both consider emotion to be an act of meaning making (the "O"), both are classified as appraisal theories (and the theory of Schachter and Singer is sometimes understood as an appraisal theory of emotion). The shifting classification of Schachter and Singer reflects a basic confusion over how psychological construction theories are distinct from appraisal theories of emotion.

Correction

Many appraisal theories (i.e., the causal appraisal theories; cf. Barrett et al., 2007; Gross & Barrett, 2011) hypothesize that meaning making (via cognitive processes called cognitive appraisals) is applied to a stimulus and an emotion results (as a unified response, or different appraisals are hypothesized to control different elements in the eventual response). The process is usually linear, but recursive. Psychological construction theories, by contrast, assume that changes in a body (experienced in the self or observed in others) are made meaningful by relating them to the surrounding context (resulting in an experience of emotion or a perception of emotion, respectively). Emotions are situated representations of bodily changes. The hypothesized processes are usually not linear, but unfold via constraint satisfaction or dynamical systems. In most psychological constructionist theories, then, the emphasis is on making an internal sensory or affective information meaningful: An emotion emerges when a person's internal state changes are understood in some way as being related to or caused by the situation. In appraisal theories, in contrast, it is the situation, not the internal state of the body, that is the target of the meaning analysis; internal state changes are assumed to result from and reflect this meaning analysis. The conceptual act theory (Barrett et al., Chapter 4, this volume), for example, proposes that the entire sensory array (sensations from the body and from the world) is subject to a meaning analysis. The processes that contribute to this analysis are not specific to the domain of emotion or special in any way; they are just the normal meaning-making processes that the brain uses to construct perceptions, memories, and the many mental events that constitute the human mind. This is in contrast to most appraisal theories which assume that appraisal processes are specific to the domain of emotion, psychological In summary, then, causal appraisal theories differ from psychological construction theories in three ways: (1) the meaning-making mechanisms that are involved in creating emotions; (2) the target of meaning making (the situation vs. the whole stimulus array of body in context); and (3) the causal flow (linear and recursive vs. nonlinear and emergent).

It should be noted, however, that some appraisal theories are strongly consistent with psychological construction theories (e.g., the Ortony, Clore, and Collins (OCC) model, outlined in Ortony & Clore, Chapter 13, this volume; also see Barrett, 2013; Clore & Ortony, 2008). In the OCC appraisal model, for example, appraisals are descriptions of how the world is experienced during emotions, rather than the literal cognitive mechanisms that produced those experiences. Emotion categories are conceived of as cognitive types that reflect the structure of recurring situations that people find important and meaningful within their own cultural context. Emotions are "embodied, enacted, and experienced representations of situations" (Clore & Ortony, 2013, p. 337). They are situated affective states. Until now, the OCC model focused mainly on describing the whole (emphasizing emergentism), whereas psychological construction theories, like the conceptual act theory, for example, concentrate on describing how interacting systems produce the emergent emotional instances (emphasizing holism); but really the two approaches are more productively considered as two sides of the same emotional coin (cf. Barrett, Mesquita, et al., 2007).

Metanarrative Element: Essentialism

If two phenomena are labeled by the same word, then they are the same thing.

Why Psychological Construction Is Misunderstood

The term "appraisal" has a common-sense meaning: an evaluation or estimation of something's value or nature. It also has several scientific meanings (as a specific set of cognitive mechanisms: e.g., Scherer [2009], Frijda [1986], Roseman [2011]; or as a description of how situations are experienced during emotions: Ortony & Clore, Chapter 13, this volume). Not all meaning-making processes are "appraisal" processes.

Correction

Different psychological constructionist theories hypothesize that internal sensory or affective cues become meaningful as emotions using a variety of different meaning-making mechanisms. Those who propose that this meaning analysis is the result of ideas (Wundt, 1897) or of social affiliation or referencing (Schachter & Singer, 1962) seem to be implying a more deliberate and conscious attempt at meaning making. Those who hypothesize that the meaning analysis results from categorization (Barrett, 2006b), from attribution (Russell, 2003), or from perceptions of the stimulating situation (Harlow & Stanger, 1932, 1933) as situations that are important to the perceiver (Dunlap, 1932; Duffy, 1941) imply that the meaning-making process is automatic. These different constructs are not meant as mere redescriptions of appraisal processes—they represent very different hypotheses about how sensory input from the body is made meaningful by binding it to events and objects in the world.

MISCONCEPTION 6. Emotions are nothing more than "core affect." All emotions can be explained with just two dimensions (valence and arousal).

Metanarrative Element: Reductionism.

Psychological theories are, for the most part, reductionistic. A mental event or a behavior is nothing more than the sum of its parts and therefore can be redefined as (or ontologically reduced to) its parts. Each part can be studied separately from every other part in a contextless way. The assumption is that reductionism will lead to a better and more complete scientific understanding of any phenomenon.

Why Psychological Construction Is Misunderstood

From a reductionistic stance, the psychological construction hypothesis that emotions are created as the interpretation of affective changes is misunderstood as the goal to decompose emotions and redefine them as their most basic elements: valence and arousal. Standard emotion theories (e.g., basic emotion theories) are reductionist, and there is historical precedent for reinterpreting psychological construction theories through a reductionist lens (e.g., Dewey's [1895] reinterpretation of James).

Correction

As far as I know, no psychological constructionist theories (except perhaps Dewey's reinterpretation of James and Titchener's theory) have suggested that emotions should be ontologically reduced to their parts (i.e., that physical sensations or affect alone provides a sufficient characterization for emotion). Instead, most psychological construction theories characterize emotions as phenomena that *emerge* from the interaction of more basic ingredients. Emergence implies that the product (the emotional instance as a whole) is more than the sum of its parts, and has properties that the core systems (the individual contributing parts) do not, making reductionism impossible. (A further implication is that each system cannot be manipulated and studied independently, because the state of any one system depends on the state of the whole. Therefore, the workings of each system cannot be studied alone, like bits and pieces of a machine, but must be holistically understood within the momentary state of the brain, body, and the surrounding context.) As a consequence, most psychological construction theories are not "dimensional" theories per se. Instead, they integrate traditional dimensional and categorical perspectives. The dimensional aspect can be found in the suggestion that all emotional events, at their core, can be described as having psychologically primitive affective properties. The categorical aspect can be found in the suggestion that people automatically and effortlessly use some type of meaning analysis to bind these affective changes to objects and events in the world, and in so doing create the experience of a discrete emotional event.

It is probably also important to point out that affective circumplex (Barrett, 2004; Russell, 1980; Russell & Barrett, 1999) is not an explanatory model of emotion and was never intended as one. It is a low dimensional, descriptive map that represents two properties or common features of emotional experiences. Since these are properties or features of experience, valence and arousal, themselves, cannot be mechanistically reduced either, and are most likely emergent properties of more basic processes.

MISCONCEPTION 7. Emotions are not products of evolution.

Metanarrative Element: Nature versus Nurture

By and large, psychological theories still tend to assume that psychological events (a mental state or a behavior) are either biologically caused or experientially learned. Of course, every act of learning cannot occur without some biological event supporting it, so this is a false dichotomy. A more subtle distinction is between biological endowment and learning (e.g., what wiring and chemistry is an organism born with and what is acquired through experience; although some experience is acquired in-utero so even this is a false dichotomy to some extent). Although every one acknowledges that nervous systems show plasticity, this insight has not yet dislodged the idea that "nature" can be equated with biology and "nurture," with learning. Scientists still ask questions about whether a phenomenon or process is "hardwired", by which they mean endowed, without realizing that learning also "hardwires" a brain. They still ask how learning modifies evolutionary endowments, without realizing that the ability to engage in certain kinds of learning is itself an evolutionary endowment.

Why Psychological Construction Is Misunderstood

Basic emotion theories propose that emotions are evolved adaptations that are homologous in all mammalian species. Because they explicitly label themselves as "evolutionary" theories, to deny their validity, as psychological construction theories do, is mistakenly seen as rejecting evolution altogether. The nature versus nurture dichotomy is largely responsible for the mistaken assumption that psychological construction theories either ignore or deny evolutionary considerations. This metanarrative element is also responsible for pitting cultural and social constructionist views against evolutionary considerations, as if they are competing explanations for behavior.

Correction

Many books and articles have been written about how the nature versus nurture dichotomy is false. It is now well accepted that culture is a major adaptive advantage in the evolution of hominids, that environmental conditions turn gene expression and protein transcription on and off, and that learning wires the brain. This means that many universal phenomena are hardwired into the brain via learning (e.g., face perception, language, and certain visual illusions). With these findings in mind, then, it should not be difficult to entertain the idea that hypotheses about the psychological construction of emotions can also be hypotheses about emotions as the products of evolution.

So, to be very clear, psychological construction does not deny an evolutionary explanation for emotions—it just *denies a certain type of evolutionary explanation* for emotion. Natural kind theories of emotion (like basic emotion theories) assume that natural selection sculpted one domain-specific mechanism corresponding to each emotion word, presumably to deal with specific, recurring environmental challenges to survival and fitness (Shariff & Tracy, 2011), and that these mechanisms endow human and nonhuman animals alike with emotional capacities. This evolutionary story, which suffers from the weaknesses of the "adaptationist programme" (discussed by Gould & Lewontin, 1979), is not the only evolutionary game in town, however. For example, the conceptual act theory (Barrett et al., Chapter 4, this volume) hypothesizes that the brain's functional architecture contains domain-general processes that interact and from which emotions emerge. In principle, domain-general processes are favored by evolution for their efficiency and flexibility (Laland & Brown, 2002). This theory hypothesizes that emotional episodes can contain species-general elements (actions that all species share; e.g., behavioral adaptations such as freezing, fleeing, or fighting), but that these are neither necessary nor sufficient for an emotion to be constructed. They are not necessary, because there is no one-to-one mapping between a specific behavioral adaptation (e.g., freezing) and an emotion category (e.g., *fear*) (Barrett, 2012; see also Gross & Canteras, 2012). Species-general processes are not sufficient, because they must be made meaningful by species-specific processes that exist only in humans (or perhaps in limited form in great apes), such as abstract emotion concepts and language.

The conceptual act theory of emotion, in particular, is inspired by Darwin's insights in *On the Origin of Species* (1859/1964). This book contains several conceptual innovations that transformed biology into a modern science (Mayr, 1988). Before On the Origin of Species, animal species were assumed to be physical "types" whose members shared certain defining properties (essences) that distinguished them from all other types. Deviations within a type were due to error or accident. Scientific study meant reducing every phenomenon to mathematics of physical, mechanical laws. Darwin, and the biologists who further developed the conceptual framework for evolution in the following century, changed all of this. They replaced the essentialist, typological thinking with population-based thinking, in which a species is a biopopulation, and individuals within a population are unique; individual variation within a species was meaningfully tied to variations in the environment. Variation within a species was the result not of species-specific processes but instead of species-general mechanisms. And perhaps most importantly, they expanded the definition of science by offering nonreductionist, analytic approaches to understanding the natural world. These conceptual advances are directly mirrored in our psychological construction approach (Barrett, 2013; Barrett et al., Chapter 4, this volume).

The Expression of Emotions In Man and Animals (Darwin, 1872/2005), written more than a decade after *On the Origin of Species*, is the book that most traditional emotion theorists claim as their intellecual inspiration. Ironically, *The Expressions* contains only one of the five conceptual innovations mentioned in the *Origins* (the idea of common decent). It does not mention important ideas like population-based thinking (instead proposing an emotion typology). Nor does it mention natural selection (instead discussing Lamarkian evolution). These two ideas are, admittedly, Darwin's greatest conceptual achievements and the very ideas that created a paradigm shift in biology. From this perspective, *The Expression of Emotions In Man and Animals* is a conceptual throwback when compared with *On the Origin of Species*.

Psychological construction approaches allow researchers to ask a broad set of evolutionary questions. For example, perhaps the evolutionary legacy to the newborn is not a set of modular emotion circuits that are hardwired into the subcortical features of the mammalian brain but instead a set of domain-general systems that involve learning, categorization, and affective responding. The ability to categorize, for example, is not a specifically human ability—many animals can categorize. It confers adaptive advantage, so it is likely biologically preserved, even if the specific categories are not. Perhaps specific categories are more likely culture-sensitive solutions to common problems that derive from our major adaptive advantage as a species: living in complex social groups.

Finally, humans' major adaptive advantage is to live in social groups and to engage in the kind of social learning that allows for the development and maintenance of culture. As a consequence, perhaps we have evolved the kind of minds that attempt to infer the internal states of others (so that we can better predict their behavior), as well as communicate our own internal states to others when it is advantageous to do so. Psychological constructionist accounts can be considered evolutionary in those terms.

MISCONCEPTION 8. Psychological construction occurs inside the head; therefore, the social context is irrelevant.

Metanarrative Element: Nature versus Nurture

The false dichotomy between nature and nurture is grounded in the common psychological assumption that forces occur either inside the person or outside in the world, with the skin as a reified boundary that separates the two. Attention, for example, is said to be directed outside to events in the world or inside to thoughts and feelings, and there are even networks in the brain that have been ascribed the function of switching from one focus to the other. Some processes are thought to be totally inside us (mental processes), and others are totally outside us (social processes). It is presumed that the processes going on inside and outside might cause other processes, or they might interact, but that they are inherently separate.

Why Psychological Construction Is Misunderstood

If emotions are constructed as interpretations of internal sensory or affective changes, then this can seem like an isolated process that occurs entirely inside the mind and, as such, denies the importance and potency of what goes on outside the skin, such as social relationships and context.

Correction

From the 1920s to the 1950s, when scientists were struggling with mounting observations that emotion categories did not seem to align with specific patterns of physical response, they proposed that measuring and understanding physical changes in the body provided an insufficient scientific account of emotions. Therefore, they concluded, emotions must be the result of interpreting those physical changes in light of the surrounding context (for a review, see Gendron & Barrett, 2009). Their articles did not outline intact theories of emotion as much as suggest how theory building in the science of emotion should proceed by incorporating the surrounding situation or context. Subsequently, some theoretical approaches tended to emphasize the psychological mechanisms by which the interpretation process took place, but were largely silent on the contexts and situations that provided constraints and influence on interpretation (i.e., psychological construction). Other theoretical approaches emphasized the social conditions during which particular emotions occurred, without specifying the mechanisms by which emotions emerged (i.e., social construction).

Modern constructionist approaches, by and large, perpetuate this fault line, not by stipulation, but by oversight. Psychological constructionist theories, for example, do not deny the importance of the social interaction as a dynamically unfolding process that shapes the construction of an emotional event; but they have not specified or emphasized the importance of situational constraints either. The reverse can be said for social constructionist theories. Nonetheless, there are several notable exceptions in this volume (Barrett et al., Chapter 4; Boiger & Mesquita, Chapter 15; Ortony & Clore, Chapter 13; also see Clore & Ortony, 2013; Solomon, 1976). These psychological constructionist theories acknowledge that the dichotomy between the person and the situation is a false one. They discuss, for example, how situations constitute the mind (e.g., children learn emotion concepts, and therefore how to construct emotions, within a matrix of social interactions). If emotion concepts are tools for regulating homeostasis (Barrett et al., Chapter 4, this volume) that are acquired in a culture-sensitive matrix of social learning, and they prepare a person for or predict situated action, then this effectively breaks down the barrier between inside and outside the skin. This makes every emotional episode a cultural artifact as much as it is a biological event.

Psychological construction also highlights how there is no "environment" that is independent of the "person" (e.g., Ortony & Clore, Chapter 13, this volume). People do not experience an environment: They construct it via their perceptions of their physical surroundings and their actions (Boiger & Mesquita, Chapter 15, this volume). Other animals also can be said to "construct" their environment by actively responding to some elements in their physical surroundings but ignoring others. Richard Lewontin, the evolutionary biologist, describes how an "environment" should be understood as the physical surroundings that are relevant to an animal's behaviors and activities. For example, he notes that two kinds of birds (phoebes and thrushes) live in the same physical surroundings within the Northeastern United States, but their ecological niches are very different (for a detailed discussion of this example, see Lewontin, 2000). The relevant niche, or situation, for each kind of bird is determined by its activities. A phoebe needs grass to build nests, so grass is part of its situation or niche.

A thrush requires rocks to crack open seeds, so rocks are part of its situation. Both birds occupy the same physical surroundings that contain grass and rocks, but the potent aspects for each—that is, each bird's situation—are different. Some aspects are physically present but unnoticed. Similarly, it is possible that within a common physical surrounding there exists different "situations" for different people (or for a single individual at different points in time). It is also consistent with the idea that the mind determines the "active ingredients" or psychological features of the situation (Shoda, Mischel, & Wright, 1994; Wright & Mischel, 1988). In essence, the mind determines the nature of the situation, so that a "situation" does not exist separately from the person. In this way, it cannot be said that the situation causes emotion in a way that is independent of the mind. The construction of an emotion might, in fact, be an element in how situations are constructed (e.g., if one person categorizes his or her high-arousal negative affective change as anger (vs. fear), then this prescribes his or her power and dominance in an interaction relative to his or her interaction partner in a particular cultural context; Solomon, 1976).

MISCONCEPTION 9. Any evidence for the biological basis of emotion is evidence that emotions are biologically basic.

Metanarrative Element: Essentialism

Biological explanations for a psychological category will, necessarily, reveal their essence. Nonessentialist views have no grounding in the physical world.

Why Psychological Construction Is Misunderstood

It is difficult to imagine a theory of emotion (or of any other psychological event) that is grounded in nature without it being a nativist theory.

Correction

Every human thought, feeling, and behavior must be causally reduced to the firing of neurons in the human brain, informed by events in the body (when the two are normally functioning). Prior experiences and learning are encoded in the human brain; even a strict constructionist approach must therefore have a strong grounding in nature. As a consequence, a neuroscience approach to emotion need not be a basic emotion approach, and it need not make the modular, essentialist assumption that distinct brain regions or circuits are dedicated to instantiating psychological categories such as *anger, sadness,* and *fear.*

It should be noted that basic emotion theories make very specific predictions about the biological bases of emotion. Each emotion, for example, must be consistently and specifically localized to an anatomically constrained and homologous circuit or network within the brain (i.e., that is inheritable and homologous in other animals). Biological evidence that distinguishes emotion categories from one another, but does not follow these predictions, does not support a basic emotion view (e.g., Kassam, Markey, Cherkassky, Loewenstein, & Just, 2013; Vytal & Hamann, 2010).

Psychological constructionist theories, in contrast, make very different predictions about how, at the biological level of analysis, instances of the same emotion category might be different, different emotion categories might differ, and instances of different emotion categories might be similar (e.g., Barrett & Satpute, 2013; Barrett et al., Chapter 4, this volume; Cunningham et al., Chapter 7, this volume; Oosterwijk et al., Chapter 5, this volume; Touroutoglou et al., 2014; Wilson-Mendenhall, Barrett, Simmons, & Barsalou, 2011; Wilson-Mendenhall, Barrett, & Barsalou, 2013).

Furthermore, psychological constructionist theories caution scientists to resist the lure of essentializing when interpreting biological data. This is important, because temptations are everywhere. Most recently, it is possible to see essentialistic thinking in interpretations of pattern classification techniques (see Barrett, 2013). It is tempting to believe that the patterns distinguishing different emotions within a single study are *the patterns* to distinguish emotion categories, rather than the patterns that distinguish those particular instance of emotions (therefore, the patterns might not generalize across experiments). As noted earlier in this chapter, two recent pattern classification studies that used similar methods and stimuli did not replicate each other in the reported patterns that distinguished between emotions in each study (Kragel & LaBar, 2013; Stephens et al., 2010). Similarly, our meta-analytic pattern classification of brain activity distinguishing different emotions (Wager et al., 2014) does not replicate a recent study that also reported patterns of distinctiveness (Kassam et al., 2013). From a psychological constructionist perspective, these are not surprising results, because experiments elicit emotional instances (even though the data are often interpreted as if they reveal truths about emotion types).

MISCONCEPTION 10. Psychological construction theories suffer from the same problems as basic emotion theories. Both attempt to localize a set of categories to brain networks in a one-to-one manner.

Metanarrative Elements: Essentialism and Reductionism

For much of psychology's history, it has been assumed that modularity was necessary for science to proceed. A psychological process must be localized to a discrete packet of brain tissue, making it possible to redefine a mental process as the specific function of a brain circuit or network.

Why Psychological Construction Is Misunderstood

The basic idea that emotions are physical types that can be localized to specific brain regions or networks is a textbook case of faculty psychology, associated with a view of the mind as comprising innate, neural modules, each with a distinct function (what Fodor [1983] called "vertical" modules; Lindquist & Barrett, 2012). Psychological construction, in contrast, hypothesizes that emotions can be described as emerging from the interactions of a set of more psychologically basic ingredients (affect, categorization, attention, language) that themselves can be understood as arising from within the brain's domain-general core systems. The idea is that the brain functions like a neural "ecosystem" from which mental states, such as instances of emotion, emerge. The metanarrative elements of essentialism and reductionism make it tempting to try and localize each psychological ingredient to a specific brain network (e.g., affect is located within the salience network; language within the language network; conceptualization within the memory network; and so on; for discussion, see Herschbach & Bechtel, Chapter 2, this volume).

Correction

The brain is a complex collection of neurons. There is no single true way to organize these neurons into functional groupings; a brain does not speak for itself in this regard. Depending on a scientist's goals, the brain's functional properties can be understood differently at different time scales and levels of organization. The brain's function must be understood in terms of the concepts and categories that we use to represent the human mind. This endeavor necessarily involves construct validity (Cronbach & Meehl, 1955).

In neuroanatomical research, when two neurons are wired together, are they part of the same circuit, or is one neuron modulating the circuit to which the other neuron belongs? When a distributed network is identified in brain imaging research, it is rarely observed to include exactly the same voxels on each occasion (meaning that it does not involve the exact same neurons each time). Is this evidence of instability in the network, or is this just a normal property of how distributed networks function? These are questions that cannot be answered anatomically; they are part of the construct validity of the psychological functions assigned to the neurons in question. Some scientists believe that we can sidestep this complexity and study the brain without appealing to psychology, but this is a mistake. The study of the brain without appealing to mental categories is just the study of neurons. The problem is that traditional approaches to construct validity (e.g., using classical measurement theory) are essentialistic in nature. They imply that there is a single underlying cause for a set of measurements (i.e., the construct), and assume that this must correspond to a specific set of neurons that is activated every single time the construct is in evidence (Barrett, 2011).

Certain psychological constructionist theories attempt to understand the brain basis of emotion using assumptions that are very different from the metanarrative elements of essentialism and reductionism (e.g., Barrett & Satpute, 2013; see, in this volume, Barrett et al., Chapter 4; Cunningham et al., Chapter 7; Oosterwijk et al., Chapter 5; Thagard & Schröder, Chapter 6). For example, the conceptual act theory proposes that the brain contains a set of intrinsic networks that can be understood as performing domain-general operations; these operations serve as the functional architecture for how mental events and behaviors are constructed. We are not suggesting that all neurons within a network have exactly the same (general) receptive field, or that all neurons within a network fire every time the network is engaged. Instead, we are suggesting that, at the level of brain imaging, a neuron's function can be understood in the context of neural responses within the network (i.e., the function is distributed across the assembly of neurons within the network that are active at a given point in time), and this function is domain-general. Each of these "core systems" in the brain does not produce one distributed pattern of response. Instead, instance by instance, the function of the core system corresponds to a set of "functional motifs" arising from the "structural motif" that undergirds each network (for a discussion of motifs, see Sporns & Kötter, 2004). A theoretical framework like ours relies on assumptions of supervenience (see Barrett, 2011), degeneracy (Barrett et al., Chapter 4, this volume), and holism (see Barrett, 2013) rather than essentialism and reductionism. The goal is to shift the empirical emphasis from the search for mental faculties as unified neurobiological categories toward development of a more componential, constructionist functional architecture of the human brain, on the expectation that such a shift will deliver a more empirically justifiable theory of how emotions are created. One thing we can say for sure is that there is no strict one-to-one correspondence between a psychological ingredient like affect or categorization and a domain general brain network.

Summary

Because the human mind's ability to assimilate new ideas into an existing metanarrative framework is so much easier than its ability to build a new framework for a novel theory, metanarrative elements have a very powerful undertow in scientific storytelling, particularly when they are unexamined or unacknowledged. Hopefully, this chapter has illuminated at least a few of the metanarrative elements that make certain emotion theories seem obvious, while making others seem preposterous.

Standard emotion theories, such as basic emotion theories, and traditional "causal" appraisal theories, have a much easier job telling stories about the nature of emotion with their data because they routinely employ the dominant metanarrative structure of psychology, which itself derives from basic assumptions within the Western philosophy of mind that have been with us since ancient times. This structure provides a simple set of hypotheses (e.g., each emotion is a biological type) that prescribes a straightforward experimental method (e.g., expose any subject to an anger-inducing stimulus of any type and *the* anger response will be triggered, assuming the correct appraisals have been employed). These hypotheses and their associated experimental procedures are used in the hope of revealing particular insights about human nature (e.g., we are animals, and emotions are part of our animal nature). Such simple and powerful ideas make for good storytelling, good careers, good press, and for some, even a lucrative consulting business. It is rather more difficult to tell a scientific story about emotion that violates these themes—that emotions are complicated, stochastic, and dependent on context, and that no simple law or force will explain every instance of a particular emotion category. These are the kinds of stories that psychological constructionist approaches offer to the science of emotion, however, as illustrated in many of this volume's chapters.

NOTES

1. Essentialism is a widespread folk theory that biological categories are natural kinds waiting to be discovered rather than human constructions, and that these categories possess an underlying (often unseen or unknown) causal force (the essence) that is responsible for category members sharing so many properties. Categories are thought to be immutable (or to change at glacial speeds) with boundaries that are sharp and strict ("cutting nature at its joints"; Gelman & Rhodes, 2012).

2. If behavioral adaptations do not map to emotion categories one-to-one, there are several ways to solve the problem. One popular way is for scientists just to stipulate that emotions correspond to individual behaviors. Freezing = fear. Aggression = anger. Behaviorists, then behavioral neuroscientists, tried this maneuver. If fear is defined as the state that accompanies freezing, then whatever we learned about the circuitry for freezing would apply to all cases of fear, by definition. In such a scenario, all the nonfreezing instances that used to be categorized as fear would now be categorized something else (so that the *fear* category would become more homogeneous). You might imagine, then, that other categories for subtypes of *fear* would pop up, so that we end up with a variety of *fear* categories, each bearing its own distinctive name ("fear 1," "fear 2," "fear 3," etc.). In fact, philosophers (Scarantino, Chapter 14, this volume) and behavioral neuroscientists (Gross & Canteras, 2012) are attempting to go the route of "fear 1," "fear 2," "fear 3," and so forth. The advantage of this approach is that such categories permit the accumulation of scientific knowledge, but why not just call them behavioral categories? Why

call all of them fear? Anyway, this strategy does not really work, probably because the category *fear* serves social functions, in addition to its scientific functions, and those social functions are not well served by having a bunch of subtype categories (Barrett, 2012). So, what actually happens is the category *fear* remains heterogeneous, but, with the help of essentialist thinking, we imagine the category to be homogeneous. What scientists learn about the instances of fear involving freezing is mistakenly thought to generalize to all instances, when a creature is not freezing. Any concerns about illegitimate generalizability can be solved by imagining that fear instances without overt freezing must involve *some tendency to freeze*, even if the behavior never actually materializes and therefore cannot be observed (i.e., an action tendency). Perhaps this is why the circuitry for learning to freeze in response to a conditioned stimulus is seen as key for understanding PTSD (see Suvak & Barrett, 2011). Of course, another way out of this quandary is to just admit that not all instances that we categorize as fear involve freezing, so that the circuitry for freezing is not the fear circuit. We might even discover that freezing can occur in instances that we might categorize as other emotions, such as anger, surprise, or awe, or even as a non-emotional state such as uncertainty. This approach, of course, requires the search for mechanisms that allow freezing to contribute to fear in certain instances, that allow instances of fear to materialize without freezing, and that allow freezing to contribute to other mental states that are not fear.

ACKNOWLEDGMENTS

Many thanks to Eliza Bliss-Moreau, Paul Condon, Maria Gendron, Paul Hamilton, Ian Kleckner, Kristen Lindquist, and Suzanne Oosterwijk for their helpful input. Preparation of this chapter was supported by a National Institutes of Health Director's Pioneer Award (No. DP1OD003312); by grants from the National Institute on Aging (No. R01AG030311), the National Institute of Mental Health (No. R21MH099605), and the National Science Foundation (No. BCS-1052790); and by contracts from U.S. Army Research Institute for the Behavioral and Social Sciences (Contract Nos. W5J9CQ-11-C-0046 and W5J9CQ-12-C-0049) to Lisa Feldman Barrett. The views, opinions, and/or findings contained in this article are solely those of the author(s) and should not be construed as an official Department of the Army or Department of Defense position, policy, or decision.

REFERENCES

Adams, R. A., Shipp, S., & Friston, K. J. (2013). Predictions not commands: Active inference in the motor system. *Brain Structure and Function, 218*, 611–643.

Bargh, J. A. (1994). The four horsemen of automaticity: Awareness, efficiency, intention, and control in social cognition. In R. S. Wyer, Jr. & T. K. Srull (Eds.), *Handbook of social cognition* (2nd ed., pp. 1–40). Hillsdale, NJ: Erlbaum.

Barrett, L. F. (2004). Feelings or words?: Understanding the content in self-report ratings of emotional experience. *Journal of Personality and Social Psychology, 87*, 266–281.

Barrett, L. F. (2006a). Emotions as natural kinds? *Perspectives on Psychological Science, 1,* 28–58.

Barrett, L. F. (2006b). Solving the emotion paradox: Categorization and the experience of emotion. *Personality and Social Psychology Review, 10,* 20–46.

Barrett, L. F. (2009). The future of psychology: Connecting mind to brain. *Perspectives in Psychological Science, 4,* 326–339.

Barrett, L. F. (2011). Bridging token identity theory and supervenience theory through psychological construction. *Psychological Inquiry, 22,* 115–127.

Barrett, L. F. (2012). Emotions are real. *Emotion, 12,* 413–429.

Barrett, L. F. (2013). Psychological construction: A Darwinian approach to the science of emotion. *Emotion Review, 5,* 379–389.

Barrett, L. F., & Bar, M. (2009). See it with feeling: Affective predictions in the human brain. *Philosophical Transactions of the Royal Society B, 364,* 1325–1334.

Barrett, L. F., Mesquita, B., Ochsner, K. N., & Gross, J. J. (2007). The experience of emotion. *Annual Review of Psychology, 58,* 373–403.

Barrett, L. F., & Satpute, A. B. (2013). Large-scale brain networks in affective and social neuroscience: Towards an integrative architecture of the human brain. *Current Opinion in Neurobiology, 23,* 361–372.

Barrett, L. F., Tugade, M. M., & Engle, R. W. (2004). Individual differences in working memory capacity and dual-process theories of the mind. *Psychological Bulletin, 130,* 553–573.

Barrett, L. F., Wilson-Mendenhall, C. D., & Barsalou, L. W. (2014). A psychological construction account of emotion regulation and dysregulation: The role of situated conceptualizations. In J. J. Gross (Ed.), *The handbook of emotion regulation* (2nd ed., pp. 447–465). New York: Guilford Press.

Bastos, A. M., Usrey, W. M., Adams, R. A., Mangun, G. R., Fries, P., & Friston, K. J. (2012). Canonical microcircuits for predictive coding. *Neuron, 76,* 695–711.

Cacioppo, J. T., Berntson, C. G., Larsen, J. T., Poehlmann, K. M., & Ito, T. A. (2000). The psychophysiology of emotion. In M. Lewis & J. M. Haviland-Jones (Eds.), *Handbook of emotions* (pp. 173–191). New York: Guilford Press.

Clark, A. (2013). Whatever next?: Predictive brains, situated agents, and the future of cognitive science. *Behavioral and Brain Sciences, 36,* 181–253.

Clore, G. L., & Ortony, A. (2008). Appraisal theories: How cognition shapes affect into emotion. In M. Lewis, J. M. Haviland-Jones, & L. F. Barrett (Eds.). *Handbook of emotions* (3rd ed., pp. 628–642). New York: Guilford Press.

Clore, G. L., & Ortony, A. (2013). Psychological construction in the OCC model of emotion. *Emotion Review, 5,* 335–343.

Cronbach, L. J., & Meehl, P. E. (1955). Construct validity in psychological tests. *Psychological Bulletin, 52,* 281–302.

Danziger, K. (1997). *Naming the mind: How psychology found its language.* London: Sage.

Darwin, C. (1964). *On the origin of species* [Facsimile of 1st ed.]. Cambridge, MA: Harvard University Press. (Original work published 1859)

Darwin, C. (2005). *The expression of emotion in man and animals.* New York: Appleton. (Original work published 1872)

Dewey, J. (1895). The theory of emotion: II. The significance of emotions. *Psychological Review, 2,* 13–32.

Dewey, J. (1896). The reflex arc concept in psychology. *Psychological Review, 3,* 357–370.

Duffy, E. (1941). An explanation of "emotional" phenomena without use of the concept "emotion." *General Journal of Psychology, 25,* 283–293.

Duffy, E. (1957). The psychological significance of the concept of "arousal" or "activation." *Psychological Review, 64,* 265–275.

Dunlap, K. (1932). Are emotions teleological constructs? *American Journal of Psychology, 44,* 572–576.

Ekman, P. (1992) An argument for basic emotions. *Cognition and Emotion, 6,* 169–200.

Fodor, J. A. (1983). *The modularity of mind: An essay on faculty psychology.* Cambridge, MA: MIT Press.

Frijda, N. H. (1986). *The emotions.* New York: Cambridge University Press.

Friston, K. (2002). Beyond phrenology: What can neuroimaging tell us about distributed circuitry? *Annual Review of Neuroscience, 25,* 221–250.

Gelman, S. A., & Rhodes, M. (2012). "Two-thousand years of stasis": How psychological essentialism impedes evolutionary understanding. In K. S. Rosengren, S. Brem, E. M. Evans, & G. Sinatra (Eds.), *Evolution challenges: Integrating research and practice in teaching and learning about evolution* (pp. 3–21). New York: Oxford University Press.

Gendron, M., & Barrett, L. F. (2009). Reconstructing the past: A century of ideas about emotion in psychology. *Emotion Review, 1,* 316–339.

Golshani, P., Liu, X.-B., & Jones, E. G. (2001). Differences in quantal amplitude reflect GluR4-subunit number at corticothalamic synapses on two populations of thalamic neurons. *Proceeding of the National Academy of Sciences USA, 98,* 4172–4177.

Gould, S. J., & Lewontin, R. C. (1979). The spandrels of San Marco and the Panglossian Paradigm: A critique of the adaptationist programme. *Proceedings of the Royal Society of London B, 205,* 581–598.

Greene, J. (2013). *Moral tribes: Emotion, reason, and the gap between us and them.* New York: Penguin.

Gross, C. T., & Canteras, N. S. (2012). The many paths to fear. *Nature Reviews Neuroscience, 13,* 651–658.

Gross, J. J., & Barrett, L. F. (2011). Emotion generation and emotion regulation: One or two depends on your point of view. *Emotion Review, 3,* 8–16.

Harlow, H. F., & Stagner, R. (1932). Psychology of feelings and emotions: I. Theory of feelings. *Psychological Review, 39,* 570–589.

Harlow, H. F., & Stagner, R. (1933). Psychology of feelings and emotions: II. Theory of emotions. *Psychological Review, 40,* 184–195.

Helmholtz, H. von. (1925). *Treatise on psychological optics* (J. P. C. Southall, Trans.) (3rd ed., Vol. 3). Menasha, WI: Banta. (Original work published 1910)

Hohwy, J. (2013). *The predictive mind.* New York: Oxford University Press.

Hunt, W. A. (1941). Recent developments in the field of emotion. *Psychological Bulletin, 38,* 249–276.

James, W. (1884). What is an emotion? *Mind, 9,* 188–205.

James, W. (1950). *The principles of psychology.* New York: Dover. (Original work published 1890)

Kahneman, D. (2011). *Thinking, fast and slow.* New York: Farrar, Straus and Giroux.

Kassam, K. S., Markey, A. R., Cherkassky, V. L., Loewenstein, G., & Just, M.

A. (2013). Identifying emotions on the basis of neural activation. *PLos One*, *8*(6), e66032.

Kragel, P. A., & LaBar, K. S. (2013). Multivariate pattern classification reveals autonomic and experiential representations of discrete emotions. *Emotion*, *13*(4), 681–690.

Kreibig, S. D. (2010). Autonomic nervous system activity in emotion: A review. *Biological Psychology*, *84*, 394–421.

Laland, K. N., & Brown, G. R. (2002). *Sense and nonsense: Evolutionary perspectives on human behavior*. New York: Oxford University Press.

Lewontin, R. C. (2000). *The triple helix: Gene, organism and environment*. Cambridge, MA: Harvard University Press.

Lindquist, K., A., & Barrett, L. F. (2012). A functional architecture of the human brain: Insights from the science of emotion. *Trends in Cognitive Sciences*, *16*, 533–540.

Mandler, G. (1975). *Mind and emotion*. New York: Wiley.

Marshall, J. C. (1984). Multiple perspectives on modularity. *Cognition*, *17*, 209–242.

Mayr, E. (1988). *Toward a new philosophy of biology: Observations of an evolutionist*. Cambridge MA: Harvard University Press.

Obrist, P. A. (1981). *Cardiovascular psychophysiology: A perspective*. New York: Plenum.

Obrist, P. A., Webb, R. A., Sutterer, J. R., & Howard, J. L. (1970). The cardiac-somatic relationship: Some reformulations. *Psychophysiology*, *6*, 569–587.

Ortony, A., & Turner, T. J. (1990). What's basic about basic emotions? *Psychological Review*, *97*, 315–331.

Roseman, I. J. (2011). Emotional behaviors, emotivational goals, emotion strategies: Multiple levels of organization integrate variable and consistent responses. *Emotion Review*, *3*, 1–10.

Russell, J. A. (1980). A circumplex model of affect. *Journal of Personality and Social Psychology*, *39*, 1161–1178.

Russell, J. A. (2003). Core affect and the psychological construction of emotion. *Psychological Review*, *110*, 145–172.

Russell, J. A., & Barrett, L. F. (1999). Core affect, prototypical emotional episodes, and other things called emotion: Dissecting the elephant. *Journal of Personality and Social Psychology*, *76*, 805–819.

Schachter, S. (1959). *The psychology of affiliation*. Stanford, CA: Stanford University Press.

Schachter, S., & Singer, J. (1962) Cognitive, social, and physiological determinants of an emotional state. *Psychological Review*, *69*, 379–399.

Scherer, K. R. (2009). The dynamic architecture of emotion: Evidence for the component process model. *Cognition and Emotion*, *23*, 1307–1351.

Searle, J. R. (1995). *The construction of social reality*. New York: Free Press.

Searle, J. R. (2010). *Making the social world: The structure of human civilization*. New York: Oxford University Press.

Seth, A. K. (2013). Interoceptive inference, emotion, and the embodied self. *Trends in Cognitive Sciences*, *17*, 565–573.

Seth, A. K., Suzuki, K., & Critchley, H. D. (2012). An interoceptive predictive coding model of conscious presence. *Frontiers in Psychology*, *2*, 1–16.

Shariff, A. F., & Tracy, J. L. (2011). What are emotion expressions for? *Current Directions in Psychological Science, 20,* 395–399.

Shipp, S., Adams, R. A., & Friston, K. J. (2013). Reflections on agranular architecture: Predictive coding in the motor cortex. *Trends in Neurosciences, 36*(12), 706–716.

Shoda, Y., Mischel, W., & Wright, J. C. (1994). Intra-individual stability in the organization and patterning of behavior: Incorporating psychological situations into the idiographic analysis of personality. *Journal of Personality and Social Psychology, 65,* 674–687.

Sillito, A. M., & Jones, H. E. (2002). Corticothalamic interactions in the transfer of visual information. *Philosophical Transactions of the Royal Society of London B, 357,* 1739–1752.

Skinner, B. F. (1971). *Beyond freedom and dignity.* New York: Knopf.

Solomon, R. C. (1976). *The passions: Emotions and the meaning of life.* New York: Doubleday.

Sporns, O., & Kötter, R (2004). Motifs in brain networks. *PLoS Biology, 2*(11), e369.

Stephens, C. L., Christie, I. C., & Friedman, B. H. (2010). Autonomic specificity of basic emotions: Evidence from pattern classification cluster analysis. *Biological Psychiatry, 84,* 463–473.

Suvak, M. K., & Barrett, L. F. (2011). The brain basis of PTSD: A psychological construction analysis. *Journal of Traumatic Stress, 24,* 3–24.

Touroutoglou, A., Lindquist, K. A., Hollenbeck, M., Dickerson, B. C., & Barrett, L. F. (2014). *Intrinsic connectivity in the human brain does not reveal networks for "basic" emotions.* Manuscript under review.

Tracy, J. L., & Randles, D. (2011). Four models of basic emotions: A review Ekman and Cordaro, Izard, Levenson, and Panksepp and Watts. *Emotion Review, 3,* 397–405.

Vytal, K., & Hamann, S. (2010). Neuroimaging support for discrete neural correlates of basic emotions: A voxel-based meta-analysis. *Journal of Cognitive Neuroscience, 22,* 2864–2885.

Wager, T. D., Kang, J., Johnson, T. D., Nichols, T. E., Satpute, A. B., & Barrett, L. F. (2014). *A Bayesian model of category-specific emotional brain responses.* Manuscript under review.

Wilson-Mendenhall, C., Barrett, L. F., & Barsalou, L. W. (2013). Neural evidence that human emotions share core affective properties. *Psychological Science, 24,* 947–956.

Wilson-Mendenhall, C. D., Barrett, L. F., Simmons, W. K., & Barsalou, L. W. (2011). Grounding emotion in situated conceptualization. *Neuropsychologia, 49,* 1105–1127.

Wright, J. C., & Mischel, W. (1988). Conditional hedges and the intuitive psychology of traits. *Journal of Personality and Social Psychology, 55,* 454–469.

Wundt, W. (1897) *Outlines of psychology* (C. H. Judd, Trans.). Leipzig, Germany: Engelmann.

Xu, F., & Kushnir, T. (2013). Infants are rational constructivist learners. *Current Directions in Psychological Science, 21,* 28–32.

PART II

PSYCHOLOGICAL CONSTRUCTION THEORIES

CHAPTER 4

The Conceptual Act Theory

A Roadmap

LISA FELDMAN BARRETT
CHRISTINE D. WILSON-MENDENHALL
LAWRENCE W. BARSALOU

Over many centuries, philosophers and psychologists have assumed that the mind is structured as a typology, containing Platonic emotional types such as anger, sadness, fear, and so forth. Emotions are presumed to be basic elements (i.e., biologically and psychologically primitive). Scientists have searched for the corresponding physical essences for these emotion types in patterns of peripheral nervous system response, in facial muscle movements, and in the structure or function of the mammalian brain, attempting to identify the "natural joints" that distinguish different one emotion type from another. This approach, aptly termed the *natural kind* approach (Barrett, 2006a), has its roots in the 17th-century mental philosophy of *faculty psychology* (e.g., see works by Wolff as discussed in Klein, 1970; works by Gall and Spurzheim discussed by Harrington, 1987; cf. Lindquist & Barrett, 2012). When viewed as mental faculties, emotions are considered to be adaptations in the teleological sense (as natural processes that evolved to serve a specific end goal).

Faculty psychology has not been without its critics over the centuries, and criticisms have laid the groundwork for an alternative approach to understanding the mind's structure, termed *psychological construction*, or sometimes just *construction*. In this chapter, we present an overview of our psychological construction model of emotion, named the conceptual act model, and later, the conceptual act theory. The conceptual act theory of

1. *If emotions are psychological events constructed from more basic ingredients, then what are the key ingredients from which emotions are constructed? Are they specific to emotion or are they general ingredients of the mind? Which, if any, are specific to humans?*

The key ingredients for emotion are not specific to emotion but are domain-general ingredients from which experiences emerge more generally. The nature of the ingredients will vary, depending on whether they are specified at the psychological or biological level. The conceptual act theory was first formulated at the psychological level, specifying ingredients as psychological processes, such as sensory processing, including interoception, category knowledge, language, executive function, and so on. We then moved to a more brain-based epistemological approach, attempting to specify the processes within the body and the brain from which emotions emerge. At this moment in time, for example, intrinsic networks within the human brain are good candidates for the functional architecture from which emotions emerge. We are not proposing a strict one-to-one correspondence between the psychological ingredients that have been proposed in constructionist theories and these brain networks. However, the network functions must be described in psychological terms (otherwise we do not have a model of how the brain creates the mind—we just have a model of how neurons fire). The bottom line is that we employ the general strategy of taking a brain-based approach to discovering the ingredients of emotion, and to describing them in psychological terms, although the specifics of what the ingredients are will likely change as more is learned about how the brain functions.

Taking a brain-based approach to discovering ingredients allows for more specific evolutionary hypotheses about the construction of emotion, as well as speculations about which ingredients are species-general and which are species-specific. For example, many intrinsic brain networks can be found in other mammals, although several show human-specific adaptation (e.g., the default mode/mentalizing network, the language network) and several exist in other great apes but not in monkeys (e.g., the frontoparietal control network and the salience network; Mantini, Corbetta, Romani, Orban, & Vanduffel, 2013). As a consequence, humans (and perhaps in a more limited way, great apes) have the capacity to symbolically represent sensory changes as emotion, and to be sufficiently aware of these products of construction to use them more deliberately in the service of behavioral regulation. Some humans can even become aware of the process of construction itself (e.g., via meditation), thereby having flexibility about when (and when not) to construct an emotion in the first place.

2. *What brings these ingredients together in the construction of an emotion? Which combinations are emotions and which are not (and how do we know)?*

Because the brain is a large, interconnected neural net, individual neurons, circuits, and networks do not function in insolation and independently of one another, like the bits and pieces of a machine. Instead, there is continual and

(continued)

spontaneous neural activation, coordinating over time (in a normal functioning brain); incoming sensory input modulates this activity, as do modulatory networks such as the frontopartietal control network. As a consequence, nothing "brings the ingredients together"; as neurons fire, they influence and constrain each other as a normal part of how the brain functions. The networks might work together via constraint-satisfaction logic (Barrett, Ochsner, & Gross, 2007; Cunningham et al., Chapter 7, this volume). Nothing biological distinguishes an emotion from a non-emotion (i.e., there are no networks that are specific for emotion). Emotion-cognition-perception distinctions are phenomenological and are not respected by the brain.

3. *How important is variability (across instances within an emotion category, and in the categories that exist across cultures)? Is this variance epiphenomenal or a thing to be explained? To the extent that it makes sense, it would be desirable to address issues such as universality and evolution.*

Variation is a key feature that must be explained in any theory of emotion. From an evolutionary standpoint, variation is the key to survival. In the conceptual act theory, an emotion word refers to a conceptual category that is populated with variable instances. So our theory, like most psychological construction theories, takes variation seriously as part of the phenomenon to be explained. We hypothesize that emotions are constructed as tools for helping humans get along and get ahead as they live in social groups; to the extent that emotion concepts solve similar problems across cultures, they will be similar across cultures (cf. Barrett, 2006b, 2012).

4. *What constitutes strong evidence to support a psychological construction to emotion? Point to or summarize empirical evidence that supports your model or outline what a key experiment would look like. What would falsify your model?*

The conceptual act theory would be falsified if it were shown that conceptual knowledge is not required for an emotional episode to emerge or for emotion perception to proceed. Studies that purportedly find such evidence (e.g., congentially blind athletes showing critical components of pride expressions) do not falsify the conceptual act theory unless it can be shown that results cannot stem from conceptual processing (e.g., representations of color are similar in congenitally blind, color-blind, and normally sighted individuals, implying that some kind of conceptual knowledge is involved; Shepard & Cooper, 1992).

For many years, it was believed that any evidence for the biological distinctiveness of emotions was evidence for a "basic emotion" view and against a "constructionist" view. But evidence of biological distinctiveness between instances of two different emotion categories does not necesarily falsify the conceptual act theory per se (see Barrett, Chapter 3, this volume). In fact, the conceptual act theory makes very specific predictions about how, at the biological level of analysis, instances of the same emotion category might be different, and how instances of different emotion categories might be similar.

(continued)

The strongest evidence supporting the conceptual act theory comes from neuroscience studies showing that the same domain-general brain networks configure differently in different varieties of the same emotion category, in instances of other emotion categories, and even in non-emotional instances (of memory, perception, social cognition, etc.). That being said, the science of emotion has been too prescriptive (stipulating what emotions are) in the absence of careful observation. Careful observational work is needed to document the variety of instances, including their contexts, for each emotion category within a given culture. Only then can we discover (rather than prescribe) any regularities in the phenomena to be explained.

emotion was introduced in 2006 and has been elaborated through a series of theoretical and empirical articles (Barrett, 2006b, 2009a, 2009b, 2011, 2012, 2013; Barrett & Bar, 2009; Barrett & Bliss-Moreau, 2009; Barrett, Lindquist, & Gendron, 2007; Barrett, Mesquita, Ochsner, & Gross, 2007; Barrett, Ochsner, & Gross, 2007; Barrett & Satpute, 2013; Barrett, Wilson-Mendenhall, & Barsalou, 2014; Duncan & Barrett, 2007; Lindquist & Barrett, 2008, 2012; Lindquist, Wager, Kober, Bliss-Moreau, & Barrett, 2012; Wilson-Mendenhall, Barrett, Simmons, & Barsalou, 2011). In this chapter, we present a summary of the main ideas within these articles.

To introduce the conceptual act theory, we first discuss the hypothesis that mental states emerge as the consequence of an ongoing, continually modified constructive process during which stored knowledge within an experiencer (as reactivation and recombination of prior experience, referred to as "top-down" influence) makes incoming sensory inputs meaningful as *situated conceptualizations*. This discussion sets the stage for an overview of four major hypotheses of the conceptual act theory.

First, emotion words (like words for all mental states) are not assumed to be Platonic, physical types but are instead hypothesized to be abstract categories populated with variable instances (Hypothesis 1: Variability). Variability is created when physical responses (e.g., from behavioral adaptations) are optimized for a particular situation or context because sensory inputs (from the body and the world) are made meaningful using highly context-dependent and culturally dependent conceptual information about emotion derived from past learning or experience.

Second, the brain's architecture can be thought of as a situated conceptualization generator producing the individual brain states that correspond to each individual instance of an emotion (Hypothesis 2: Core Systems). Each category of conceptualized instances does not share an essence but instead arises from the interaction of core systems within the brain's architecture that are domain-general (which means that the systems are not specific to the traditional domains of emotion, cognition, or perception). These core systems can be characterized both at the psychological level and at the level of brain networks.

Third, instead of redefining (or reducing) mental phenomena into these core systems, the goal of the conceptual act theory is to analyze how mental states emerge from their interaction (Hypothesis 3: Constructive Analysis).

Fourth, from this viewpoint, emotions exist as conceptualized instances of sensation based on functional (rather than teleological) considerations (Hypothesis 4: Social Ontology). The idea is that conceptual knowledge is embodied and enactive, producing novel features during an instance of emotion via inference, such that emotional episodes take on functions that the physical sensations do not have on their own during the trajectory of a situated conceptualization. At the chapter's conclusion, we briefly consider how the conceptual act theory provides a unified framework for studying emotional experience, emotion perception, and emotion regulation, and more generally provides a novel approach to the functional architecture of the human brain.

Conceptual Knowledge Combines with Sensory Inputs to Construct Human Experiences

Take a look at Figure 4.1. Most of you, right now, are in a state called "experiential blindness" (e.g., Fine et al., 2003). You are taking in visual input, but your brain cannot make sense of it, so you do not see an object— you see black and white blobs. Normally, in the blink of an eye, your brain is able to integrate this sensory stimulation seamlessly with its vast amount of stored knowledge (from prior experience, referred to as "top-down" contributions), allowing you to construct a visual experience of the object. In fact, it is well accepted, now, that this is how normal vision works (Gilbert

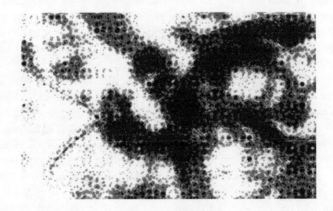

FIGURE 4.1. An illustration of experiential blindness. From Barrett, Wilson-Mendenhall, and Barsalou (2014). Copyright 2014 by The Guilford Press. Reprinted by permission.

& Li, 2013). This occurs via the process of predictive coding (Adams, Shipp, & Friston, 2013; Bastos et al., 2012; Clark, 2013; Friston, 2002; Hohwy, 2013; Shipp, Adams, & Friston, 2013). Your brain continually generates hypotheses based on past experience in a top-down fashion and tests them against incoming data. Such knowledge is not merely helpful—it is necessary to normal perception. With this knowledge, you normally categorize incoming information to construct a visual representation of the object in Figure 4.1. Your current instance of experiential blindness unmasks what you brain normally does so automatically and effortlessly. Without prior experience, sensations are meaningless, and you would not know how to act in the world.

To cure your experiential blindness, please look at the figure on the last page of this chapter, then look back at Figure 4.1. If you now see a fully formed object, several important things just happened. First, you *categorized the sensory input* using conceptual knowledge from past experience. No matter how hard you try, you cannot gain introspective access to how your brain accomplished this feat of making incoming sensations from Figure 4.1 a meaningful visual experience. Also, once the conceptual knowledge is applied, it should now be virtually impossible to "unsee" the object—to deconstruct the experience by the sheer force of will. The process of combining incoming sensory input with stored knowledge is ongoing, obligatory, and automatic (which means that you have no sense of agency, effort, or control in constructing your visual experience). Experimental methods are necessary to unmask its workings (or exercises such as the one we are engaged in right now). To you, it feels as if the act of seeing is passive, that seeing is merely the reflexive detection of visual information from the page. You are unaware of the extent to which *your prior knowledge contributes to your own experiences.*

Second, in viewing the image, it is now probably not that hard to infer extra experiential detail—to imagine the soft drone of buzzing, or to feel the delicate flutter of wings. In your mind's eye, you might see the object fly around as it searches for pollen. You might even be able to smell the sweet fragrance of the flower, or see the yellow petals swaying the light breeze. Perhaps you feel the sun warming your skin. The knowledge you bring to bear (as reactivation and recombination of prior experience that is represented in modal systems of the brain) to perceive this bee is *enactive*—as a consequence of predictive coding, your brain performs a *perceptual inference*. Inferring elements that are not immediately present in the visual input (e.g., the lines that link the black and white blobs together into the shape of a bee) creates your visual experience. Inference is considered one of the primary purposes of memory, and it is how experiences of the past inform situated action in the present. You could not survive in the world without this capacity. Some scientists refer to this inference process as *simulation* (e.g., Barsalou, 1999, 2009), in which you connect immediate sensory input with vast amounts of sensory, motor, affective, and other related information stored in memory. Others refer to it prediction (e.g., Clark, 2013). Still others simply call it *categorization* (Barrett, 2006b). Categorization typically is viewed as comprising two processes: (1) accessing and activating a relevant category representation and binding it to a perceived instance, and (2) drawing inferences from knowledge associated with the category and applying them to the instance.

Third, because the primary purpose of categorization is to produce inferences, it *prepares you for situated action*. For people who have experienced bees as part of a beautiful garden and/or as producing a sweet, tasty delight (honey), the image of a bee is calming and bucolic. For these people, seeing a bee might mean moving in to get a closer look, with an associated reduction in heart rate, blood pressure, and skin conductance. For other people who have been stung, with resultant pain and swelling, the image of a bee is terrifying. For these people, seeing a bee might mean freezing, with an associated increase in heart rate, blood pressure, and skin conductance. Or they might wave their arms or run away, with an increase in heart rate and skin conductance but a decrease in blood pressure. These are the sorts of physiological changes that we scientists record when we show study participants images from the International Affective Picture System (IAPS; Lang, Bradley, & Curthbert, 2008) stimulus set (e.g., Bradley, Codispoti, Cuthbert, & Lang, 2001). They arise when your brain predicts how the body should respond in a specific situation (what we have previously referred to as an "affective prediction"; Barrett & Bar, 2009, and what Seth, Suzuki, & Critchley [2012; Seth, 2013] call "interoceptive predictive coding").

Fourth, because categorization is enactive and prepares you for a specific action, it always produces *some kind of automatic change in your physical state*, impacting the internal sensations that contribute to your pleasant or unpleasant core affective tone (Barrett & Bliss-Moreau, 2009; Russell, 2003; Wundt, 1897). The concepts that are used during categorization can be thought of as tools used by the human brain to modify and regulate the body (i.e., homeostasis and allostasis, metabolism, and/or inflammatory processes), to create feelings, and to create dispositions toward action. The actual visceral changes are not necessary for feeling, although some representation of them in the brain (i.e., prediction) is required. In the same way that your brain used prior experience to predict and make meaning of the visual sensations in Figure 4.1, it uses such knowledge to predict and make meaning of bodily sensations. These two meaning-making achievements (of external and internal sensations) are not happening sequentially; they are occurring transactively and simultaneously, as a function of how the brain understands the current sensory array to create a unified conscious moment (cf. Barrett, 2009a). They are not occurring in a single instant, but they comprise a conceptual act that is evolving over time.

Fifth, this process of meaning making rarely happens because of a deliberate, conscious goal to figure things out; more often it occurs as instantaneously, continuously, and effortlessly for internal sensations as it does for external sensations. This is how the brain creates the mind. Whether you experience the situation as a perception or as an emotion depends on your attentional focus. When your brain is foregrounding visual sensations while viewing the bee, you experience a perception—the bee is friendly or dangerous because you are using the affective feelings that correspond to your physical response as information about the state of the world (e.g., Zadra & Clore, 2011; Anderson, Siegel, White, & Barrett, 2012). When your brain is foregrounding sensations from your body, and when these sensations are particularly intense (because such focus has been useful and reinforced in a prior situation like this one, or because you focus explicitly on the sensations), you experience tranquility or distress. In each case, information from the world, the body, and prior experience was present—what differed was the attentional focus within the dynamic conceptualization.

Sixth, prior experiences *seed* the construction of present and future experiences by predicting and therefore shaping the meaning of momentary, incoming sensory input. Why might you automatically experience the calm of a bee buzzing in a bucolic garden, whereas another person might automatically experience the terror of a bee attacking and stinging the body? The answer lies in the nature of prior experience. Actual experiences with bees, movie scenes that involve bees, stories, or simply instruction about bees constitute the knowledge that is used to make sensations meaningful. Your learning history predisposes you to experience sensations from the world and from your own body in particular ways. All things being equal, you have developed experiential "habits"—what you have experienced in the past is very likely what you will experience in the present, because stored representations of the past help to constitute the present (hence, the phrase "the remembered present"; Edelman, 1998). With additional learning or training, it should be possible to change your experiential habits. By deliberately cultivating certain types of experiences, it should be possible to modify the population of representations that are available for use in the present.

Finally, the bee example also illustrates that *states* and *processes* are easy to confuse when it comes to meaning making. Regardless of whether you automatically experience the calm of a bee buzzing in a bucolic garden or the terror of a bee attacking and stinging the body, it is possible to retrieve different concepts related to bees in the next instance, which in turn has the capacity to change the sensations that your brain predicts from your body. The same processes that were engaged during the initial instance of meaning making (creating tranquility or fear) are engaged again, and again, and again. When your bodily response changes, along with the feelings and actions to which you easily have access, you experience this as emotion regulation. If this is correct, then what we call "emotion regulation" does not occur via a special set of emotion-specific processes but instead occurs via the more basic meaning-making processes that are operating all the time to create the flow of mental states that constitute your mind.

Reappraisal, distraction, and other terms might not refer to processes at all, but are descriptions of changes that occur as one mental state flows into another (and one physical state transitions to another) as meaning changes. A series of sequential mental states that are experientially distinct are easy to understand as distinct psychological processes, even though scientists have known for a long time that experiences do not reveal the processes that make them.

To summarize these insights: During the brain's normal process of predictive coding, it performs a continual stream of *conceptual acts* when it applies prior knowledge to incoming sensory input. This was illustrated with you were presented with visual input to construct the visual experience of the bee. It was an "act" on your part rather than a passive event, because you are not merely detecting and experiencing what it is out there in the world or what is going on inside your body—your prior experiences (i.e., knowledge) played a role in creating momentary experience. (To call this construction an "act" does not imply anything deliberate, special, or effortful about the process.) Any conceptual act is embodied, because prior experience, in the form of category knowledge, comes "online" as the activation of sensory and motor neurons, thereby *reaching down* to influence bodily activations and/or their representations and sensory processing. Conceptual acts are also self-perpetuating, such that experiences created today *reach forward* to shape the trajectory of future experiences. Our hypothesis is that this is the way the mind works: The act of seeing the bee was at once a perception, a cognition, and a feeling. All mental states are, in fact, *conceptualizations* of internal bodily sensations and incoming sensory input. These conceptualizations are *situated* in that they use highly context-dependent representations that are tailored to the immediate situation.

There are four broad hypotheses that derive from this view of mental states as situated conceptualizations:

1. Emotions, like other mental state categories, are populations of instances that are tailored to the environment.
2. Each instance of emotion is constructed within the brain's functional architecture for creating situated conceptualizations, involving domain-general core systems.
3. Emotional episodes cannot be deconstructed and reduced into these domain-general systems but instead emerge from their interaction; therefore, the workings of each system cannot be studied alone and must be holistically understood within the momentary state of the brain and body.
4. Emotional episodes, because they are emergent states, have functional features that physical states, alone, do not have.

We address each hypothesis in turn.

Hypothesis 1: Variation

Whereas the faculty psychology approach to emotion is a textbook case of classical typological thinking (in which emotions are simply organized as a limited number of physical or morphological types), the conceptual act theory makes the more complex assumption that emotion words such as "anger," "sadness," "fear," and so forth, refer to abstract categories that contain a variety of unique instances. Within each abstract category, say, *anger*, or *fear*, instances (emotional episodes) vary in their physical manifestations (heart rate can go up or down, there can be avoidance or approach, etc.) that reflect different avenues of coping with particular kinds of situations. In this view, emotional episodes are situated affective states that are tailored to the immediate situation (for congruent views, see Cunningham, Dunfield, & Stillman, Chapter 7, and Ortony & Clore, Chapter 13, this volume). If each emotion category represents a population of instances, then experiments can be designed to model and capture the fully variety in those instances (rather than attempting to evoke only the most typical instance in the laboratory, which, ironically still produces variation that then has to be explained after the fact). For example, in our lab, we explicitly studied how neural responses differ during fearful instances of social threat and physical danger, as well as how neural responses during fear and anger are similar when experienced in a similar context (e.g., social threat) (Wilson-Mendenhall et al., 2011). In fact, a growing number of studies are designed explicitly to capture heterogeneity within emotion categories, both within individuals and across cultures (e.g., Ceulemans, Kuppens, & Van Mechelen, 2012; Hortensius, Schutter, & Harmon-Jones, 2012; Kuppens, Van Mechelen, & Rijmen, 2008; Kuppens, Van Mechelen, Smits, De Boeck, & Ceulemans, 2007; Nezlek & Kuppens, 2008; Stemmler, Aue, & Wacker, 2007).

There appear to be at least five sources of the variation within a category of emotion: (1) behavioral adaptations that serve as affective predictions about how best to act in a particular situation, (2) concepts that develop for emotion, (3) vocabulary used for emotions, (4) the types of situations that arise in different cultures, and (5) stochastic processes. Each of these is discussed briefly in turn.

Behavioral Adaptations

As a human, you have a variety of "behavioral adaptations" that help you "survive and thrive." Like other animals, you can flee, freeze, fight, and so on. Many of these adaptations are preserved options for dealing with threat and achieving safety (LeDoux, 2012). Upon the presentation of new sensory input, your brain quickly and efficiently predicts which action will be optimal given the current situation, constituting an affective prediction (Barrett & Bar, 2009). In humans, these adaptations are neither necessary nor sufficient for emotion: You do not routinely freeze, flee, or fight in emotion, and when you do, it is not always in the way prescribed by emotion stereotypes (e.g., people can withdraw during anger or fight during fear). Even in a rat, there is no necessary one-to-one correspondence between a particular behavioral adaptation and an emotion category (e.g., Barrett, 2012; LeDoux, 2012); depending on the context, a rat will flee, freeze, or defensively tread (i.e., aggress) in a threatening situation.

Concepts That Develop for Emotions

The brain state corresponding to an emotional episode is not just whatever happens in the body, in the subcortical neurons responsible for fighting, fleeing, freezing, or mating, and so forth, or in the brain regions that represent or regulate the body (e.g., the insula, amygdala, and orbitofrontal cortex). Our hypothesis is that the brain state for an emotional instance is a representation of the state of affairs in the world in relation to that physical state; both sensations from the world and from the body are made meaningful by information stored in the brain from past instances, and so include a neural representation of whatever portion of that information is being used. Thus, the second source of variation within an emotion category derives from the conceptual knowledge that it contains.

A concept can be viewed as aggregated memories that accumulate for a category across experiences with its instances. By focusing attention on some aspect of experience repeatedly, you develop a concept over time from instances of the respective category experienced across situations (Barsalou, 1999; Barsalou & Hale, 1993; Murphy, 2002; Schyns, Goldstone, & Thibaut, 1998). The concept of *bee*, for example, aggregates diverse information about the category of bees across a variety of situations into a loosely organized representation that includes properties (e.g., yellow and black, with wings), relations (e.g., flowers), rules (e.g., for something to be a bee, it must have black and yellow stripes, it must fly, etc.), and exemplars (instances of honey bees, carpenter bees, a queen bee, etc.).[1] Concepts develop for all aspects of your experience related to *bee*, including objects, settings, and actions (e.g., *flowers, honey, gardens, freezing, running, swatting, flying, buzzing, stinging*). From simpler concepts, more complex concepts emerge for events (e.g., *strolling in a garden, fear of the bee*). You also develop concepts for a wide variety of internal states (e.g., *aroused, quiet*), and for the properties and relations that describe instances of concepts (e.g., *yellow, fast, sweet, above, after, cause*). Although concepts reflect experience to a considerable extent, they undoubtedly have biological bases that scaffold learning (Barsalou, 1999, 2008; Carey, 2009; Rips, 2010; Simmons & Barsalou, 2003).

Category instances (e.g., a bee) are never encoded alone into conceptual knowledge, even though their context may not explicitly be the focus of attention. Initially, when encoding a category instance of a bee, for example, from actual prior experience with bees, observational learning about bees, hearing stories about bees, being told rules about bees, your brain captures the elements of the setting in which the bee occurs (i.e., other agents and objects), internal sensory (i.e., somatovisceral) cues from the body, as well as actions, instructions from others (in the form of rules) and words (e.g., the phonological form for "bee"). Over time, these situated conceptualizations create a heterogeneous population of information that is available for you to represent new instances of the category *bee*.[2] Later, when your brain requires conceptual knowledge to process some incoming sensory input, it samples from the populations of situated conceptualizations associated with relevant concepts to create a novel situated conceptualization, integrating current sensory input and retrieved (modal) conceptual knowledge (Barsalou, 2009). In this way, a situated conceptualization allows you to interpret incoming information and draw inferences that go beyond the information given.

Once concepts become established in memory, they play central roles throughout cognition and perception (e.g., Barsalou, 2003; Murphy, 2002), and, as we suggest, emotion. As you experience incoming sensory input from the world and the body, you use prior experience to categorize the agents, objects, setting, behaviors, events, properties, relations, and interoceptive inputs that are present. As described in Wilson-Mendenhall et al. (2011), a situated conceptualization is the conceptualization of the current situation across parallel streams of conceptual processing for all of these elements. As information from the current situation registers simultaneously in these processing streams, local concepts in each of these streams categorize the respective information and draw inferences. At a more global level, abstract relational concepts, such as *emotions*, integrate conceptualizations produced by local concepts on the individual processing streams into a coherent representation of the situation, which is constructed to interpret what is happening in the world in relation to the body and mind. Categorical inferences (i.e., predictions) follow, including inferences about how an object or entity is likely to behave, how you can best interact with it, the likely value to be obtained from interacting with it, and so forth, and on a temporal scale, about how situations may unfold during an event. From the perspective of grounded cognition, situated conceptualizations are responsible for producing the action, internal states, and perceptual construals that underlie goal-related activity in the current situation. Because modalities for action, internals states, and perceptual construals are typically active when you learn a concept, situated conceptualizations generate activity in these systems as they become active on later occasions to interpret experience. When the concept for *bee* becomes active in your brain, the situated conceptualization might include representations of situation-specific approach–avoidance actions (e.g., swatting the bee), representations of internal states (e.g., pleasure or displeasure), and perceptual construals. Not only does *bee* represent perceptual instances of the concept, it also controls interactions and predicts the resultant events.

We have hypothesized that concepts and categories for emotion work in essentially the same way as other kinds of abstract concepts in the conceptual system, where each individual's situated conceptualizations for an emotion (e.g., fear or anger) refer to an entire situation, including both the internal and external sensations (Wilson-Mendenhall et al., 2011). Initially, when your brain is encoding an instance of an emotion category in memory, say, *anger*, we hypothesize that your brain captures the elements of the setting in which the anger occurs (i.e., other agents and objects), internal sensory (i.e., somatovisceral) cues from your body, as well as actions, instructions from others (in the form of rules), and words (e.g., the phonological form for "anger" or "angry"). Over time, these situated conceptualizations create a heterogeneous population of information that is available for you to represent new instances of the category *anger*.

No single situated conceptualization for the concept *anger* need give a complete account of your category for *anger*. There is not one script for *anger* or one abstract representation for *anger*.[3] Consider the actions you might take upon experiencing anger in the following situations. When another driver cuts you off in traffic, you might shout as you slam on the breaks. When your child picks up a sharp knife, you might calmly take it away or ask your child to put it down. When you hear a news report about a bombing or a hurricane, you might turn up the radio. When a colleague criticizes you in front of a group, you might sit very still and perhaps even nod your head and smile. You may tease a friend who threatens your view of yourself, and so on. During these instances, your blood pressure might go up or down, or stay the same—whatever will allow you to prepare for the situated action. Sometimes you will feel your heart beating in your chest, and other times you will not. Your hands might become clammy, or they might remain dry. Sometimes your eyes will widen, but other times your brow will furrow, or you may even smile. On any given occasion, the content of a situated conceptualization for *anger* will be constructed to contain mainly those properties of *anger* that are contextually relevant, and it therefore contains only a small subset of the knowledge available in long-term memory about the category *anger*.[4] Later, when your brain requires conceptual knowledge to construct an instance of *anger*, it samples from the populations of situated conceptualizations, associated with relevant concepts, to create a novel situated conceptualization that integrates current sensory input and retrieved conceptual knowledge. In a given instance, then, the situated conceptualization for *anger* has the potential to change the internal state of the perceiver, because when retrieving information about *anger*, sensory, motor, and interoceptive states are partially reinstated in the relevant aspects of cortex, simulating an instance. The consequence is that accumulating conceptual knowledge for *anger*, for example, will vary within a person over instances as context and situated action demand.

Emotion Vocabulary

According to the conceptual act theory, emotion categories (i.e., the instances that populate them) vary as a function of learning, and in particular, how emotion words shape concept learning. Accumulating evidence shows that words are powerful in concept learning. Words facilitate learning novel categories (Lupyan, Rakison, & McClelland, 2007) and activate conceptual information effectively and efficiently (Lupyan & Thompson Shill, 2012). As early as 6 months of age, words guide an infant's categorization of animals and objects by directing the infant to focus on the salient and inferred similarities shared by animals or by objects with the same name (Fulkerson, & Waxman, 2007; Booth & Waxman, 2002). Words even allow infants to go beyond perceptual features and group things together that look and sound nothing alike (Dewar & Xu, 2009; Plunkett, Hu, & Cohen, 2008). Words also allow infants to extend their working memory span, taking a larger number of objects and chunking them into smaller units that can be more efficiently stored in memory (Feigenson & Halberda, 2008). Xu, Cote, and Baker (2005) refer to words as "essence placeholders," because a word allows an infant to categorize a new object as a certain kind, and to make inductive inferences about the new object based on prior experiences with other objects of the same kind.

Initially, young children are exposed to instances in which caregivers and other adults use emotion words to label and communicate changes in physical sensations and actions (either the child's or other people's), setting the stage for statistical learning of the emotion concept. So when developing a concept of *anger*, for example, the child's brain encodes instances in which the word "anger" or "angry" is used. When an emotion word (e.g., "angry") is explicitly uttered (e.g., by a caregiver or teacher), the brain captures the elements of the setting in which anger occurs (i.e., including the other agents and objects), the internal sensory (i.e., somatovisceral) cues from the child's body, the child's actions and the actions of others, instructions from others (in the form of rules), and words (e.g., the phonological form for "angry"). Our hypothesis is that across unique instances involving different feelings, physiology, and actions, the phonological form of the word becomes the statistical regularity that holds the concept together across instances (cf. Barrett, Lindquist, et al., 2007).

There is evidence that in infants, conceptual learning proceeds via the rational, constructive form of statistical inference (also called *rational constructivism*; e.g., Xu & Kushnir, 2013) that supports inferences about the world and guides behavior. Because emotions are abstract (i.e., emotions are not specific, concrete things in the world that one can point to), language most likely guides selective attention to the changes in internal states that characterize an emotion in a given situation. For example, each time your parent (or some other person) labeled your internal state or behavior with an emotion term when you were a child, or you observed the emotion term being used to label someone else's behavior, you extracted information about that instance (including the phonological form of the word) and integrated it with past information associated with the same term in memory. In this way, the phonological form for the emotion word becomes a perceptual regularity that, when repeeded across situations, underlies formation of the concept for that emotion, even if there are no strong physical similarities in the internal body states or actions from instance to instance within that emotion category (cf. Barrett, 2006b).

The Structure of Situations

Linked to variation within the conceptual system for a given emotion category is variation in the recurring situations that people find important and meaningful for a given emotion within a cultural context. If the conceptual system for emotion is constituted out of past experience, and if past experience is largely structured by people within a cultural context, then both the emotion categories that develop and the population of instances within each category will be culturally relative. Such ideas integrate the conceptual act theory with social construction approaches, positing that interpersonal situations "afford" certain emotions (or certain varieties of an emotion category; see Boiger & Mesquita, Chapter 15, this volume), and with the Ortony–Clore–Collins (OCC) model, in which the structure of emotion categories is thought to represent the structure of recurrent, important situations (see Ortony & Clore, Chapter 13, this volume). The word "affordance" here is meant to convey the idea that as an emotional episode is constructed, and that the construction process is dynamic, proceeding not only within the brain of a single perceiver but also in the transaction with surrounding circumstances. As practices and reinforcements differ within a cultural context, so do the emotional episodes that unfold. In this way, the practices and reinforcements structuring interpersonal situations come from the concepts that people share within a common cultural context; to the extent that concepts are enactive in the moment, they lead people to act in certain ways toward each other. To the extent that these practices and reinforcements shape the immediate emotional episode, they further seed the conceptual system for emotion. Concepts, then, are the carriers of culture.

The word "affordance" might also have a more literal Gibsonian meaning in social construction (i.e., to mean "given by the sensory properties of the world"). For example, conceptualization leads one person to modulate the acoustics of his or her vocalizations while talking to another person, the frequency with which he or she touches another person, or the frequency of certain facial movements (e.g., widening of the eyes). Each of these changes influences the affective state of the other person (i.e., the perceiver) in an immediate way, making certain emotional episodes in that person more or less likely.

Stochastic Variability

A final source of variation in the population of instances for an emotion category is the idea that incoming sensory input and conceptual knowledge do not combine in a deterministic way to create emotional episodes. Instead, they are probabilistic and combine stochastically (which means that there is not one, and only one, behavioral adaptation or conceptual representation for a given situation). Other influences (some of which are random), such as the state of the body or the prior state of the brain, might influence the specific emotional episode that is constructed in a given instance.

Hypothesis 2: Core Systems

According to the conceptual act theory, the brain's architecture can be thought of as a situated conceptualization generator producing the sequences of brain states that correspond to the mental features that a person experiences. As such, an emotion category does not have a single physical essence, such as brain circuit, or a psychological essence, such as an affect program or a pattern of appraisals, to determine the identity of an instance. Although there might be a stereotype, or a schema or script for a category prototype, it is misleading to believe that this represents the most typical instance of each category in an arithmetic sense (cf. Barrett, 2006b; Clore & Ortony, 2013). William James (1890, p. 195), one of the original psychological constructionists (cf. Gendron & Barrett, 2009; but see Scarantino, Chapter 14, this volume), described the danger of essentialism when he wrote, "Whenever we have made a word . . . to denote a certain group of phenomena, we are prone to suppose a substantive entity existing beyond the phenomena, of which the word shall be the name."

Instead of essences (either as a domain-specific system for each emotion type or as a general emotion-specific system such as that in certain accounts of the limbic system), we hypothesize that each situated conceptualization (as a series of brain states) can be understood as a construction that derives from the interaction of more basic, domain-general operations. These operations can themselves be characterized at the psychological level (e.g., Barrett, 2006b, 2012) and are supervenient on (emerging from) different combinations of brain networks that emerge from neural integration across time and space within the brain (e.g., Barrett & Satpute, 2013; Lindquist & Barrett, 2012; Oosterwijk et al., Chapter 5, this volume). Such basic operations are akin to the "mental state variables" (see Salzman & Fusi, 2010), facets, or core systems that describe the brain state. Rather than presuming that each network functions in a modular, mechanistic way, each operation can be thought of as arising as a family of "functional motifs" (i.e., patterns of activation) within the structural motif (i.e., the anatomical connectivity) that undergirds each network (e.g., Sporns & Kotter, 2004). Moreover, if these operations are the functional architecture for the mind, then the science of emotion should focus on modeling emotions as high-dimensional brain states within this architecture (reflecting the engagement of domain-general networks, their internal operations, and their interactions).

At the psychological level of description, the conceptual act theory hypothesizes that an instance of emotion is constructed when physical changes in the body (or their corresponding affective feelings) are made psychologically meaningful because they are related to or caused by a situation in the world. Physical changes are occurring all the time in your body: Blood pressure is going up and down, breathing rates speed and slow, voluntary muscles contract so that limbs move. Your affective feelings of pleasure and displeasure with some level of arousal, which in part are based on your body's moment-to-moment homeostatic and energy changes, are ever-present and always changing. However, only sometimes do you perceive these changes as being causally related to surrounding events, and when this happens, an emotion is constructed (this occurs whether or not you are aware that it is happening and whether or not you experience effort or agency, or have an explicit goal to make sense of things). To put it more formally, emotional episodes, no matter the category, are created with at least two domains of core systems: a system (or systems) for representing sensations related to the body (which is usually referred to as "affective"), and a system (or systems) for conceptually making sense of these sensations and/or feelings in relation to the situation (including the language network). Categorization is not specifically directing the construction of emotional episodes—it is necessary for every mental event. If you are awake, you are categorizing.

The conceptual act theory also proposes that the brain's matrix of attentional networks is an additional domain-general core system that supports constructing emotions (including the endogenous attention that is linked to goals and values) (Barrett, Tugade, & Engle, 2004; see also Cunningham et al., Chapter 7, this volume). In our view, an individual is more likely to experience an emotion when conceptual knowledge for emotion is reactivated, because attention foregrounds ongoing affective changes that are occurring in relation to a specific situation in the world (in contrast, an individual is more likely to experience a perception when attention is directed to events in the world; Barrett, 2009a). Although affective changes are always ongoing, it is only when they are foregrounded that they are experienced as emotional.

As we noted earlier, other systems important to constructing emotional episodes also include the circuits for basic behavioral adaptations such as freezing, fleeing, and fighting, although no one-to-one correspondence is necessary between a behavior and an emotion category (e.g., Barrett, 2012; LeDoux, 2012). When your brain predicts that one of these behavioral adaptations might be necessary in the immediate situation, you may experience affective changes even when the prediction is modified and the action is not realized (Barrett & Bar, 2009; Clark, 2013).

Hypothesis 3: Constructive Analysis

Instead of reducing situated conceptualizations to these core systems, the conceptual act theory directs scientists to take a constructive analytic approach to understanding how situated conceptualizations arise from their ongoing interaction over time. Reductionism is impossible, because any situated conceptualization (as a sequence of brain states) contains properties that emerge at a different level of integration from the individual networks that construct them (referred to as *emergentism*). The idea is that a composite whole has properties not evident in its individual parts. The concept of emergentism has long been a key assumption of psychological constructionist accounts; emotions have been described as "psychical compounds" (Wundt, 1897), "unanalyzable wholes" (Harlow & Stagner, 1932), and "emotional gestalts" (Barrett, Mesquita, et al., 2007). The conceptual act theory highlights the importance of analyzing and understanding emotions as integrated wholes.

The idea that emotional episodes are emergent has become popular over the past decade. Nearly all psychological construction approaches to emotion make this assumption, as evidenced throughout this volume. The conceptual act theory is somewhat unique, however, in also proposing that reductionism is ill-advised, because the function of each network within the brain's functional architecture is conditional on the whole system in that instance (referred to as *holism*; for a discussion of holism, see Harrington, 1987). Holism is the other side of the coin from emergentism. If emergentism is the idea of studying properties of a whole system that no part alone can produce, then holism is the idea of studying the interacting parts in a complex system, or never studying a part alone, out of context (also called *contextualism* or *compositionalism*). Holistic thinking means that it is not possible to know how a part of a system works without considering its role in the whole system. To be clear, the problem is not in attempting to break a mechanism down into its smallest definable bits; the problem is that those bits cannot be studied independently of one another like parts of a machine.

In the conceptual act theory, the core systems of the brain's intrinsic architecture are the neural "ecosystem" that creates brain representations that transition through time, from which a mental event, such as an instance of emotion, emerges. These ideas are very consistent with the hypothesis that the brain is a predictive organ that creates mental states by a process called "predictive coding." It continually generates hypotheses based on past experience in a top-down fashion and tests them against incoming data (e.g.,Adams et al., 2013; Bastos et al., 2012; Clark, 2013; Friston, 2002; Hohwy, 2013; Shipp et al., 2013). As a result, an analytic strategy of constructive analysis, rather than reductionism, is preferred. Understanding how emotions are constructed does not require ontologically reducing them out of existence. Instead, it requires understanding the dynamics of how core systems interact and influence each other through time. This represents a serious analytic challenge for psychological constructionism at the moment, however, since most data-analytic and modeling strategies are based on reductionist mathematical models (for alternatives, see Herschbach & Bechtel, Chapter 2, and Coan & Gonzalez, Chapter 9, this volume; Coan, 2010; but then see Barrett, 2011).

Theoretical need often spurs methodological development, however. For example, in a recent article, Raz et al. (2012) reported the development of a network cohesion index that can be used to investigate how the dynamics of interacting brain networks over time are related to self-reported emotional experience and to peripheral nervous system arousal. Subjects passively watched movies during functional magnetic resonance imaging (fMRI) scans, then after the scan, watched the films again, continuously rating the intensity of their emotional experiences. The fMRI blood-oxygen-level-dependent (BOLD) signal collected during movie watching was used to compute the connectivity between brain networks across time using a sliding time window of each movie (i.e., what the authors refer to as a network cohesion index). The dynamic changes in network cohesion during the movie clips predicted the moment-to-moment self-reported changes in the intensity of emotional experience during the clip.

Unlike constructive analysis, most analytic approaches applied within the science of emotion are stimulus driven and assume some version of the Stimulus → Organism → Response model, in which the causal mechanism for an emotion is "off" until it is switched "on" by the properties of a stimulus (whether physical or appraised). This assumption uses the logic of an experimental trial as a metaphor for how the mind works. In contrast, the conceptual act theory is, to a large extent, unmoored from the exteroceptive stimulus as the triggering event for the unfolding emergence of an emotional episode. The state of core systems within the brain before the onset of the stimulus (and perhaps even the process of deciding between stimulus and nonstimulus) is as important to the scientific explanation of emotion as the subsequent perturbations of the systems. The mind is understood as brain and body in context (usually in the context of other brains and bodies), transitioning from one state to another over time, with conceptualization creating emotional episodes that reflect a series of these state transitions.

Hypothesis 4: Social Ontology

When emotions are viewed as mental faculties that correspond to physical types, they are often said to have evolved to solve a specific functional need. Shariff and Tracy (2011, p. 396), for example, believe that emotions have evolved specifically to deal with "recurrent environmental events that pose fitness challenges." This view of emotion (along with similar typological views) are explicitly called "evolutionary," leading to the unfortunate and mistaken implication that psychological constructionist views are not consistent with the principles of evolution. At issue is *what* evolved, however, not *whether* emotions emerged in an evolutionary context. In our view, the emotion faculty approach to emotion suffers from the weaknesses of the "adaptationist programme" discussed out by Gould and Lewontin (1979), not the least of which is that natural selection is presumed to be teleological. Emotions are thought to have evolved to serve specific functions because a need for those functions existed (but for a discussion of how this view of emotions exemplifies the error of arbitrary aggregation, see Barrett, 2006c).

The conceptual act theory instead proposes that a neural architecture supporting situated conceptualizations evolved as the ability to conceptualize physical states in a context-specific fashion, and that it underlies other mental phenomena besides emotions. As such, it is possible to discuss *what* functions situated conceptualizations serve (the utility question) without answering the question of *why* they came to exist (which itself is a very interesting and important question with multifaceted and complicated answers). In our view, the utility of emotions does not necessarily reveal anything about their ultimate reason for existing.

Our hypothesis is that when physical sensations, such as one's own interoceptive state, and others' movements and vocalizations, are conceptualized as emotions, those sensations take on functions that they would not normally have on their own (i.e., by virtue of their physical structure alone; for a full discussion, see Barrett, 2012). They are what philosophers call "social reality." Conceptualization supports five functions that are necessary for getting along and getting ahead in social life: (1) It prescribes specific, situated actions (over and above approaching and avoiding); (2) it allows communication about many aspects of experience and the situation efficiently, with a word or two; (3) it creates meaning about the social value of the physical sensations, over and above their immediate sensorial valence and arousal; (4) it provides an avenue for social influence (as a bid to control the mental states and actions of another person) over and above the valence and arousal of vocal prosody or facial actions; and (5) it represents a way to use prior experience (including cultural learning) to influence momentary homeostasis, glucose metabolism, and inflammatory responses, over and above the immediate properties of any physical stimulation.

To say that emotional episodes exist in the domain of social reality does not deny that an instance of emotion exists in nature. Instead, it highlights the hypothesis that their physical nature involves not only the parts of the brain that are involved in homeostasis, interoception, and motor movements (limbic and motor tissue), but *also* those parts of the brain (often in concert with other brains) that are necessary for making meaning of those physical changes. Said another way, an emotional episode corresponds to a series of brain states that include both parts of the brain that represent and regulate the body (limbic tissue, motor cortex) and the additional information necessary for creating the new functions that create emotions from physical sensations—that is, the parts that are crucial for creating the conceptualizations necessary for emotional gestalts.

Evolution has endowed humans with the capacity to shape the microstructure of our own brains, in part via the complex categories that we transmit to one another within the social and cultural context. This means that even though emotions are real in the social world, they both cause and are caused by changes in the natural world. They can be causally reduced, but not ontologically reduced, to the brain states that create them. To more fully explain how humans get to social reality (e.g., emotions) from the properties of the natural world—that is, to explain social reality in physical terms—it will probably be necessary to study a human brain in context (including in the context of other functioning human brains in real time).

In our view, then, changes in heart rate or blood pressure, facial actions such as smiles or frowns, and behaviors such as crying or freezing in and of themselves are not evidence of emotions, and the fact that these behavioral adaptations are shared with nonhuman animals is not evidence that emotions are shared with other animals. Instead, these physical changes become part of an emotional episode when they take on a certain meaning in a certain situation. The adaptations, themselves, might be species-general, but the capacity to make additional meaning of them is a species-specific adaptation that evolves in humans (Barrett, 2006a, 2012). And with this meaning-making came additional flexibility in deploying these adaptations that is also likely species specific for humans. But the basic point is that via situated conceptualizations, physical changes acquire the ability to perform functions that they do not have on their own (creating social meaning, prescribing actions, allowing communication, aiding social influence). In this view, category knowledge about emotions does not *cause* emotions per se; it *constitutes* emotions by adding epistemologically novel functions to sensory input and action. Put another way, an emotion is constructed when embodied conceptual knowledge is enacted to shape the perception of sensory information from the body and the world, binding a physical state to an event in the world (as opposed to being merely a physical sensation or action). A bodily state or an action has a certain physical function (e.g., changes in respiration might regulate autonomic reactivity or widened eyes increase the size of the visual field), but neither event intrinsically has certain functions *as an emotion*; events acquire those functions in the act of categorizing them as emotion during the construction of a situated conceptualization.

Concluding Remarks

Given that the conceptual act theory is about a decade old, it is not surprising that many of its key formulations represent hypotheses yet to be tested. Perhaps its main value at present is to prescribe a different scientific paradigm for the design and interpretation of experiments (to seek out explicitly and model variation *within* each emotion category rather than attempting to aggregate across instances to find the essence of each category, and to engage in complex analysis of interacting domain-general systems over the time that an emotional episode unfolds). But the conceptual act theory holds other insights for the science of emotion. Its use of population logic and constructive analysis brings it closer to a Darwinian approach to emotion than the basic emotion models that usually claim Darwin as their intellectual heir (cf. Barrett, 2013). The conceptual act model also unites emotional experience and emotion perception within a single theoretical framework, with a single set of common domain-general mechanisms involved in mind–perception (Barrett, 2006a), suggesting, for example, that one's state as a perceiver is as important during an act of emotion perception as during an act of emotional experience (Anderson et al., 2012). The conceptual act theory also represents a set of hypotheses for how the phenomena that we refer to as *emotion* and *emotion regulation* are derived within a common mechanistic framework (Barrett, Wilson-Mendenhall, & Barsalou, 2014). Specifically, we view emotion regulation as occurring in the more basic meaning-making processes that are operating all the time. As such, reappraisal, distraction, and other terms do not refer not to processes but to changes that occur from one mental state to another (and from one physical state to another) as meaning changes.

   Finally, the conceptual act theory also represents an opportunity to unify theories of how the brain creates the mind. Faculty psychology traditions carved up human brain imaging research into at least three sister disciplines—affective, social, and cognitive neuroscience—but we unite social, affective, and cognitive neuroscience within one constructionist functional brain architecture (Barrett & Satpute, 2013). Emotions, social cognitions, and nonsocial cognitions (and perceptions, which for this chapter we include in the category "cognition") are better thought of as mental events (prompted by specific experimental tasks, or arising as naturally occurring states) that are constructed from interactions within and between these networks that compute domain-general functions. There is no "affective" brain, "social" brain, or "cognitive" brain. Each human has one brain whose functional properties can be understood differently for different timescales and levels of organization.

ACKNOWLEDGMENTS

Preparation of this chapter was supported by a National Institutes of Health Director's Pioneer Award (No. DP1OD003312); by grants from the National Institute on Aging (No. R01AG030311), the National Institute of Mental Health (No. R21MH099605), and the National Science Foundation (No. BCS-1052790); and by contracts from the U.S. Army Research Institute for the Behavioral and Social Sciences (Contract Nos. W5J9CQ-11-C-0046 and W5J9CQ-12-C-0049) to Lisa Feldman Barrett. The views, opinions, and/or findings contained in this chapter are solely those of the author(s) and should not be construed as an official Department of the Army or Department of Defense position, policy, or decision.

NOTES

1. Throughout this chapter, we use italics to indicate a concept (e.g., *car*) and quotes to indicate the word or phrase associated with it (e.g., "car").

2. Theory and research strongly suggest that concepts do not have conceptual cores (i.e., information that is necessary and sufficient for membership in the associated category). Instead, concepts are represented with loose collections of situated exemplars that are related by family resemblance. Exemplar theories of categorization further illustrate that loose collections of memories for category members can produce sophisticated classification behavior, demonstrating that abstractions for prototypes and rules are not necessary. Neural net systems similarly demonstrate that only loose statistical coherence is necessary for sophisticated categorization. To the extent that abstraction does occur for a category, it may only occur partially across small sets of category instances, reflect the abstraction of nondefining properties and relations that can be used to describe category members in a dynamcial manner, or reflect an online abstraction at retrieval, rather than stored abstractions in memory. Nevertheless, people often believe mistakenly that categories do have cores, perhaps because a word can lead people to essentialize.

3. As goal-directed categories that develop to guide action, the most typical member of a category such as fear is not the one that is most frequently encountered,

but rather the one that maximally achieves the theme or goal of the category (Barsalou, 2003). As a result, the most typical instances of a category contain properties that represent the ideal form of the category—that is, whatever is ideal for meeting the goal around which the category is organized—not those that most commonly appear as instances of the category. From a situated conceptualization viewpoint, prototypes do not exist as stored representations in memory, but they can be constructed (or simulated) when needed (Barsalou, Niedenthal, Barbey, & Ruppert, 2003).

4. Highly different instances for the same category can become integrated over time, and become available to construct novel simulations that have never been experienced before. This, in part, may help to explain why people believe that emotions such as anger, sadness, fear, and so on, have specific response signatures, even though the available data do not support this view. A simulation of *fear* could allow a person to go beyond the information given to fill in aspects of a internal sensation that are not present at a given perceptual instance. In such a case, the simulation essentially produces an illusory correlation between response outputs, helping to explain why researchers continue to search for coordinated autonomic, behavioral, and experiential aspects of a *fear* response.

REFERENCES

Adams, R. A., Shipp, S., & Friston, K. J. (2013). Predictions not commands: Active inference in the motor system. *Brain Structure and Function*. E pub.

Anderson, E., Siegel, E. H., White, D., & Barrett, L. F. (2012). Out of sight but not out of mind: Unseen affective faces influence evaluations and social impression. *Emotion, 12*, 1210–1221.

Barrett, L. F. (2006a). Emotions as natural kinds? *Perspectives on Psychological Science, 1*, 28–58.

Barrett, L. F. (2006b). Solving the emotion paradox: Categorization and the experience of emotion. *Personality and Social Psychology Review, 10*, 20–46.

Barrett, L. F. (2006c). Valence as a basic building block of emotional life. *Journal of Research in Personality, 40*, 35–55.

Barrett, L. F. (2009a). The future of psychology: Connecting mind to brain. *Perspectives on Psychological Science, 4*(4), 326–339.

Barrett, L. F. (2009b). Variety is the spice of life: A psychologist constructionst approach to understanding variability in emotion. *Cognition and Emotion, 23*, 1284–1306.

Barrett, L. F. (2011). Bridging token identity theory and supervenience theory through psychological construction. *Psychological Inquiry, 22*, 115–127.

Barrett, L. F. (2012). Emotions are real. *Emotion, 12*(3), 413–429.

Barrett, L. F. (2013). Psychological construction: A Darwinian approach to the science of emotion. *Emotion Review, 5*, 379–389.

Barrett, L. F., & Bar, M. (2009). See it with feeling: Affective predictions in the human brain. *Philosophical Transactions of the Royal Society B, 364*, 1325–1334.

Barrett, L. F., & Bliss-Moreau, E. (2009). Affect as a psychological primitive. *Advances in Experimental Social Psychology, 41*, 167–218.

Barrett, L. F., Lindquist, K. A., & Gendron, M. (2007). Language as context for the perception of emotion. *Trends in Cognitive Science, 11*(8), 327–332.

Barrett, L. F., Mesquita, B., Ochsner, K. N., & Gross, J. J. (2007). The experience of emotion. *Annual Review of Psychology, 58*, 373–403.

Barrett, L. F., Ochsner, K. N., & Gross, J. J. (2007). On the automaticity of emotion. In J. Bargh (Ed.), *Social psychology and the unconscious: The automaticity of higher mental processes* (pp. 173–218). New York: Psychology Press.

Barrett, L. F., & Satpute, A. B. (2013). Large-scale brain networks in affective and social neuroscience: Towards an integrative architecture of the human brain. *Current Opinion in Neurobiology, 23*(3), 361–372.

Barrett, L. F., Tugade, M. M., & Engle, R. W. (2004). Individual differences in working memory capacity and dual-process theories of the mind. *Psychological Bulletin, 130*, 553–573.

Barrett, L. F., Wilson-Mendenhall, C. D., & Barsalou, L. W. (2014). A psychological construction account of emotion regulation and dysregulation: The role of situated conceptualizations. In J. J. Gross (Ed.), *Handbook of emotion regulation* (2nd ed., pp. 447–465). New York: Guilford Press.

Barsalou, L. W. (1999). Perceptual symbol systems. *Behavioral and Brain Sciences, 22*(4), 577–609; discussion 610–560.

Barsalou, L. W. (2003). Situated simulation in the human conceptual system. *Language and Cognitive Processes, 18*, 513–562.

Barsalou, L. W. (2008). Grounded cognition. *Annual Review of Psychology, 59*, 617–645.

Barsalou, L. W. (2009). Simulation, situated conceptualization, and prediction. *Philosophical Transactions of the Royal Society B, 364*(1521), 1281–1289.

Barsalou, L. W., & Hale, C. R. (1993). Components of coceptual representation: From feature lists to recursive frames. In I. Mechelen, J. Hampton, R. Michalski, & P. Theuns (Eds.), *Categories and concepts: Theoretical views and inductive data analysis* (pp. 97–144). San Diego, CA: Academic Press.

Barsalou, L. W., Niedenthal, P. M., Barbey, A., & Ruppert, J. (2003). Social embodiment. In B. Ross (Ed.), *The psychology of learning and motivation* (Vol. 43, pp. 43–92). San Diego, CA: Academic Press.

Bastos, A. M., Usrey, W. M., Adams, R. A., Mangun, G. R., Fries, P., & Friston, K. J. (2012). Canonical microcircuits for predictive coding. *Neuron, 76*, 695, 711.

Booth, A. E., & Waxman, S. R. (2002). Object names and object functions serve as cues to categories in infants. *Developmental Psychology, 38*, 948–957.

Bradley, M. M., Codispoti, M., Cuthbert, B. N., & Lang, P. J. (2001). Emotion and motivation: I. Defensive and appetitive reactions in picture processing. *Emotion, 1*(3), 276–298.

Carey, S. (2009). *The origin of concepts*. New York: Oxford University Press.

Ceulemans, E., Kuppens, P., & Van Mechelen, P. (2012). Capturing the structure of distinct types of individual differences in the situation-specific experience of emotions: The case of anger. *European Journal of Personality, 26*, 484–495.

Clark, A. (2013). Whatever next?: Predictive brains, situated agents and the future of cognitive science. *Behavioral and Brain Sciences, 36*, 181–253.

Clore G., & Ortony, A. (2013). Psychological construction in the OCC model of emotion. *Emotion Review, 5*, 335–343.

Coan, J. A. (2010). Emergent ghosts of the emotion machine. *Emotion Review, 2,* 274–285.

Dewar, K. M., & Xu, F. (2009). Do early nouns refer to kinds or distinct shapes?: Evidence from 10-month old infants. *Psychological Science, 20,* 252–257.

Duncan, S., & Barrett, L. F. (2007). Affect as a form of cognition: A neurobiological analysis. *Cognition and Emotion, 21,* 1184–1211.

Edelman, G. M. (1998). *The remembered present: A biological theory of consciousness.* New York: Basic Books.

Feigenson, L., & Halberda, J. (2008). Conceptual knowledge increases infants' memory capacity. *Proceedings of the National Academy of Sciences, 105,* 9926–9930.

Fine, I., Wade, A. R., Brewer, A. A., May, M. G., Goodman, D. F., Boynton, G. M., et al. (2003). Long-term deprivation affects visual perception and cortex. *Nature Neuroscience, 6,* 915–916.

Friston, K. (2002). Beyond phrenology: What can neuroimaging tell us about distributed circuitry? *Annual Review of Neuroscience, 25,* 221–250.

Fulkerson, A. L., & Waxman, S. R. (2007). Words (but not tones) facilitate object categorization: Evidence from 6- and 12-month-olds. *Cognition, 105,* 218–228.

Gilbert, C. D., & Li, W. (2013). Top-down influences on visual processing. *Nature Reviews Neuroscience, 14,* 350–363.

Gould, S. J., & Lewontin, R. C. (1979). The spandrels of San Marco and the Panglossian paradigm: A critique of the adaptationist programme. *Proceedings of the Royal Society of London B, 205,* 581–598.

Harlow, H. F., & Stagner, R. (1932). Psychology of feelings and emotions: I. Theory of feelings. *Psychological Review, 39*(6), 570–589.

Harrington, A. (1987). *Medicine, mind, and the double brain: A study in 19th century thought.* Princeton, NJ: Princeton University Press.

Hohwy, J. (2013). *The predictive mind.* New York: Oxford University Press.

Hortensius, R., Schutter, D. J. L. G., & Harmon-Jones, E. (2012). When anger leads to aggression: Induction of relative left frontal cortical activity with transcranial direct current stimulation increases the anger-aggression relationship. *Social Cognitive Affective Neuroscience, 7,* 342–347.

James, W. (1890). *The principles of psychology* (Vol. 1). New York: Holt.

Klein, D. B., (1970). *A history of scientific psychology: Its origins and philosophical backgrounds.* New York: Basic Books.

Kuppens, P., Van Mechelen, I., & Rijmen, F. (2008). Towards disentangling sources of individual differences in appraisal and anger. *Journal of Personality, 76,* 1–32.

Kuppens, P., Van Mechelen, I., Smits, D. J. M., De Boeck, P., & Ceulemans, E. (2007). Individual differences in patterns of appraisal and anger experience. *Cognition and Emotion, 21,* 689–713.

Lang, P. J., Bradley, M. M., & Curthbert, B. N. (2008). *International Affective Picture System (IAPS): Affective ratings of pictures and instruction manual.* Gainsville: University of Florida.

LeDoux, J. (2012). Rethinking the emotional brain. *Neuron, 73,* 653–676.

Lindquist, K., & Barrett, L. F. (2008). Emotional complexity. In M. Lewis, J. M. Haviland-Jones, & L. F. Barrett (Eds.), *Handbook of emotions* (3rd ed., pp. 513–530). New York: Guilford Press.

Lindquist, K. A., Wager, T. D., Kober, H., Bliss-Moreau, E., & Barrett, L. F. (2012). The brain basis of emotion: A meta-analytic review. *Behavioral and Brain Sciences, 35*(3), 121–143.

Lindquist, K. A., & Barrett, L. F. (2012). A functional architecture of the human brain: Insights from the science of emotion. *Trends in Cognitive Sciences, 16*, 533–540.

Lupyan, G., Rakison, D. H., & McClelland, J. L. (2007). Language is not just for talking: Labels facilitate learning of novel categories. *Psychological Science, 18*, 1077–1083.

Luypan, G., & Thompson Schill, S. L. (2012). The evocative power of words: Activation of concepts by verbal and non-verbal means. *Journal of Experimental Psychology: General, 141*, 170–186.

Mantini, D., Corbetta, M., Romani, G. L., Orban, G. A., & Vanduffel, W. (2013). Evolutionary novel functional networks in the human brain? *Journal of Neuroscience, 33*, 3259–3275.

Murphy, G. L. (2002). *The big book of concepts*. Cambridge, MA: MIT Press.

Nezlek, J. B., & Kuppens, P. (2008). Regulating positive and negative emotions in daily life. *Journal of Personality, 76*, 561–580.

Plunkett, K., Hu, J.-F., & Cohen, L. B. (2008). Labels can override perceptual categories in early infancy. *Cognition, 106*, 665–681.

Raz, G., Winetraub, Y., Jacob, Y., Kinreich, S., Maron-Katz, A., Shaham, G., et al. (2012). Portraying emotions at their unfolding: A multilayered approach for probing dynamics of neural networks. *NeuroImage, 60*, 1448–1461.

Rips, L. J. (2010). *Lines of thought*. New York: Oxford University Press.

Russell, J. A. (2003). Core affect and the psychological construction of emotion. *Psychological Review, 110*, 145–172

Salzman, C. D., & Fusi, S. (2010). Emotion, cognition, and mental state representation in amygdala and prefrontal cortex. *Annual Review of Neuroscience, 33*, 173–202.

Schyns, P. G., Goldstone, R. L., & Thibaut, J. P. (1998). The development of features in object concepts. *Behavioral and Brain Sciences, 21*(1), 1–17; discussion 17–54.

Seth, A. K. (2013). Interoceptive inference, emotion, and the embodied self. *Trends in Cognitive Sciences, 17*, 565–573.

Seth, A. K., Suzuki, K., & Critchley, H. D. (2012). An interoceptive predictive coding model of conscious presence. *Frontiers in Psychology, 2*, 1–16.

Shariff, A. F., & Tracy, J. L. (2011). What are emotion expressions for? *Current Directions in Psychological Science, 20*, 395–399.

Shepard, R. N., & Cooper, L. A. (1992). Representation of colors in the blind, color-blind, and normally sighted. *Psychological Science, 3*, 97–104.

Shipp, S., Adams, R. A., & Friston, K. J. (2013). Reflections on agranular architecture: Predictive coding in the motor cortex. *Trends in Neurosciences, 36*(12), 706–716.

Simmons, W. K., & Barsalou, L. W. (2003). The similarity-in-topography principle:

Reconciling theories of conceptual deficits. *Cognitive Neuropsychology,* *20*(3), 451–486.

Sporns, O., & Kotter, R. (2004). Motifs in brain networks. *PLoS Biology, 2,* e369.

Stemmler, G., Aue, T., & Wacker, J. (2007). Anger and fear: Separable effects of emotion and motivational direction on somatovisceral responses. *International Journal of Psychophysiology, 66,* 141–153.

Wilson-Mendenhall, C. D., Barrett, L. F., Simmons, W. K., & Barsalou, L. W. (2011). Grounding emotion in situated conceptualization. *Neuropsychologia, 49,* 1105–1127.

Wundt, W. (1897). *Outlines of psychology* (C. H. Judd, Trans.). Leipzig, Germany: Engelmann.

Xu, F., Cote, M., & Baker, A. (2005). Labeling guides object individuation in 12-month-old infants. *Psychological Science, 316,* 372–377.

Xu, F., & Kushnir, T. (2013). Infants are rational constructivist learners. *Current Direction in Psychological Science, 21,* 28–32.

Zadra, J. R., & Clore, G. L. (2011). Emotion and perception: The role of affective information *Wiley Interdisciplinary Reviews: Cognitive Science, 2*(6), 676–685.

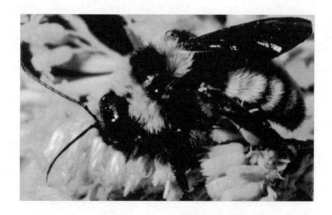

CHAPTER 5

The Neuroscience of Construction

What Neuroimaging Approaches Can Tell Us about How the Brain Creates the Mind

SUZANNE OOSTERWIJK
ALEXANDRA TOUROUTOGLOU
KRISTEN A. LINDQUIST

One of the most defining characteristics of mental life is that it changes from moment to moment. One can ponder the groceries needed for dinner and in the next moment feel angry because an important ingredient is sold out, or vividly remember the last time the same recipe was prepared. These mental events are experienced with different subjective qualities. Anger is experienced differently than thinking about a grocery list, and emotions and thoughts are experienced differently than remembering a previous moment in time. This subjective quality of emotions and other mental states is one of the central phenomena that psychological science seeks to measure and explain (Barrett, 2012).

For many years, psychologists took a "faculty psychology approach" (cf. Lindquist & Barrett, 2012; Uttal, 2001; Barrett, Wilson-Mendenhall, & Barsalou, Chapter 4, this volume) to the mind, assuming that the subjective quality of different mental states gives evidence of separate and distinct psychological processes, such as emotion, cognition, memory, and perception. In modern neuroscience, scientists have tried to map these faculties to specific locations in the brain (e.g., Barrett, 2009; Lindquist & Barrett, 2012). For example, neuroscientists have sought the neural modules of mental constructs, such as "fear" (e.g., Whalen et al., 1998), "theory of mind" (Saxe & Kanwisher, 2003), "episodic memory" (Rugg, Otten, & Henson, 2002), and "face perception" (e.g., Kanwisher, McDermott, &

1. *If emotions are psychological events constructed from more basic ingredients, then what are the key ingredients from which emotions are constructed? Are they specific to emotion or are they general ingredients of the mind? Which, if any, are specific to humans?*

The hypothesis that emotions are psychological events constructed from more basic ingredients is central to our psychological constructionist approach. According to our constructionist view the brain can be described as engaging in three basic psychological processes that combine in different patterns to produce myriad different mental states. These three processes are *exteroception*, or representing basic sensory information from the world; *core affect*, or representing basic interoceptive sensations from the body; and *conceptualization*, or making meaning of internal and external sensations utilizing stored representations of prior experience. Our constructionist perspective hypothesizes that these ingredients contribute not only to the experience of specific emotions (e.g., anger, fear, disgust, joy) but also to the experience of other mental states, such as memories, thoughts, and perceptions. Furthermore, we argue that these ingredients are basic to recognizing and understanding mental states in other people (see Oosterwijk & Barrett, 2014).

We do not believe that it is useful to talk about these basic processes as strictly human specific versus species general. Since we hypothesize that these processes correspond to the basic functional architecture of the mind (Lindquist & Barrett, 2012), we expect that there will be both similarities and differences in these networks across the phylogenetic scale. For instance, core affective circuitry is clearly conserved in other mammalian species (Barrett & Bliss-Moreau, 2009). Much of this circuitry supports the basic adaptive behaviors that contribute to survival in nonhuman animals (LeDoux, 2012). Despite overall similarities in the regions that comprise core affect, important differences exist, however. Humans exclusively seem to possess aspects of the anterior insular cortex that are linked to being consciously aware of body states (see Craig, 2009). We hypothesize that this ability to represent core affective states in awareness is central to the ability to generate a second-order conscious experience of emotion.

In addition, there is some evidence for the conservation of circuitry supporting conceptualization across nonhuman animals. For instance, a network resembling the default network has been identified in the monkey brain (Kojima et al., 2009). Yet, since we argue that concepts represented in language are an important ingredient in the experience of reified discrete mental states (Barrett, 2009; Lindquist & Gendron, 2013) and most nonhuman animals do not possess this type of symbolic conceptual representation, it is likely that animals do not experience subjective states as humans do. For example, since a rat cannot conceptualize the meaning of its internal state using symbolic representations of abstract concepts (e.g., "anger"), it is not likely to experience a state like human anger when it aggresses against another

(continued)

rat (Barrett, 2012; Barrett et al., 2007; LeDoux, 2012). It remains a possibility, however, that animals with relatively sophisticated conceptual systems (e.g., dolphins and great apes) might have mental states that more closely resemble those experienced by humans.

2. *What brings these ingredients together in the construction of an emotion? Which combinations are emotions and which are not (and how do we know)?*

According to our framework, ingredients come together during the experience of an emotion via the domain-general process of executive control. In our model, the network supporting executive control modulates activity in other networks, helping to determine which sensory and conceptual information is prioritized, and which information is inhibited in a given context. For example, when a person is walking on a grassy path in a bustling wood and a snake moves in the grass, executive control prioritizes certain exteroceptive sensations (e.g., biological motion of the snake) and inhibits others (e.g., a bird moving in the trees) for conscious awareness. Similarly, certain core affective sensations (e.g., arousal) are prioritized for conscious awareness, while others (e.g., thirst) are inhibited in the moment. Executive attention further selects and inhibits the conceptual representations from memory that are best suited to make meaning of exteroceptive and interoceptive sensations in that situational context (e.g., the concept of surprise is selected as opposed to fear, because the snake is small and not dangerous). Due to the involvement of executive control, the mental state that emerges from the combination of ingredients is experienced as unified, rather than as a dysregulated array of affective, exteroceptive, and conceptual representations (for discussion, see Barrett et al., 2004; Lindquist et al., 2012). Disorders in which executive control is impaired, such as schizophrenia (Krabbendam, Arts, Van Os, & Aleman, 2005), are a testament to the important role of this ingredient in maintaining unified conscious states; patients with schizophrenia characteristically experience fractionated and dysregulated sensory and affective states. Sleep is another example in which impairment of executive attention (due to sleep cycles) results in mental states that comprise dysregulated and odd combinations of affective and conceptual information (as is often the case in dreams) (see Lindquist et al., 2012, for discussion).

The question of which combinations of basic ingredients are emotions and which are not is a matter of custom, cultural norms, and personal opinion, and not of mechanism. First, there are strong cultural and individual differences in the states that people call emotions. Different cultures might have different norms that drive which "recipes" of ingredients are experienced as anger, fear, or happiness. Furthermore, some cultures do not draw a distinction between emotion and cognition (Wikan, 1990), implying that individuals from those cultures may experience great similarity between states that Western people experience as subjectively different. Second, the lines between mental state

(continued)

categories are equally fuzzy from the standpoint of the brain. Neuroimaging evidence cannot identify brain states that are consistently and specifically (i.e., uniquely) linked to emotions versus cognitions. Instead, brain patterns associated with emotions strongly overlap with other psychological processes such as memory, internal mentation, and social cognition (see Barrett & Satpute, 2013; Lindquist & Barrett, 2012). Based on these insights, it is unlikely that we can identify a single brain pattern that reliably distinguishes emotions from other discrete mental states.

3. How important is variability (across instances within an emotion category, and in the categories that exist across cultures)? Is this variance epiphenomenal or a thing to be explained? To the extent that it makes sense, it would be desirable to address issues such as universality and evolution.

In our constructionist framework, variability is a defining quality of emotional experience and mental life in general. Despite the essentialist tendency to assume that emotions are entities with clear essences in the brain and body (e.g., Lindquist, Gendron, Oosterwijk & Barrett, 2013), we do not believe that emotion categories have a biological (Barrett, 2006; Barrett et al., 2007; Lindquist et al., 2012) or even conceptual core (see Wilson-Mendenhall et al., 2011). In our model, emotions are *situated conceptualizations:* instances of the mind that vary dynamically depending on the conceptualization that is tuned to the context. During conceptualization, the brain merges sensations in the moment with representations of previous experience, categorical knowledge, situational predictions, regulation rules, and so forth. Since these activated representations differ depending on the personal history of an individual, his or her cultural background, or the demands of the situation, instances of emotions will be highly variable. For instance, our approach predicts that instances from the same emotion category (e.g., two instances of fear) might be just as different from one another as instances from two different emotion categories (e.g., an instance of fear versus anger) (see Wilson-Mendenhall et al., 2011). Cultural variability, individual variability, and variability in experience within the same individual across different contexts are thus core phenomena to be explained and measured by scientists, not errors to be ignored. Therefore, if we want to understand the basic mechanisms that underlie emotions, it may be more informative to focus on individual variability and contextual variability than on the categorical label of the subjective mental state itself. For instance, studies that treat emotions as situated conceptualizations by modeling contextual variation have been far more successful at identifying the peripheral physiological (Kreibig, 2010) or neural (Wilson-Mendenhall et al., 2011) basis of emotions than attempts that treat emotions as having biological essences (see Barrett, 2006; Cacioppo, Berntson, Larsen, Poehlmann, & Ito, 2000; Lindquist et al., 2012; Mauss & Robinson, 2009).

(continued)

4. *What constitutes strong evidence to support a psychological construction to emotion? Point to or summarize empirical evidence that supports your model or outline what a key experiment would look like. What would falsify your model?*

In this chapter, we emphasize neuroscientific evidence from our own body of work that supports a psychological constructionist approach to emotion. Recent years have seen a surge in psychological constructionist approaches to emotion (as indicated by this book), and we believe this surge is in no small part due to ongoing efforts to understand the brain basis of emotions. Although behavioral evidence has demonstrated that emotions are decomposable into more basic parts (Gendron Lindquist, Barsalou, & Barrett, 2012; Lindquist & Barrett, 2008; Lindquist, Barrett, Bliss-Moreau, & Russell, 2006; Oosterwijk, Topper, Rotteveel, & Fischer, 2010, 2012; Russell & Widen, 2002; Widen & Russell, 2008), neuroimaging techniques uniquely allow scientists to "peer inside" the mind of healthy humans as they experience emotions in real time.

Neuroimaging methods convincingly support the idea that emotions emerge from domain-general psychological operations. For instance, meta-analyses of brain activity during anger, disgust, fear, happiness, and sadness do not reveal consistent and specific neural modules for those categories, but instead reveal networks supporting more basic processes, such as affect generation and representation, conceptualization, and attention (Kober et al., 2008; Lindquist et al., 2012; Vytal & Hamann, 2009). Furthermore, recent research demonstrated that there are no intrinsic, anatomically defined functional networks for distinct emotion categories in the brain (Touroutoglou et al., in press), but there are domain-general networks that support basic functions across emotional, cognitive, and affective mental states (Barrett & Satpute, 2013; Lindquist & Barrett, 2012). Finally, growing neuroimaging evidence demonstrates activity in these networks in real time as individuals experience emotions (and other mental states) in the scanner (Oosterwijk et al., 2012; Satpute, Shu, Weber, Roy, & Ochsner, 2013; Wilson-Mendenhall et al., 2011). These findings are consistent with systems neuroscience accounts that emphasize that psychological function (e.g., anger, fear, disgust, autobiographical memory, visual perception) emerges from the dynamic interplay of distributed neuronal assemblies across the brain. Moreover, research emphasizing the roles of neural context (e.g., Basole, White, & Fitzpatrick, 2003; Izhikevich, Desai, Walcott, & Hoppensteadt, 2003; also see McIntosh, 2004) and neural reuse (Anderson, 2010) specifically point to the idea that mental states emerge from the dynamic interplay of neurons that flexibly code for different psychological content. Although this research does not focus on emotions per se, it bolsters support for constructionist views of emotion by pointing out that the biological machinery underlying all mental states ultimately relies on principles of constructionism.

Chun, 1997). Faculty psychology beliefs are specifically striking in the field of emotion. Descartes (1985) believed that emotions emerge from the pineal gland, a small gland in the middle of the brain. Cannon (1927) argued that the thalamus is the neural center for emotion. Later, Papez (1937/1995) and MacLean (1952) argued that emotions emerge from the limbic system, a set of phylogentically "old" subcortical and allocortical structures. In recent years, scientists have carried faculty psychology forward, particularly in the domain of neuroimaging, in which they sought evidence for emotion modules in the brain, not only for fear, (Sprengelmeyer et al., 1999; Whalen et al., 1998) but also disgust (the insula; Wicker et al., 2003). Twenty years of neuroimaging research has revealed, however, that the brain does not respect common-sense emotion categories, or any faculty psychology categories for that matter (Barrett, 2009; Barrett & Satpute, 2013; Duncan & Barrett, 2007; Gonsalves & Cohen, 2010; Lindquist & Barrett, 2012; Lindquist, Wager, Kober, Bliss, & Barrett, 2012; Pessoa, 2008; Poldrack, 2010; Uttal, 2001). In this chapter, we discuss how neuroscience data, and in particular, neuroimaging data, are beginning to yield evidence for a constructionist approach to emotion, and more broadly, to mind–brain correspondence. We begin our chapter by elaborating on specific constructionist hypotheses for mind–brain correspondence. Then we discuss how these hypotheses are supported by meta-analyses of the neuroimaging literature, by studies revealing the brain's intrinsic functional networks, and by individual neuroimaging studies that explicitly have tested constructionist hypotheses. We close with a discussion of how these findings might shape the way scientists understand how the brain creates the mind.

Constructionist Hypotheses for Mind–Brain Correspondence

Unlike a faculty psychology approach, constructionist models of the mind propose that emotions, thoughts, memories, and perceptions are mental states constructed out of more basic, domain-general psychological processes. This framework moves away from an attempt to localize mental events to specific areas or networks and instead aims to understand mental events by focusing on the interaction of large-scale distributed brain networks that support basic psychological processes (Barrett, 2009, 2011; Barrett & Satpute, 2013; Lindquist & Barrett, 2012; for a similar view, see Fox & Friston, 2012; Fuster, 2006; Mesulam, 1998). According to our constructionist view of the mind, the brain can be described as engaging in three domains of basic mental processes at any given point in time: (1) representing basic sensory information from the world; (2) representing basic interoceptive sensations from the body; and (3) making meaning of internal and external sensations by activating stored representations of prior experience. We refer to these three processes as "core affect," "exteroception," and "conceptualization," respectively. (For further discussions of core affect in this volume, see Barrett et al., Chapter 4; Russell, Chapter 8; Kleckner & Quigley, Chapter 12; and Ortony & Clore, Chapter 13. For discussions of conceptualization and acts of meaning in this volume, see Barrett et al., Chapter 4; Cunningham, Dunfield, & Stillman, Chapter 7; and Ortony & Clore, Chapter 13.)

We hypothesize that these basic processes combine in different patterns to generate specific mental content—for instance, when people experience a specific emotion, think about their plans for the day, remember an event, focus on a sensation, ruminate on someone's intentions, or attend to their bodily state. A person experiences a different mental state depending on the relative weight given to these processes in any given instance, and on which source of information is being represented in conscious awareness. As a result, executive control is another important basic psychological process that shapes mental experiences, because it helps to determine which information is prioritized and which is inhibited for representation in conscious experience. The result is that a mental state is experienced as unified (for a discussion see Barrett, Tugade, & Engel, 2004; Lindquist et al., 2012).

According to our constructionist model, whichever source of information is at the forefront of attention in a given moment is made meaningful by using the two other sources of information (Barrett, 2009). For instance, when a shift in core affect is at the forefront of attention and made meaningful using exteroceptive sensations and conceptualization, a person is said to be experiencing an emotion (e.g., fear or anger). When exteroceptive sensations are at the forefront of attention and made meaningful using core affect and conceptualization, a person is said to be experiencing a perception. Finally, when representations of prior experiences are at the forefront of attention and comprise representations of exteroceptive sensations and core affect, a person is said to be having a memory about past core affective and exteroceptive sensations, or a thought about future core affective and exteroceptive sensations. All three sources of information are present all the time; it is the relative weight given to the processes depending on contextual and situational factors that gives rise to unique subjective experiences.

Brain-Based Hypotheses of Constructionism

According to our constructionist view, we hypothesize that each of these basic "domains of processing" maps on to a distributed network (or networks) in the brain. We focus on broadscale, distributed networks, since growing evidence indicates that brain regions do not act in isolation; rather, the psychological function of a set of brain regions exists as the interaction of those regions (see McIntosh, 2000, 2004). Table 5.1 lists seven networks identified within the brain's intrinsic architecture (Yeo et al., 2011;

TABLE 5.1. Overview of Seven Intrinsic Networks

Brain regions	Task domains	Psychological description
	"Limbic network" (Yeo et al., 2011)	
Bilateral anterior temporal lobe, medial temporal lobe, subgenual anterior cingulate cortex, medial and lateral orbitofrontal cortex (although Yeo et al.'s network only covers the cortex, we also hypothesize that the basal ganglia, including the caudate, putamen, globus pallidus, and central nucleus of the amygdala will be a part of this network).	• Emotion and affect (Lindquist et al., 2012; Andrews-Hanna et al., 2010) • Autobiographical memory (Spreng & Grady, 2010)	*Core affect generation:* engaging visceromotor control of the body to create core affective feelings of pleasure or displeasure with some degree of arousal.
	"Salience network" (Seeley et al., 2007) or "ventral attention network" (Yeo et al., 2011; Corbetta & Shulman, 2002) or "cingulo-opercular network" (Vincent et al., 2008)	
Bilateral anterior midcingulate cortex (aMCC), anterior insula (AI) and midinsula, frontal operculum, and parts of the pars opercularis and temporoparietal junction	• Cognitive control (Cole & Schneider, 2007) • Stimulus-driven control of attention (Corbetta & Shulman, 2002) • Set maintenance (Dosenbach et al., 2006) • Maintaining subgoals (Fincham, Carter, van Veen, Stenger, & Anderson, 2002) • Anxiety (Seeley et al., 2007) • Representation of the body (Craig, 2009) • Pain (Lamm, Decety, & Singer, 2010)	*Body-directed attention:* using representations from the body to guide attention and behavior. This ingredient might make use changes in the homeostatic state of the body to signal salient events in the environment and regulate behavioral responses.
	"Default network" (Dosenbach et al., 2008; Vincent et al., 2008; Yeo et al., 2011)	
Medial prefrontal cortex, parts of the pars triangularis, retrosplenial area, posterior cingulate cortex/precuneus, medial temporal lobe (hippocampus, entorhinal cortex), bilateral superior temporal sulcus, parts of the anterior temporal lobe (ATL), and angular gyrus.	• Autobiographical memory (Spreng & Grady, 2010) • Prospection (Spreng & Grady, 2010) • Theory of mind (Spreng & Grady, 2010) • Moral reasoning (Greene, Sommerville, Nystrom, Darley, & Cohen, 2001) • Context-sensitive visual perception (Bar, 2004) • Spontaneous thought (Andrews-Hanna et al., 2010)	*Conceptualization:* representing prior experiences (i.e., memory or category knowledge) to make meaning of sensations from the body and the world in the moment.

Brain regions	References	Psychological description
	• Emotion (Lindquist et al., 2012; Andrews-Hanna et al., 2010) • Semantics, phonology, sentence processing (Binder et al., 2009)	
"Frontoparietal network" (Dosenbach et al., 2008; Vincent et al., 2008; Yeo et al., 2011) or "executive control network" (Seeley et al., 2007)		
Bilateral dorsolateral prefrontal cortex (dlPFC), inferior parietal lobe, inferior parietal sulcus, and aspects of the middle cingulate cortex (mCC).	• Task switching (Crone, Wendelken, Donohue, & Bunge, 2006) • Alerting to a stimulus after a cue (Fan et al., 2005) • Planning (Fincham et al., 2002) • Rule-specific processing (Sakai & Passingham, 2006) • Working memory (Sakai & Passingham, 2003)	*Executive attention:* modulating activity in other ingredients to create a unified conscious field during the construction of a mental state (e.g., selecting some conceptual content when meaning is made of sensations and inhibiting other content; selecting some sensations for conscious awareness and inhibiting others).
"Dorsal attention network" (Corbetta & Shulman, 2002; Yeo et al., 2011)		
Bilateral frontal eye fields, dorsal posterior parietal cortex, fusiform gyrus, area MT+.	• Top-down control of visuospatial attention (Corbetta et al., 2002)	*Visuospatial attention:* modulating activity in an ingredient for processing visual content in particular (e.g., selecting which visual sensations are selected for conscious awareness and inhibiting others).
"Somatomotor network" (Yeo et al., 2011)		
Precentral and postcentral gyri (sensorimotor cortex), Heschl's gyrus (primary auditory cortex), posterior insula.	• Audition (Morosan et al., 2001) • Somatovisceral sensation (Eickhoff et al., 2006)	*Exteroceptive sensory perception:* representing auditory and tactile sensations.
"Visual network" (Yeo et al., 2011)		
Occipital lobe	• Vision (Engel et al., 1994)	*Exteroceptive sensory perception:* representing visual sensations.

Note. The table lists the brain regions that are found to comprise each network across studies (column 1), the references that contribute to a functional understanding of each network (column 2), and the psychological *description* that is supported by the network as hypothesized by a constructionist framework (see further in Lindquist & Barrett, 2012).

see also Seeley et al., 2007; Vincent, Kahn, Snyder, Raichle, & Buckner, 2008; Dosenbach, Fair, Cohen, Schlaggar, & Petersen, 2008; Corbetta & Shulman, 2002; Fox & Raichle, 2007) that are likely candidates to support the basic building blocks of the mind. We hypothesize that emotions (and all mental states, for that matter) are constructed from the moment-to-moment interaction of these networks (cf. Barrett, 2009; Lindquist et al., 2012; Oosterwijk et al., 2012; for similar views, see Fuster, 2006; Goldman-Rakic, 1988; McIntosh, 2000; Mesulam, 1998; also see Bullmore & Sporns, 2009).

We hypothesize that one basic domain, core affect (experienced as feelings of pleasure or displeasure with some degree of arousal), is produced via a network of "limbic" tissue that is involved in visceromotor control, as well as representing visceromotor information within the brain. This "limbic network," which includes the basal ganglia, periaqueductal gray, central nucleus of the amygdala, and ventromedial prefrontal cortex, supports the brain's ability to generate and/or represent the somatovisceral changes that are experienced as the core affective tone that is common to every mental state (for a discussion, see Barrett, Mesquita, Ochsner, & Gross, 2007; Lindquist & Barrett, 2012; Oosterwijk et al., 2012). We hypothesize that this core affective function is further supported by the "salience network," which comprises regions involved in interoception (Critchley, Elliott, Mathias, & Dolan, 2000; Critchley, Wiens, Rotshtein, Ohman, & Dolan, 2004) and shifts of attention resulting from body-based signals (Corbetta, Kincade, & Shulman, 2002; Eckert et al., 2009), including the anterior insular cortex, anterior midcingulate cortex (aMCC), and the temporoparietal junction (TPJ). In particular, we hypothesize that the salience network performs the psychological function of directing attention and behavior using core affective information from the body. By contrast, networks that comprise modal sensory brain areas, their respective association cortices, and the thalamus support the brain's ability to represent exteroceptive sensations occurring outside the body (see the somatomotor and visual network in Table 5.1).

Key to our constructionist approach is the idea that both core affective and exteroceptive sensations are made meaningful in a given context when representations of prior experiences are brought online. We hypothesize that this conceptualization function is supported by the "default network," which comprises the medial prefrontal cortex (mPFC), medial temporal lobe, posterior cingulate cortex, ventrolateral prefrontal cortex (vlPFC; pars triangularis) and lateral temporal lobe (superior temporal gyrus extending into the anterior temporal lobe). In particular, we hypothesize that this network is involved in integrating activations in sensorimotor regions that support concept knowledge and memories (Barsalou, 2009) into rich, embodied representations that are specifically tied to the situation at hand. Midline posterior aspects of the default network (e.g., posterior cingulate, precuneus, hippocampus) may be involved particularly in the integration of visuospatial aspects of concept knowledge (Cavanna & Trimble, 2006); midline anterior aspects of the default network (e.g., mPFC) may be involved in integration of the affective, social, and self-relevant aspects of concept knowledge (Gusnard, Akbudak, Shulman, & Raichle, 2001); and lateral prefrontal and temporal regions may be involved in amodal aspects of concept representation (e.g., as in language; Smith et al., 2012).

Finally, we hypothesize that a "frontoparietal network" that comprises the dorsolateral prefrontal cortex (dlPFC), inferior parietal lobe, inferior parietal sulcus, and aspects of the middle cingulate cortex (mCC), supports executive function by modulating activity in other functional networks to help construct an instance of a mental state. The "dorsal attention network," which comprises the frontal eye fields, dorsal posterior parietal cortex, fusiform gyrus, and visual area MT+ appears to play a similar role by directing attention to visual exteroceptive sensations in particular. Together, these networks contribute to the executive control processes involved in foregrounding certain types of information in conscious awareness.

The hypothesized networks we have just outlined (or some variation on them) provide a fruitful avenue to understand how the brain creates emotions and other subjective mental states. In the next sections we discuss neuroscientific results indicating that these networks appear (1) across meta-analyses of neuroimaging studies on emotion, (2) as intrinsic functional networks in the brain, and (3) within individual functional neuroimaging studies.

Meta-Analyses of Emotion Give Evidence That Favors Constructionism, Not Faculty Psychology

One avenue for testing constructionist hypotheses about the brain basis of emotion is the meta-analysis. Meta-analytic summaries are useful tools for understanding mind–brain correspondence, because they can identify the brain regions that are consistently and specifically activated across many studies of a mental phenomenon. Therefore, meta-analyses weigh in on whether mental states are best conceived of as emergent events that map onto functional assemblies of brain networks that support more basic psychological processes, or as faculties that map onto specific locations or networks. In theory, this information might be gleaned from single neuroimaging studies, but there are several reasons why the meta-analytic whole is greater than the sum of its parts. First, meta-analyses can weed out false positives (which occur frequently in neuroimaging studies; see Wager, Lindquist, & Kaplan, 2007; Yarkoni, 2009); thus, interpretation focuses on activations that are *consistently* observed across a number of studies. Second, meta-analyses can provide a picture of whether the consistent activation observed across studies is general to a number of mental states or *specific* to a single mental state. Individual studies rarely, if ever, do so, because most studies do not have enough comparison conditions to allow a proper test of the specificity hypothesis. Thus, meta-analyses can compare activity that occurs consistently for two mental states within the same superordinate category (e.g., fear vs. anger within the domain of emotion) or even two mental states that are thought to be members of different superordinate categories (e.g., fear from the superordinate category of emotion vs. memory from the superordinate category of cognition). Finally, meta-analyses allow the comparison of data across methods. For instance, as we describe in the next section, the findings from a meta-analysis of task-related neuroimaging studies (in which brain activity correlates with a mental task) can be compared to the intrinsic brain networks that are derived from analyses of task-independent brain activity (when participants lay at rest in the scanner).

Recent meta-analyses of the neuroimaging literature on emotion (Kober et al., 2008; Lindquist et al., 2012; Vytal & Hamann, 2010) provide evidence that favors a constructionist view of the mind and calls into question the faculty psychology views that have dominated the emotion literature to date. First and foremost, meta-analyses of the emotion literature reveal that many of the brain regions that have a consistent increase in activity across studies of emotion are the same regions that have been associated with other mental states, such as memory (hippocampus, entorhinal cortex, medial prefrontal cortex), perception (primary and associative visual cortex, auditory cortex), attention (dlPFC) and language (vlPFC, anterior temporal lobe). These brain regions together form the "neural reference space for discrete emotion" (Lindquist et al., 2012, p. 126 ; for a visual depiction, see their Fig. 4), which is the set of brain regions that shows a consistent increase across all studies of emotion experience and perception.[1] These findings echo recent observations that the brain basis of "emotion" versus "cognition" is not as distinct as was once assumed (Barrett & Satpute, 2013; Barrett & Bar, 2009; Duncan & Barrett, 2007; Pessoa, 2008). Indeed, meta-analyses of different types of mental content (e.g., semantic judgments: Binder, Desai, Graves, & Conant, 2009; autobiographical memory, prospection about the future, theory of mind: Spreng, Mar, & Kim, 2009) produce a surprisingly similar neural reference space, suggesting that the same mental "ingredients" may contribute to a number of different types of mental states.

Another important finding from meta-analyses of the neuroimaging literature on emotion is that instances of an emotion category (e.g., *fear*) are not *consistently* and *specifically* associated with increased activity in a particular brain region (or a set of regions within an anatomically inspired network), consistent with a constructionist account and contrary to faculty psychology approaches. *Consistency* refers to the fact that a brain region shows increased activity for every instance of an emotion category (e.g., the amygdala shows increased activity each time a person experiences an instance of the category *fear*). *Specificity* refers to the fact that a given brain region is active for instances of one (and only one) emotion category (e.g., the amygdala does not show increased activity when a person is experiencing an instance of *anger, disgust, happiness,* or *sadness*). Rather than exhibiting consistency and specificity for a given emotion category, the same brain region(s) are involved in realizing instances of several emotion categories.[2] For instance, in our most recent meta-analysis (Lindquist et al., 2012), we found that the amygdala, which has been associated with fear (e.g., Whalen et al., 1998; also see Ohman & Mineka, 2000), had increased activity in not only the perception of fear but also every other type of emotion experience and perception (Lindquist et al., 2012). The insula, which has been associated with disgust (e.g., Wicker et al., 2003; also see Calder, 2003), had increased activity in not only the perception of disgust but also most other types of emotion experiences and perceptions. The anterior cingulate cortex (ACC), which has been associated with sadness (e.g., Murphy, Nimmo-Smith, & Lawrence, 2003), had increased activity in not only sadness but also several other types of emotion experiences and perceptions. This lack of specificity would have been difficult to observe in single neuroimaging studies alone, since no existing neuroimaging studies assess both the experience and perception of five different emotion categories.

Finally, and most important to a constructionist view, our meta-analytic findings revealed evidence of brain networks associated with domain-general, basic psychological functions in our constructionist account. For instance, the general activity that we observed in the basal ganglia, periaqueductal gray, ventromedial prefrontal cortex, amygdala, ACC, insula, and TPJ across different instances of emotion is consistent with the limbic and the salience network that, we hypothesize, support the psychological ingredient of "core affect." We also observed consistent increases in the medial prefrontal cortex, hippocampus and medial temporal lobe, lateral temporal lobe (superior temporal gyrus into the anterior temporal lobe), TPJ (angular gyrus) and vlPFC (pars triangularis) that comprise the default network linked to our basic ingredient of conceptualization. Finally, we observed consistent activation in areas of visual, auditory, and somatosensory cortex linked to exteroception (somatomotor network), and areas of dorsolateral and vlPFC linked to executive control.

Consistent with the constructionist view that these domain-general networks act as functional networks that together create instances of emotion, a very similar set of networks is observed when the meta-analytic data are analyzed in an inductive, theory-free manner assessing how brain regions functionally cluster together across studies (Kober et al., 2008). A series of cluster analyses and multidimensional scalings reveal functional clusters of voxels that are consistently coactivated across studies of emotion experience and perception, and provide convergent evidence for the basic psychological "ingredients" proposed by our constructionist account (for a visual depiction, see Kober et al., 2008, Fig. 7). For instance, we found a functional cluster of brain regions that comprised the amygdala, hypothalamus, ventral striatum, and periacqueductal gray, and contained aspects of the limbic network that we hypothesize is generating bodily states across studies of emotion experience and perception. A paralimbic group that comprises the anterior and midinsula, putamen, and posterior orbitofrontal cortex (OFC) contains aspects of the salience network thought to represent core affective states and to use them to guide behavior and attention. Groups in medial prefrontal cortex and medial posterior cortex together resemble the default network that we hypothesize is performing a conceptualization function. A visual group that comprises primary and secondary visual cortex is consistent with the visual network that supports exteroception in the visual modality. Finally, a group in the lateral prefrontal cortex resembles the frontoparietal network that we hypothesize is performing an attentional function. Such findings are not unique to meta-analyses of emotion; other meta-analyses show similar brain networks involved across diverse types of psychological tasks (Binder et al., 2009; Smith et al., 2009; Spreng et al., 2009; Lenartowicz, Kalar, Congdon, & Poldrack, 2010; Yarkoni, Poldrack, Nichols, Van Essen, & Wager, 2011).

Of course, it remains a possibility that the domain-general networks we observed in our meta-analyses reflect the limitations of task-related neuroimaging in which participants are asked to engage in a psychological task in the scanner that involves other psychological processes (executive attention, concepts, etc.). But there are two reasons why this interpretation is unlikely. First, even data from single-cell recordings, electrical stimulation, and lesion studies provide evidence consistent with the constructionist view that brain regions are part of networks that support more general psychological functions (for a discussion, see Lindquist et al., 2012). For instance, cells in rhesus monkey auditory cortex show increased activity in response to the screams of other monkeys (indicating threat), but they also show increased activity in response to the sounds of coos (affiliative sounds) and sounds indicating aggression (Kuraoka & Nakamura, 2007), suggesting that even individual cells do not respond to individual emotions. Electrical stimulation of the same site within the temporal lobe of the human brain produces not only emotions but also bodily sensations and cognitions; sometimes it produces no mental state at all (Halgren, Walter, Cherlow, & Crandall,1978; Sem-Jacobson, 1968; Valenstein, 1974; for a discussion, see Barrett et al., 2007). Although lesion findings have long been taken as evidence that a particular brain region serves a particular mental faculty, there is growing evidence that lesions in a given brain region impair a more general psychological function that itself contributes to a certain mental state. For instance, researchers assumed for years that the amygdala supports fear, because a patient (S. M.) with bilateral amygdala lesions could not perceive fear on the faces of others (e.g., Adolphs, Tranel, Damasio, & Damasio, 1994, 1995; Adolphs et al., 1999). Yet more recent findings demonstrate that amygdala lesions cause an inability to focus on the socially relevant features of a face. Patient S. M. is capable of perceiving fear when her attention is explicitly directed to the eyes of a face (Adolphs et al., 2005) or when viewing caricatures of fearful body postures (Atkinson, Heberlein, & Adolphs, 2007). These findings, along with lesion evidence linking the amygdala to impaired processing of novel stimuli (e.g., Bliss-Moreau, Toscano, Bauman, Mason, & Amaral, 2010) and blunted affect more generally (Bliss-Moreau, Bauman, & Amaral, 2011), are consistent with the idea that the amygdala is part of a more general network involved in detecting motivationally salient stimuli in the environment (cf. Cunningham & Brosch, 2012; Seeley et al., 2007; Touroutoglou, Hollenbeck, Dickerson, & Barrett, 2012).

Second, the domain-general networks hypothesized in a constructionist view and observed in meta-analyses of emotion studies are unlikely to reflect merely the limitations of task-related neuroimaging, because these networks are also observed as task-independent, intrinsic connectivity that is grounded by anatomical connections in healthy, functioning brains (Fox & Raichle, 2007; Vincent et al., 2008; Yeo et al., 2011). We now demonstrate how the science of intrinsic connectivity provides further evidence of the brain's basic networks and is consistent with a constructionist view of mind–brain correspondence.

Intrinsic Functional Connectivity Provides Evidence of the Brain's Basic Networks

The science of intrinsic functional connectivity is another emerging source of knowledge from cognitive neuroscience that can shed light on the basic psychological functions that comprise the mind and speak to a constructionist model of mind–brain correspondence. Intrinsic functional networks are broadscale networks that span the cortex and subcortex, and comprise brain regions that show a similar time course of activation, even when a person is "at rest" in the scanner and not engaging in an external psychological task. Methods for measuring this so-called "resting-state functional connectivity MRI" (rs-fcMRI) of regions distributed across the brain have been developed over the past decade but have undergone an explosion in the past 3–5 years. rs-fcMRI reflects the temporal correlations between low-frequency BOLD signal fluctuations of brain areas and as such provides a basis for understanding the large-scale intrinsic organization of brain networks (Buckner, 2010; Deco, Jirsa, & McIntosh, 2010; Fox & Raichle, 2007; Vincent et al., 2008). In this method, a region of interest is selected (i.e., a seed region) and low-frequency BOLD signal fluctuations are extracted within that region. Next, correlations are computed between the low-frequency signal fluctuations within the seed region and all voxels in the brain. The resulting map is an intrinsic connectivity network of functionally related regions that is present in the absence of task, that is, during resting-state conditions.

rs-fcMRI has been widely used by many different laboratories to generate large-scale neuroanatomical intrinsic networks (Smith et al., 2009; Yeo et al., 2011) subserving critical brain functions, such as visual, auditory, and language processes (Cordes et al., 2000), as well as motor function (Biswal, Yetkin, Haughton, & Hyde, 1995), episodic memory (Vincent et al., 2006), executive control and salience processing (Seeley et al., 2007), affective experience (Touroutoglou et al., 2012), and attention (Fox, Corbetta, Snyder, Vincent, & Raichle, 2006). The spatial topography of these networks is consistent across individuals and scans, resting conditions (Van Dijk et al., 2010), and levels of consciousness (Greicius et al., 2008), demonstrating the specificity and robustness of the intrinsic functional correlations within large-scale brain networks. See Table 5.1 for a functional description of seven networks identified by Yeo and colleagues (2011), derived from the largest sample of participants (1,000) in any study of intrinsic functional connectivity to date, that likely reflect the most stable estimates of intrinsic networks. Importantly, relevant to the psychology of individual differences, the magnitude of intrinsic connectivity within a given network predicts differences in behavior related to the function of that network. For example, participants with stronger intrinsic connectivity in the ventral subnetwork of the salience network (comprising ventral anterior insula (AI) and pregenual ACC, lateral OFC, thalamus, and basal ganglia) reported feeling more aroused during the viewing of negative evocative images than did individuals with weaker connectivity (Touroutoglou et al., 2012). Taken together, these findings suggest that patterns of rs-fcMRI likely represent the intrinsic functional architecture of the brain (Fox & Raichle, 2007) or regions of the brain that are commonly used together to produce a distributed function (Barrett & Satpute, 2013; Deco et al., 2010). In so doing, the intrinsic functional connectivity is particularly useful for examining psychological construction hypotheses about the mind.

In the context of rs-fcMRI, an important question, however, is how do we infer the functional interpretation of a given intrinsic connectivity network, considering that its defined independent of tasks and other experimental stimuli? Traditionally this is done by examining the tasks that either engage individual regions within a network of interest or the network as a whole during task-related fMRI studies (e.g., Barrett & Satpute, 2013). Because the intrinsic networks are independent of experimental context, they can also be compared with task-related functional connectivity networks activated during tasks across different studies. Additionally, more recently Laird et al. (2011) provided a means to assess the link between intrinsic connectivity networks and behaviors in a more direct way. By quantifying the relationship between intrinsic connectivity networks and behavioral domains coded in the BrainMap database—the largest fMRI and positron emission tomography (PET) database of task-related activation studies to date—Laird et al. were able to map intrinsic connectivity networks to specific groups of functional ontology, including reasoning, language, social cognition, attention, and emotion. For example, the connectivity within the salience network was found to be strongly related to the behavioral domain of emotion and interoception. Other projects that map distributed brain activity to functional categories are the Neurosynth database (Yarkoni et al., 2011) and the Cognitive Atlas Project (Poldrack et al., 2011). These projects will no doubt prove useful as research in this area continues.

More recently, our laboratory used rs-fcMRI to gain insight into the nature of emotion, contributing to the long-standing scientific debate between psychological construction and basic emotion approaches to emotion. Basic emotion accounts hypothesize that happiness, sadness, anger, disgust, and fear arise from innate, culturally universal neural modules in the brain (Panksepp, 1998), which leads to the prediction that there are intrinsic connectivity networks specific to each distinct emotion category. In contrast, our psychological constructionist hypothesis that emotions (like all other complex mental states) are constructed from more basic core systems that correspond to functional networks in the brain predicts that domain-general intrinsic connectivity networks, such as salience detection, language, or executive control networks, would subserve all different emotions. Intrinsic connections are influenced by the anatomy and activation history of a given network (Buckner, 2010; Deco & Corbetta, 2011; Fox & Raichle, 2007), and some intrinsic connections are also homologous in other primate species (Hayes & Northoff, 2011; Vincent et al., 2007; Kojima et al., 2009; Rilling et al., 2007). The science of intrinsic connectivity therefore has the potential to enhance our understanding of a fundamental question: Do inherited emotion networks really exist in the brain?

To answer the question whether anger, disgust, fear, sadness and happiness are each associated with an anatomically given intrinsic brain network, Touroutoglou, Lindquist, Dickerson, and Barrett (2014) used meta-analytic peaks of these emotion categories (Vytal & Hamann, 2010) as rs-fcMRI seeds and generated a whole-brain rs-fcMRI map for each seed. Each seed, then, was a location of voxels that was consistently activated at levels greater than chance during that emotion. Using a spatial similarity index between every pair of rs-fcMRI maps, the study showed very low similarity between maps within each emotion category (i.e., the maps anchored by all anger seeds were not found to be part of the same spatially similar map), indicating that there was no intrinsic connectivity network specific to each emotion. Consistent with a psychological construction approach, intrinsic networks identified in other studies (Shirer, Ryali, Rykhlevskaia, Menon, & Greicius, 2012) instead accounted for variance in the derived rs-fcMRI maps, indicating that domain-general intrinsic networks are important for all emotions. Furthermore, the rs-fcMRI maps anchored in seeds that are commonly considered to be specifically related to distinct emotions (i.e., amygdala for fear, basal ganglia for happiness, insula for disgust, OFC for anger) were found to converge in regions of the ventral portion of the salience network (Touroutoglou et al., 2012). These results support the psychological construction hypothesis that emotions are not subserved by heritable anatomical networks; instead the voxels that are consistently active during a given emotion are part of a variety of large-scale intrinsic networks that are important, but not limited, to emotions. In addition, and consistent with a constructionist account, Laird and colleagues (2011) found that the intrinsic connectivity between AI and ACC, two major nodes of the salience network (Seeley et al., 2007), is linked to a variety of general psychological processes, such as language, executive function, and affective and interoceptive processes, thus calling into question the traditional distinction between emotion and cognition. Similarly, both Seeley et al. and Touroutoglou et al. (2012) found that parts of the AI and ACC overlapped with both the executive function and salience network.

These analyses provide an example of how the science of intrinsic connectivity has the potential to identify the functional architecture of the brain that corresponds to the basic core operations of the mind. However, intrinsic connectivity MRI cannot determine how basic psychological processes combine in a given instance to produce the variety of mental states that characterize human life. To this end, task-related fMRI studies, carefully designed to manipulate the basic ingredients of the mind, are better suited to examine relationships between the interaction of neural networks supporting these ingredients and the emergence of mental states. In the next section, we report on two recent neuroimaging studies that examined how large-scale distributed networks in the brain combine when people construct different mental states in the fMRI scanner.

Functional Neuroimaging as an Explicit Tool to Test Constructionist Hypotheses

Based on the research reviewed thus far, it is possible to formulate and test specific hypotheses about the relative involvement of domain-general networks when mental states are constructed in real time. Although individual behavioral studies have explicitly tested a constructionist approach by manipulating the ingredients hypothesized to produce emotions and testing the behavioral outcome (e.g., Lindquist & Barrett, 2008), individual neuroimaging studies are perhaps even better suited for testing constructionist hypotheses for several reasons. First of all, mental states are emergent phenomena. This means that when a subjective experience has manifested itself in consciousness, it cannot be subjectively reduced to its underlying parts (cf. Barrett, 2011, 2012; Coan & Gonzalez, Chapter 9, this volume). That is, people cannot report on the underlying processes that shape their mental state, just as they cannot report on the underlying processes that create a conscious percept (e.g., the visual features of contrast, color, edges, etc., that contribute to the perception of a red vase). Furthermore, the processes that combine to form emergent states typically operate unconsciously and automatically (Barrett, 2006; Wilson-Mendenhall, Barrett, Simmons, & Barsalou, 2011). Since functional neuroimaging is not restricted by conscious or volitional report, this technique is particularly suitable to study how these processes combine in real time. Second, individual neuroimaging studies can explicitly test hypotheses that have been formulated (based in part on the data reviewed earlier) about the regions and networks involved in conceptualization, core affect, and other basic processes that create mental states (see Barrett, 2009; Lindquist et al., 2012; Kober et al., 2008; Touroutoglou et al., 2014).

In a recent experiment (Oosterwijk et al., 2012), we tested a constructionist model of the mind using fMRI by asking participants to generate three categories of mental states (emotions, body feelings, or thoughts) while examining similarities and differences in patterns of network activity. We used a scenario immersion method developed in our laboratory (Wilson-Mendenhall et al., 2011) to immerse participants in sensory-rich, vivid scenarios of unpleasant situations. Critically, before each scenario was presented, participants were asked to experience the situation as a body feeling (e.g., increased heartbeat, touch of an object against the skin, smells, unpleasantness), as an emotion (e.g., fear, anger, guilt) or as a thought (e.g., plan, reflection). Each trial started with a cue, followed by the scenario (the "immersion" phase), followed by an "experience" phase in which participants could further construct and elaborate on the body feeling, emotion, or thought (see also Addis, Wong, & Schacter, 2007). Taking a network-based model of the mind as our starting assumption, we hypothesized that body feelings, emotions, and thoughts are constructed from the interaction of large-scale distributed networks (Fox & Friston, 2012; Fuster, 2006; Goldman-Rakic, 1988; McIntosh, 2000; Mesulam, 1998; also see Bullmore & Sporns, 2009). In our study we focused specifically on the previously discussed intrinsic networks identified by Yeo and colleagues (2011). For a functional description of each of these networks see Table 5.1.

First, we found experimental support for the hypothesis that body feelings, emotions, and thoughts, although subjectively distinct, each involve participation of the same distributed brain networks. Most notably, a conjunction analysis that reveals overlapping patterns of brain activation across different tasks demonstrated common engagement of the salience network. We hypothesize that this network is involved in directing attention and behavior using core affective information from the body (Barrett & Satpute, 2013; Lindquist & Barrett, 2012; see also Seeley et al., 2007). The finding that the salience network was commonly active during the experience of a variety of mental states involving negative information is consistent with the role for this network in stress (Hermans et al., 2011), the experience of unpleasant affect (Hayes & Northoff, 2011), and tasks requiring the allocation of attention to evocative or behaviorally relevant stimuli (Corbetta, Patel, & Shulman, 2008; Corbetta & Shulman, 2002; Nelson et al., 2010; Seeley et al., 2007). Moreover, several regions within the salience network, specifically the AI and the aMCC have been associated in the literature with interoception (Critchley et al., 2003, 2004) and subjective experiences more generally (Craig, 2002, 2009). The finding in our study that the salience network was engaged across all mental states suggests that representations of body sensations play a role when people experience body states or emotions *and* when they objectively think about a negative situation. This is consistent with several suggestions in the literature that cues from the body are a fundamental component of all mental life, including perception (Barrett & Bar, 2009; Cabanac, 2002), judgment (Clore & Huntsinger, 2007), tasks involving effort (Critchley et al., 2003), and consciousness more generally (Barrett & Bliss-Moreau, 2009; Craig, 2009; Damasio, 2000; Russell, 2003; Wundt, 1897).

In addition to the salience network, our results also suggest a common role for several other networks during the construction of subjective mental experiences, most notably the default network and the frontoparietal network. The finding that the default network is commonly active during the experience of mental states is consistent with the hypothesis that this network is involved in the process of conceptualization—in which representations of prior experiences are brought to bear to construct representations of the past, the future, or the present moment (for discussion, see Oosterwijk et al., 2012; Lindquist et al., 2012). The common engagement of the frontoparietal network across body states, emotions, and thoughts suggests that all these mental states involve executive control (Seeley et al., 2007; Dosenbach et al., 2008; Vincent et al., 2008). This network may modulate activity in other functional networks to help construct an instance of a mental state. Finally, although our analyses focused on the cortical surface of the brain, we also examined common activation in subcortical areas during emotions, body states, and thoughts. We found common activations within subcortical regions such as the pallidum, putamen, and cerebellum across bodily feelings, emotions, and thoughts. These regions may be part of the limbic network (Yeo et al., 2011) that we hypothesize generates and/

or represents somatovisceral changes that are experienced as the core affective tone that is common to every mental state (also see Oosterwijk et al., 2012).

Although the same distributed brain networks were implicated in body feelings, emotions, and thoughts, we also found evidence that different network profiles were associated with each mental state category. First, as we predicted, the salience network was engaged significantly more during body feelings than during thoughts in the "immersion" phase. This pattern of activation was present across multiple regions of the salience network, including the dorsal AI, the vlPFC (pars opercularis), and the aMCC. Emotions also demonstrated increased activation in the salience network compared to thoughts, including in the left vlPFC (pars opercularis), the right aMCC and the right TPJ. Additionally, subcortical regions hypothesized to be involved in core affective generation, such as the thalamus, pallidum, and caudate, were more engaged during body feelings than during thoughts. Together, these results suggest that core affect, as supported by the salience network, plays a relatively more important role in emotions and body feelings than in thoughts.

During the "experience" phase of the experiment we found that the salience network was equally engaged during all mental states. The default network, however, showed stronger engagement during thoughts than during emotions and bodily states. This result is consistent with previous findings that show the default network's robust involvement in spontaneous thought (Andrews-Hanna, Reidler, Huang, & Buckner, 2010), predicting the future (Spreng & Grady, 2010; Addis et al., 2007) and mental state attribution or theory of mind (Spreng & Grady, 2010; Mitchell, Banaji, & Macrae, 2005). Together, these findings suggest that conceptualization plays a larger role in mental states in which the representation of prior experiences is used to guide plans, associations, and reflections about a situation.

Together, these findings demonstrate that body feelings, emotions, and thoughts, although subjectively distinct, cannot be localized to distinct regions (or even networks) within the human brain. Instead, body feelings, emotions, and thoughts each involve a relatively different combination of the same set of distributed brain networks. Recent evidence demonstrates that even instances of the same superordinate category (e.g., emotion) involve relatively different combinations of the same set of distributed brain networks. In a neuroimaging experiment, Wilson-Mendenhall and colleagues (2011) examined which distributed brain circuits engaged when people conceptualized different situations as instances of a discrete emotion (e.g., anger or fear). Based on a constructionist view on the mind, Wilson-Mendenhall and colleagues hypothesized that this distributed circuitry would not be specific to anger or fear, but it would support basic psychological processes such as conceptualization, core affect, and executive control. This study is particularly important because it illustrates how the situation in which an emotion is experienced shapes the way the brain is engaged during that emotion.

Using the scenario immersion method, participants were cued to conceptualize situations describing physical danger (e.g., being lost in the woods) or social evaluation (e.g., being unprepared during a meeting at work) as an instance of an emotion (i.e., fear or anger) or as an instance of a non-emotional mental state (i.e., planning or observing). The results showed that the same emotion was associated with very different brain states across different situations. For example, the brain state representing fear in physical danger situations shared only 47% of the active voxels with the brain state representing fear in social evaluation situations. Furthermore, consistent with the network account proposed in this chapter, both anger and fear demonstrated engagement of regions in the salience network (e.g., posterior insula, midcingulate) in situations where physical harm was anticipated. Social evaluation situations, in contrast, demonstrated activation of the ventromedial prefrontal cortex, which is part of the default network and specifically associated with self-related, evaluative processes (see Amodio & Frith, 2006; Mitchell, Heatherton, & Macrae, 2002; Northoff et al., 2006). Together, these data highlight a basic premise of our constructionists account: A mental state cannot be understood separately from the context in which it is experienced.

To our knowledge, these two neuroimaging studies are the first to test explicitly a constructionist functional architecture of the mind by assessing both similarities and relative differences in distributed brain patterns during the experience of different mental states. The findings are consistent with the reviewed evidence from meta-analyses and analyses of intrinsic connectivity that mind–brain correspondence may be best understood by examining relative differences in the engagement of distributed networks that support basic psychological processes. Moreover, these findings directly call into question the faculty psychology view that different classes of mental states differ categorically at the level of brain organization.

Conclusion

In this chapter, we have presented a constructionist functional framework of mind–brain correspondence, with the basic premise that mental states emerge from the combination of more basic core systems, or psychological "ingredients" that map to the functional states of broadscale brain networks. Despite the fact that the first two decades of neuroimaging used a faculty psychological viewpoint as their guiding framework, the research we reviewed here demonstrates clearly that faculty psychology should be discarded. Instead, the meta-analyses, intrinsic network studies, and individual neuroimaging studies reviewed in this chapter point to a constructionist model of the mind in which not only emotions but also other mental states emerge from the combination of broadscale brain networks that support basic psychological functions.

It is important to note that our constructionist approach does not explain subjectively different mental states out of existence (see also Barrett, 2012), nor does it argue that all subjective experiences look the same in the brain. Take fear as an example. An individual brain state for one instance of fear in a given context is distinguishable from the brain state of, say, anger, concentration, or curiosity. The point is that the similarities and differences between these brain states are best understood not by focusing on the unique subjective experience that they represent at a given moment in time, but by focusing instead on the interaction between broad, domain-general processes that cause the subjective experience to emerge. Specificity in subjective experience (e.g., a specific feeling of fear when preparing for a job talk vs. a specific feeling of fear when bleeding from a deep finger cut) occurs because each instance of an emotion is tailor made to a given context by a unique situated conceptualization supported by a pattern of brain activity that engages general psychological processes (Barrett, 2012; Wilson-Mendenhall et al., 2011). Specificity is not caused by the activation of a module or dedicated network for fear, however. Although there might be some brain pattern that characterizes all instances of fear (which further research must still discern), we argue that this pattern is a combination of intrinsic networks and not an anatomically prescribed, inheritable network. Thus, our constructionist view accounts for the heterogeneity of mental states by assuming that each mental state is represented by a unique brain state that involves networks supporting general psychological processes such as language, conceptualization, interoception, exteroception, and executive control. Furthermore, we argue that the context in which the mental state occurs may be more informative in guiding the interpretation of the engaged psychological processes than the categorical label of the subjective mental state itself.

The evidence presented in this chapter has important scientific implications. First of all, the presented findings challenge the assumption that subjective experiences (i.e., how we experience our mental states as qualitatively different) reveal in a one-to-one fashion how the brain works (i.e., that different mental states must be associated with functionally specific brain activation). These data instead contribute to a new understanding of how mental states, including emotions, are realized by the brain. Rather than states that differ in kind from one another, mental states might instead be considered complex "recipes" that reflect the relative weighting of a number of domain-general "ingredients" of the mind.

Second, the data presented in this chapter challenge traditional views on a strict separation of different mental faculties, such as perception, cognition, and emotion (or seeing, feeling, and thinking; see also Barrett, 2009; Barrett & Bar, 2008; Pessoa, 2008; Duncan & Barrett, 2007). In the literature, scientists still refer to cognitive, social, and affective neuroscience as different domains of inquiry. Nevertheless, the networks discussed in this chapter are important not only in emotion but also other domains, such as decisions (Kringelbach & Rolls, 2004), attention (Corbetta & Shulman, 2002; Lenartowicz et al., 2010), memory (Spreng et al., 2009), semantic processing (Binder et al., 2009), mentalizing (Spreng et al., 2009), and consciousness more generally (also see Craig, 2009; Nelson et al., 2010).

In future research, it will be important to model the interaction of the networks hypothesized to support basic psychological processes when examining a person's mental state. For instance, already there is some evidence that is consistent with the idea that brain regions supporting conceptualization (i.e., the default network) combine with brain regions supporting core affect (e.g., aspects of the limbic and salience networks) during the experience of emotion. One recent study found that a correlation between the default network and networks supporting core effect (e.g., thalamus, basal ganglia, insula) significantly predicted participants' ratings of valence as they watched evocative movies in the scanner (Viinikainen et al., 2012). Another recent study found a similar interactive pattern between the default network and aspects of the salience network (e.g., insula, aMCC) when participants mentalized about both the self and others (Lombardo et al., 2009).

We hope that with more incremental research, experimental support for a constructionist view of the mind will contribute to the identification of a set of neural "common denominators" that link a range of findings across psychological domains that appear very different on the surface (e.g., emotions vs. thoughts vs. perceptions). It is often argued that psychology is not useful in the age of the brain; similarly, it is sometimes argued that neuroimaging cannot offer much beyond being a form of new phrenology. In our constructionist framework, psychology and neuroimaging can be used to inform and constrain one another as we attempt to understand how the brain constructs the mind.

ACKNOWLEDGMENTS

The writing of this chapter was supported by a Marie Curie International Outgoing Fellowship (No. 275214) awarded by the European Union's Seventh Framework Programme to Suzanne Oosterwijk, a National Institute on Aging grant (No. AG030311) that funds Alexandra Touroutoglou, and a Harvard University Mind/Brain/Behavior Postdoctoral Fellowship to Kristen A. Lindquist.

NOTES

1. The neural reference spaces reported in both Vytal and Hamann (2010) and Kober et al. (2008) were surprisingly similar to those reported by Lindquist et al. (2012), especially given that the Lindquist et al. meta-analysis included a slightly different sample of studies than the others, and that Lindquist et al. (2012) and Kober et al. (2008) used a different method than Vytal and Hamann (2010).

2. Vytal and Hamann (2010) claim to have found evidence of specific patterns for discrete emotions, but upon further inspection, their meta-analytic findings look quite similar to our own. They report clusters with peaks that have relatively greater activity for one emotion than all others, but these peaks are part of clusters that overlap between different emotions. That is, they fail to show the kind of specificity that would be necessary to claim evidence for the anatomical basis of discrete emotions in the brain. It is beyond the scope of this chapter to discuss the methodological differences between the Vytal and Hamann meta-analysis and our own, but for a discussion, see Lindquist et al. (2012).

REFERENCES

Addis, D. R., Wong, A. T., & Schacter, D. L. (2007). Remembering the past and imagining the future: Common and distinct neural substrates during event construction and elaboration. *Neuropsychologia, 45*, 1363–1377.

Adolphs, R., Gosselin, F., Buchanan, T. W., Tranel, D., Schyns, P., & Damasio, A. R. (2005). A mechanism for impaired fear recognition after amygdala damage. *Nature, 433*, 68–72.

Adolphs, R., Tranel, D., Damasio, H., & Damasio, A. (1994). Impaired recognition of emotion in facial expressions following bilateral damage to the human amygdala. *Nature, 372*, 669–672.

Adolphs, R., Tranel, D., Damasio, H., & Damasio, A. R. (1995). Fear and the human amygdala. *Journal of Neuroscience, 15*, 5879–5879.

Adolphs, R., Tranel, D., Hamann, S., Young, A. W., Calder, A. J., Phelps, E. A., et al. (1999). Recognition of facial emotion in nine individuals with bilateral amygdala damage. *Neuropsychologia, 37*, 1111–1117.

Amodio, D. M., & Frith, C. D. (2006). Meeting of minds: The medial frontal cortex and social cognition. *Nature Reviews Neuroscience, 7*, 268–277.

Anderson, M. L. (2010). Neural reuse: A fundamental organizational principle of the brain. *Behavioral and Brain Sciences, 33*, 245–313.

Andrews-Hanna, J. R., Reidler, J. S., Huang, C., & Buckner, R. L. (2010). Evidence for the default network's role in spontaneous cognition. *Journal of Neurophysiology, 104*, 322–322.

Atkinson, A. P., Heberlein, A. S., & Adolphs, R. (2007). Spared ability to recognise fear from static and moving whole-body cues following bilateral amygdala damage. *Neuropsychologia, 45*, 2772–2782.

Bar, M. (2004). Visual objects in context. *Nature Reviews Neuroscience. 5*, 617–629.

Barrett, L. F. (2006). Solving the emotion paradox: Categorization and the experi ence of emotion. *Personality and Social Psychology Review, 10,* 20–46.

Barrett, L. F. (2009). The future of psychology: Connecting mind to brain. *Perspectives on Psychological Science, 4,* 326–339.

Barrett, L. F. (2011). Bridging token identity theory and supervenience theory through psychological construction. *Psychological Inquiry, 22,* 115–127.

Barrett, L. F. (2012). Emotions are real. *Emotion, 12,* 413–429.

Barrett, L. F., & Bar, M. (2009). See it with feeling: Affective predictions in the human brain. *Philosophical Transactions of the Royal Society of London B: Biological Sciences, 364,* 1325–1334.

Barrett L. F., & Bliss-Moreau, E. (2009). Affect as a psychological primitive. *Advances in Experimental Social Psychology, 41,* 167–218.

Barrett, L. F., Lindquist, K., Bliss-Moreau, E., Duncan, S., Gendron, M., Mize, J., et al. (2007). Of mice and men: Natural kinds of emotion in the mammalian brain? *Perspectives on Psychological Science, 2,* 297–312.

Barrett, L. F., Mesquita, B., Ochsner, K. N., & Gross, J. J. (2007). The experience of emotion. *Annual Review of Psychology, 58,* 373–403.

Barrett, L. F., & Satpute, A. B. (2013). Large-scale brain networks in affective and social neuroscience: Towards and integrative functional architecture of the brain. *Current Opinion in Neurobiology, 23*(3), 361–372.

Barrett, L. F., Tugade, M. M., & Engle, R. W. (2004). Individual differences in working memory capacity and dual-process theories of the mind. *Psychological Bulletin, 130,* 553–573.

Barsalou, L. W. (2009). Simulation, situated conceptualization, and prediction. *Philosophical Transactions of the Royal Society of London B: Biological Sciences, 364,* 1281–1289.

Basole, A., White, L. E., & Fitzpatrick, D. (2003). Mapping multiple features in the population response of visual cortex. *Nature, 423,* 986–990.

Binder, J. R., Desai, R. H., Graves, W. W., & Conant, L. L. (2009). Where is the semantic system?: A critical review and meta-analysis of 120 functional neuroimaging studies. *Cerebral Cortex, 19,* 2767–2796.

Biswal, B., Yetkin, F. Z., Haughton, V. M., & Hyde, J. S. (1995). Functional connectivity in the motor cortex of resting human brain using echo-planar MRI. *Magnetic Resonance in Medicine, 34,* 537–541.

Bliss-Moreau, E., Bauman, M. D., & Amaral, D. G. (2011). Neonatal amygdala lesions result in globally blunted affect in adult rhesus macaques. *Behavioral Neuroscience, 125,* 848–858.

Bliss-Moreau, E., Toscano, J. E., Bauman, M. D., Mason, W. A., & Amaral, D. G. (2010). Neonatal amygdala or hippocampus lesions influence responsiveness to objects. *Developmental Psychobiology, 52,* 487–503.

Buckner, R. L. (2010). The role of the hippocampus in prediction and imagination. *Annual Review of Psychology, 61,* 27–48.

Bullmore, E., & Sporns, O. (2009). Complex brain networks: Graph theoretical analysis of structural and functional systems. *Nature Review Neuroscience, 10,* 186–198.

Cabanac, M. (2002). What is emotion? *Behavioural Processes, 60,* 69–83.

Cacioppo, J. T., Berntson, C. G., Larsen, J. T., Poehlmann, K. M., & Ito, T. A.

(2000). The psychophysiology of emotion. In M. Lewis & J. M. H. Jones (Eds.), *Handbook of emotions* (2nd ed., pp. 173–191). New York: Guilford Press.

Calder, A. J. (2003). Disgust discussed. *Annals of Neurology, 53*, 427–428.

Cannon, W. (1927). The James–Lange theory of emotions: A critical examination and alternative theory. *American Journal of Psychology, 39*, 106–124.

Cavanna, A. E., & Trimble, M. (2006). The precuneus: A review of its functional anatomy and behavioural correlates. *Brain, 129*, 564–583.

Clore, G. L., & Huntsinger, J. R. (2007). How emotions inform judgment and regulate thought. *Trends in Cognitive Sciences, 11*, 393–399.

Cole, M. W., & Schneider, W. (2007). The cognitive control network: Integrated cortical regions with dissociable functions. *NeuroImage, 37*, 343–360.

Corbetta, M., Kincade, J. M., & Shulman, G. L. (2002). Neural systems for visual orienting and their relationships to spatial working memory. *Journal of Cognitive Neuroscience, 14*, 508–523.

Corbetta, M., Patel, G., & Shulman, G. L. (2008). The reorienting system of the human brain: From environment to theory of mind. *Neuron, 58*, 306–324.

Corbetta, M., & Shulman, G. L. (2002). Control of goal-directed and stimulus-driven attention in the brain. *Nature Reviews Neuroscience, 3*, 215–229.

Cordes, D., Haughton, V. M., Arfanakis, K., Wendt, G. J., Turski, P. A., Moritz, C. H., et al. (2000). Mapping functionally related regions of brain with functional connectivity MR imaging. *American Journal of Neuroradiology, 21*, 1636–1644.

Craig, A. D. (2002). How do you feel?: Interoception: The sense of the physiological condition of the body. *Nature Reviews Neuroscience, 3*, 655–666.

Craig, A. D. (2009). How do you feel—now?: The anterior insula and human awareness. *Nature Reviews Neuroscience, 10*, 59–70.

Critchley, H. D., Elliott, R., Mathias, C. J., & Dolan, R. J. (2000). Neural activity relating to generation and representation of galvanic skin conductance responses: A functional magnetic resonance imaging study. *Journal of Neuroscience, 20*, 3033–3040.

Critchley, H. D., Mathias, C. J., Josephs, O., O'Doherty, J., Zanini, S., Dewar, B. K., et al. (2003). Human cingulate cortex and autonomic control: Converging neuroimaging and clinical evidence. *Brain, 126*, 2139–2152.

Critchley, H. D., Wiens, S., Rotshtein, P., Ohman, A., & Dolan, R. J. (2004). Neural systems supporting interoceptive awareness. *Nature Neuroscience, 7*, 189–195.

Crone, E. A., Wendelken, C., Donohue, S. E., & Bunge, S. A. (2006). Neural evidence for dissociable components of task-switching. *Cerebral Cortex, 16*, 475–486.

Cunningham, W. A., & Brosch, T. (2012). Motivational salience: Amygdala tuning from traits, needs, values, and goals. *Current Directions in Psychological Science, 21*, 54–59.

Damasio, A. (2000). *The feeling of what happens: Body and emotion in the making of consciousness*. New York: Harcourt.

Deco, G., & Corbetta, M. (2011). The dynamical balance of the brain at rest. *Neuroscientist, 17*, 107–123.

Deco, G., Jirsa, V. K., & McIntosh, A. R. (2010). Emerging concepts for the dynamical organization of resting-state activity in the brain. *Nature Reviews Neuroscience, 12,* 43–56.

Descartes, R. (1985). *The philosophical writings of Descartes* (Vol. 2). Cambridge, UK: Cambridge University Press.

Dosenbach, N. U. F., Fair, D. A., Cohen, A. L., Schlaggar, B. L., & Petersen, S. E. (2008). A dual-network architecture of top-down control. *Trends in Cognitive Sciences, 12,* 99–105.

Duncan, S., & Barrett, L. F. (2007). Affect is a form of cognition: A neurobiological analysis. *Cognition and Emotion, 21,* 1184–1211.

Eckert, M. A., Menon, V., Walczak, A., Ahlstrom, J., Denslow, S., Horwitz, A., et al. (2009). At the heart of the ventral attention system: The right anterior insula. *Human Brain Mapping, 30,* 2530–2541.

Eickhoff, S. B., Lotze, M., Wietek, B., Amunts, K., Enck, P., & Zilles, K. (2006). Segregation of visceral and somatosensory afferents: An fMRI and cytoarchitectonic mapping study. *NeuroImage, 31,* 1004–1014.

Engel, S. A., Rumelhart, D. E., Lee, A. T., Glover, G. H., Chichilnisky, E.-J., & Shadlen, M. N. (1994). fMRI of human visual cortex. *Nature, 369,* 525.

Fan, J., Bruce, T., McCandliss, D., Fossella, J. A., Flombaum, J. I., & Posner, M. I. (2005). The activation of attentional networks. *NeuroImage, 26,* 471–479.

Fincham, J. M., Carter, C. S., van Veen, V., Stenger, A., & Anderson, J. R. (2002). Neural mechanisms of planning: A computational analysis using event-related fMRI. *Proceedings of the National Academy of Sciences. 99,* 3346–3351.

Fox, M. D., Corbetta, M., Snyder, A. Z., Vincent, J. L., & Raichle, M. E. (2006). Spontaneous neuronal activity distinguishes human dorsal and ventral attention systems. *Proceedings of the National Academy of Sciences, 103,* 10046–10051.

Fox, M. D., & Friston, K. J., (2012). Distributed processing; distributed functions? *NeuroImage, 61,* 407–421.

Fox, M. D., & Raichle, M. E. (2007). Spontaneous fluctuations in brain activity observed with functional magnetic resonance imaging. *Nature Reviews Neuroscience, 8,* 700–711.

Fuster, J. M. (2006). The cognit: A network model of cortical representation. *International Journal of Psychophysiology, 60,* 125–132.

Gendron, M., Lindquist, K., Barsalou, L., & Barrett, L. F. (2012). Emotion words shape emotion percepts. *Emotion, 12,* 314–325.

Goldman-Rakic, P. S. (1988). Topography of cognition: Parallel distributed networks in primate association cortex. *Annual Review of Neuroscience, 11,* 137–156.

Gonsalves, B. D., & Cohen, N. J. (2010). Brain imaging, cognitive processes, and brain networks. *Perspectives on Psychological Science, 5,* 744–752.

Greene, J. D., Sommerville, R. B., Nystrom, L. E., Darley, J. M., & Cohen, J. D. (2001). An fMRI investigation of emotional engagement inmoral judgment. *Science, 293,* 2105–2108.

Greicius, M. D., Kiviniemi, V., Tervonen, O., Vainionpaa, V., Alahuhta, S., Reiss, A. L., et al. (2008). Persistent default-mode network connectivity during light sedation. *Human Brain Mapping, 29,* 839–847.

Gusnard, D. A., Akbudak, E., Shulman, G. L., & Raichle, M. E. (2001). Medial prefrontal cortex and self-referential mental activity: Relation to a default mode of brain function. *Proceedings of the National Academy of Sciences, 98*, 4259–4264.

Halgren, E., Walter, R. D., Cherlow, D. G., & Crandall, P. H. (1978). Mental phenomena evoked by electrical stimulation of the human hippocampal formation and amygdala. *Brain, 101*, 83–117.

Hayes, D. J., & Northoff, G. (2011). Identifying a network of brain regions involved in aversion-related processing: A cross-species translational investigation. *Frontiers in Integrative Neuroscience, 5*, 1–21.

Hermans, E. J., van Marle, H. J., Ossewaarde, L., Henckens, M. J. A., Qin, S., van Kesteren, M. T., et al. (2011). Stress-related noradrenergic activity prompts large-scale neural network reconfiguration. *Science, 334*, 1151–1153.

Izhikevich, E. M., Desai, N. S., Walcott, E. C., & Hoppensteadt, F. C. (2003). Bursts as a unit of neural information: Selective communication via resonance. *Trends in Neurosciences, 26*, 161–167.

Kanwisher, N., McDermott, J. F., & Chun, M. M. (1997). The fusiform face area: A module in human extrastriate cortex specialized for face perception. *Journal of Neuroscience, 17*, 4302–4311.

Kober, H., Barrett, L. F., Joseph, J., Bliss-Moreau, E., Lindquist, K. A., & Wager, T. D. (2008). Functional grouping and cortical-subcortical interactions in emotion: A meta-analysis of neuroimaging studies. *NeuroImage, 42*, 998–1031.

Kojima, T., Onoe, H., Hikosaka, K., Tsutsui, K., Tsukada, H., & Watanabe, M. (2009). Default mode of brain activity demonstrated by positron emission tomography imaging in awake monkeys: Higher rest-related than working memory-related activity in medial cortical areas. *Journal of Neuroscience, 29*, 14463–14471.

Krabbendam, L., Arts, B., van Os, J., & Aleman, A. (2005). Cognitive functioning in patients with schizophrenia and bipolar disorder: A quantitative review. *Schizophrenia Research, 80*, 137–149.

Kreibig, S. D. (2010). Autonomic nervous system activity in emotion: A review. *Biological Psychology, 84*, 394–421.

Kringelbach, M. L., & Rolls, E. T. (2004). The functional neuroanatomy of the human orbitofrontal cortex: Evidence from neuroimaging and neuropsychology. *Process in Neurobiology, 72*, 341–372.

Kuraoka, K., & Nakamura, K. (2007). Responses of single neurons in monkey amygdala to facial and vocal emotions. *Journal of Neurophysiology, 97*, 1379–1387.

Laird, A. R., Fox, P. M., Eickhoff, M., Turner, J. A., Ray, K. L., McKay, D. R., et al. (2011). Behavioral interpretations of intrinsic connectivity networks. *Journal of Cognitive Neuroscience, 23*, 4022–4037.

Lamm, C., Decety, J., & Singer, T. (2010). Meta-analytic evidence for common and distinct neural networks associated with directly experienced pain and empathy for pain. *NeuroImage, 54*, 2492–2502.

LeDoux, J. (2012). Rethinking the emotional brain. *Neuron, 73*, 653–676.

Lenartowicz, A., Kalar, D. J., Congdon, E., & Poldrack, R. A. (2010). Towards an ontology of cognitive control. *Topics in Cognitive Science, 2*, 678–692.

Lindquist, K. A., & Barrett, L. F. (2008). Constructing emotion: The experience of fear as a conceptual act. *Psychological Science, 19*(9), 898–903.

Lindquist, K. A., & Barrett, L. F. (2012). A functional architecture of the human brain: Insights from emotion. *Trends in Cognitive Sciences, 16,* 533–554.

Lindquist, K., Barrett, L. F., Bliss-Moreau, E., & Russell, J. A. (2006). Language and the perception of emotion. *Emotion, 6,* 125–138.

Lindquist, K. A., & Gendron, M. (2013). What's in a word?: Language constructs emotion perception. *Emotion Review, 5,* 66–71.

Lindquist, K. A., Gendron, M., Oosterwijk, S., & Barrett, L. F. (2013). Do people essentialize emotions?: Individual differences in emotion essentialism and emotional experience. *Emotion, 13,* 629–644.

Lindquist, K. A., Wager, T. D., Kober, H., Bliss-Moreau, E. & Barrett, L. F. (2012). The brain basis of emotion: A meta-analytic review. *Behavavioral Brain Sciences, 35,* 121–143.

Lombardo, M. V., Chakrabarti, B., Bullmore, E. T., Wheelwright, S. J., Sadek, S. A., Suckling, J., et al. (2009). Shared neural circuits for mentalizing about the self and others. *Journal of Cognitive Neuroscience, 22,* 1623–1635.

MacLean, P. D. (1952) Some psychiatric implications of physiological studies on frontotemporal portion of limbic system (visceral brain). *Electroencephalography and Clinical Neurophysiology, 4,* 407–418.

Mauss, I. B., & Robinson, M. D. (2009). Measures of emotion: A review. *Cognition and Emotion, 23,* 209–237.

McIntosh, A. R. (2000). Towards a network theory of cognition. *Neural Networks, 13,* 861–870.

McIntosh, A. R. (2004) Contexts and catalysts: A resolution of the location and integration of function in the brain. *Neuroinformatics, 2,* 175–181.

Mesulam, M. M. (1998). From sensation to cognition. *Brain, 121,* 1013–1052.

Mitchell, J., Banaji, M. R., & Macrae, C. N. (2005). The link between social cognition and self-referential thought in the medial prefrontal cortex. *Journal of Cognitive Neuroscience, 17,* 1306–1315.

Mitchell, J. P., Heatherton, T. F., & Macrae, C. N. (2002). Distinct neural systems subserve person and object knowledge. *Proceedings of the National Academy of Sciences, 99,* 15238–15243.

Morosan, P., Rademacher, J., Schleicher, A., Amunts, K., Schormann, T., & Zilles, K. (2001). Human primary auditory cortex: Cytoarchitectonic subdivisions and mapping into a spatial reference system. *NeuroImage, 13,* 684–701.

Murphy, F. C., Nimmo-Smith, I., & Lawrence, A. D. (2003). Functional neuroanatomy of emotions: A meta-analysis. *Cognitive, Affective, and Behavioral Neuroscience, 3,* 207–233.

Nelson, S. M., Dosenbach, N. U., Cohen, A. L., Wheeler, M. E., Schlaggar, B. L., & Petersen, S. E. (2010). Role of the anterior insula in task-level control and focal attention. *Brain Structure and Function, 214,* 669–680.

Northoff, G., Heinzel, A., de Greck, M., Bermpohl, F., Dobrowolny, H., & Panksepp, J. (2006). Self-referential processing in our brain—a meta-analysis of imaging studies on the self. *NeuroImage, 31,* 440–457.

Ohman, A., & Mineka, S. (2001). Fears, phobias, and preparedness: Toward an evolved module of fear and fear learning. *Psychological Review 108,* 483–522.

Oosterwijk, S., & Barrett, L. F. (2014). Embodiment in the construction of emotion experience and emotion understanding. In L. Shapiro (Ed.), *Routledge handbook of embodied cognition* (pp. 250–260). New York: Routledge.

Oosterwijk, S., Lindquist, K. A., Anderson, E., Dautoff, R., Moriguchi, Y., & Barrett, L. F. (2012). Emotions, body feelings, and thoughts share distributed neural networks. *NeuroImage, 62,* 2110–2128.

Oosterwijk, S., Topper, M., Rotteveel, M., & Fischer, A. H. (2010). When the mind forms fear: Embodied fear knowledge potentiates bodily reactions to fearful stimuli. *Social Psychological and Personality Science, 1,* 65–72.

Panksepp, J. (1998). *Affective neuroscience: The foundations of human and animal emotions.* New York: Oxford University Press.

Papez, J. W. (1995). A proposed mechanism of emotion. *Journal of Neuropsychiatry and Clinical Neurosciences, 7,* 103–112. (Original work published 1937)

Pessoa, L. (2008). On the relationship between emotion and cognition. *Nature Reviews Neuroscience, 9,* 148–158.

Poldrack, R. A. (2010). Mapping mental function to brain structure: How can cognitive neuroimaging succeed? *Perspectives on Psychological Science, 5,* 753–761.

Poldrack, R. A., Kittur, A., Kalar, D., Miller, E., Seppa, C., Gil, Y., et al. (2011). The Cognitive Atlas: Towards a knowledge foundation for cognitive neuroscience. *Frontiers in Neuroinformatics, 5,* 1–11.

Rilling, J. K., Barks, S. K., Parr, L. A., Preuss, T. M., Faber, T. L., Pagnoni, G., et al. (2007). A comparison of resting-state brain activity in humans and chimpanzees. *Proceedings of the National Academy of Sciences, 104,* 17146–17151.

Rugg, M. D., Otten, L. J., & Henson, R. N. (2002). The neural basis of episodic memory: Evidence from functional neuroimaging. *Philosophical Transactions of the Royal Society of London B: Biological Sciences, 357,* 1097–1110.

Russell, J. A. (2003). Core affect and the psychological construction of emotion. *Psychological Review, 110,* 145–172.

Russell, J. A., & Widen, S. C. (2002). A label superiority effect in children's categorization of facial expressions. *Social Development, 11,* 30–52.

Sakai, K., & Passingham, R. E. (2003). Prefrontal interactions reflect future task operations. *Nature Neuroscience. 6,* 75–81.

Sakai, K., & Passingham, R. E. (2006). Prefrontal set activity predicts rule-specific neural processing during subsequent cognitive performance. *Journal of Neuroscience. 26,* 1211–1218.

Satpute, A. B., Shu, J., Weber, J., Roy, M., & Ochsner, K. N. (2013). The functional neural architecture of self-reports of affective experience. *Biological Psychiatry, 73,* 631–638.

Saxe, R., & Kanwisher, N. (2003). People thinking about thinking people: The role of the temporo-parietal junction in "theory of mind." *NeuroImage, 19,* 1835–1842.

Seeley, W. W., Menon, V., Schatzberg, A. F., Keller, J., Glover, G. H., Kenna, H., et al. (2007). Dissociable intrinsic connectivity networks for salience processing and executive control. *Journal of Neuroscience, 27,* 2349–2349.

Sem-Jacobson, C. W. (1968). *Depth-electroencephalographic stimulation of the human brain and behavior.* Springfield, IL: Thomas.

Shirer, W. R., Ryali, S., Rykhlevskaia, E., Menon, V. & Greicius, M. D. (2012).

Decoding subject-driven cognitive states with whole-brain connectivity patterns. *Cerebral Cortex, 22,* 158–168.

Smith, S. M., Miller, K. A., Moeller, S., Xu, J., Auerbach, E. J., Woolrich, M. W., et al. (2009). Correspondence of the brain's functional architecture during activation and rest. *Proceedings of the National Academy of Sciences, 106,* 13040–13045.

Smith, S. M., Miller, K. L., Moeller, S., Xu, J., Auerbach, E. J., Woolrich, M. W., et al. (2012). Temporally-independent functional modes of spontaneous brain activity. *Proceedings of the National Academy of Sciences, 109,* 3131–3136.

Spreng, R. N., & Grady, C. L. (2010). Patterns of brain activity supporting autobiographical memory, prospection, and theory of mind, and their relationship to the default mode network. *Journal of Cognitive Neuroscience, 22,* 1112–1123.

Spreng, R. N., Mar, R. A., & Kim, A. S. N. (2009). The common neural basis of autobiographical memory, prospection, navigation, theory of mind, and the default mode: A quantitative meta-analysis. *Journal of Cognitive Neuroscience, 21,* 489–510.

Sprengelmeyer, R., Young, A. W., Schroeder, U., Grossenbacher, P. G., Federlein, J., Buttner, T., et al. (1999). Knowing no fear. *Proceedings of the Royal Society of London, B: Biological Sciences, 266,* 2451–2456.

Touroutoglou, A., Hollenbeck, M., Dickerson, B. C., & Barrett, L. F. (2012). Dissociable large-scale networks anchored in the anterior insula subserve affective experience and attention/executive function. *NeuroImage, 60,* 1947–1958.

Touroutoglou, A., Lindquist, K. A., Dickerson, B. C., & Barrett, L. F. (2014). *Intrinsic connectivity in the human brain does not reveal networks for "basic" emotions.* Manuscript under review.

Uttal, W. R. (2001). *The new phrenology: The limits of localizing cognitive processes in the brain.* Cambridge, MA: MIT Press.

Valenstein, E. S. (1974). *Brain control: A critical examination of brain stimulation and psychosurgery.* New York: Wiley.

Van Dijk, K. R., Hedden, T., Venkataraman, A., Evans, K. C., Lazar, S. W., & Buckner, R. L. (2010). Intrinsic functional connectivity as a tool for human connectomics: Theory, properties, and optimization. *Journal of Neurophysiology, 103,* 297–321.

Viinikainen, M., Glerean, E., Jääskeläinen, I. P., Kettunen, J., Sams, M., & Nummenmaa, L. (2012). Nonlinear neural representation of emotional feelings elicited by dynamic naturalistic stimulation. *Open Journal of Neuroscience, 2,* 1–7.

Vincent, J. L., Kahn, I., Snyder, A. Z., Raichle, M. E., & Buckner, R. L. (2008). Evidence for a frontoparietal control system revealed by intrinsic functional connectivity. *Journal of Neurophysiology, 100,* 3328–3342.

Vincent, J. L., Patel, G. H., Fox, M. D., Snyder, A. Z., Baker, J. T., Van Essen, D. C., et al. (2007). Intrinsic functional architecture in the anaesthetized monkey brain, *Nature, 447,* 83–86.

Vincent, J. L., Snyder, A. Z., Fox, M. D., Shannon, B. J., Andrews, J. R., Raichle, M. E., et al. (2006). Coherent spontaneous activity identifies a hippocampal-parietal memory network. *Journal of Neurophysiology, 96,* 3517–3531.

Vytal, K., & Hamann, S. (2010). Neuroimaging support for discrete neural correlates of basic emotions: A voxel-based meta-analysis. *Journal of Cognitive Neuroscience, 22,* 2864–2885.

Wager, T. D., Lindquist, M., & Kaplan, L. (2007). Meta-analysis of functional neuroimaging data: Current and future directions. *Social Cognitive and Affective Neuroscience, 2,* 150–158.

Whalen, P. J., Rauch, S. L., Etcoff, N. L., McInerney, S. C., Lee, M. B., & Jenike, M. A. (1998). Masked presentations of emotional facial expressions modulate amygdala activity without explicit knowledge. *Journal of Neuroscience, 18,* 411.

Wicker, B., Keysers, C., Plailly, J., Royet, J. P., Gallese, V., & Rizzolatti, G. (2003). Both of us disgusted in My insula: The common neural basis of seeing and feeling disgust. *Neuron, 40,* 655–664.

Widen, S. C., & Russell, J. A. (2008). Children acquire emotion categories gradually. *Cognitive Development, 23,* 291–312.

Wikan, U. (1990). *Managing turbulent hearts: A Balinese formula for living.* Chicago: University of Chicago Press.

Wilson-Mendenhall, C. D., Barrett, L. F., Simmons, W. K., & Barsalou, L. (2011). Grounding emotion in situated conceptualization. *Neuropsychologia, 49,* 1105–1127.

Wundt, W. (1998). *Outlines of psychology* (C. H. Judd, Trans.). Bristol, UK: Thoemmes Press. (Original work published 1897)

Yarkoni, T. (2009). Big correlations in little studies: Inflated fMRI correlations reflect low statistical power: Commentary on Vul et al. (2009). *Perspectives on Psychological Science, 4,* 294–298.

Yarkoni, T., Poldrack, R. A., Nichols, T. E., Van Essen, D. C., & Wager, T. D. (2011). Large-scale automated synthesis of human functional neuroimaging data. *Nature Methods, 8,* 665–670.

Yeo, B. T., Krienen, F. M., Sepulcre, J., Sabuncu, M. R., Lashkari, D., Hollinshead, M., et al. (2011). The organization of the human cerebral cortex estimated by functional connectivity. *Journal of Neurophysiology, 106,* 1125–1165.

CHAPTER 6

Emotions as Semantic Pointers

Constructive Neural Mechanisms

PAUL THAGARD
TOBIAS SCHRÖDER

I n this chapter we propose a new neurocomputational theory of emotions that is broadly consistent with the psychological construction view (Russell, 2009; Gross & Barrett, 2011), and that enhances it by laying out an empirically plausible set of underlying neural mechanisms. The new theory specifies a system of neural structures and processes that potentially explain a wide range of phenomena, supporting the claim that emotions are not *just* physiological perceptions or *just* cognitive appraisals, or *just* social constructions. We claim that emotions can be understood as *semantic pointers*, a special kind of neural process hypothesized by Chris Eliasmith (2013) to provide explanations of many kinds of cognitive phenomena, from low-level perceptual abilities all the way up to high-level reasoning. Our aim is to show that Eliasmith's semantic pointer architecture for neural processing has the potential to account for a wide range of phenomena that have been used to support physiological, appraisal, and social constructionist accounts of emotion. We also discuss how it can be used to provide neural mechanisms for emotions as psychological constructions. Specifically, we show how the semantic pointer hypothesis helps to specify how emotional states sometimes result from application of linguistic categories to representations of biological states, a core proposition of the psychological constructionist approach (e.g., Barrett, 2006; Lindquist

1. *If emotions are psychological events constructed from more basic ingredients, then what are the key ingredients from which emotions are constructed? Are they specific to emotion or are they general ingredients of the mind? Which, if any, are specific to humans?*

Emotions are constructed from neural processes that involve semantic pointers, binding, and control, operating on multiple brain areas to integrate physiological perception and cognitive appraisal. The basic neural processes are common to all psychological operations, but the integration operations are specific to emotion. We speculate that the social emotions are restricted to humans because they require a high-level, linguistic representation, but that other emotions are common in other mammals.

2. *What brings these ingredients together in the construction of an emotion? Which combinations are emotions and which are not (and how do we know)?*

The various physiological and cognitive ingredients in the construction of an emotion are brought together by general neural mechanisms of binding and compression. Because of substantial evidence that both physiological perception and cognitive appraisal are relevant to emotions, it is reasonable to conjecture that emotions differ from other psychological processes in that they combine neural representations of *both* physiology and appraisal. In addition, for a few species, such as humans, self-representations can be bound into the overall emotion.

3. *How important is variability (across instances within an emotion category, and in the categories that exist across cultures)? Is this variance epiphenomenal or a thing to be explained? To the extent that it makes sense, it would be desirable to address issues such as universality and evolution.*

Because of the large degree of variation in the beliefs, attitudes, and goals across different cultures, we should expect some degree of variability in emotion categories, as suggested by the linguistic evidence. This variance can be explained by the role that societies play in inculcating the cognitive–affective elements, especially attitudes and goals that are crucial for cognitive appraisal. Despite this variance, there is also the need to explain apparent commonalities deriving from biological universals in brain anatomy. Little evidence addresses the question of how much variability there is within particular emotion categories in particular societies.

4. *What consitutes strong evidence to support a psychological construction to emotion? Point to or summarize empirical evidence that supports your*

(continued)

model or outline what a key experiment would look like. What would falsify your model?

Strong evidence to support a SPA interpretation of the psychological construction of emotions would come from its ability to simulate the results of a wide variety of experiments concerning emotions (e.g., Schachter & Singer, 1962). While building POEM, we will compile a list of key experiments that will provide targets for simulation. We will strive to show that POEM behaves similarly with experiment participants at both quantitative and qualitative levels. Contrary to Karl Popper's philosophy of science, direct falsification of theory by evidence is not an important part of scientific practice (Thagard 1988, 2010a). Rather, theories compete to explain the evidence, and a theory is rejected when it is surpassed by another with greater explanatory power. The POEM model of emotions would be falsified if other researchers produced a model that explains more experimental results.

& Gendron, 2013; Russell, 2009; Barrett, Wilson-Mendenhall, & Barsalou, Chapter 4, this volume).

We begin with a quick review of the semantic pointer architecture (SPA), introducing its key ideas: neural representation, semantic pointers, binding, and control. These ideas have natural applications to emotions in ways that provide a unified account of their physiological, cognitive, and social aspects. Since SPA was designed as a framework for creating biologically plausible models of cognitive processes in general, its application to a theory of emotion is a contribution to "unifying the mind" (e.g., Barrett, 2009; Duncan & Barrett, 2007): The basic mechanisms governing emotion generation are no different from the mechanisms governing other aspects of human cognition. We sketch a neurocomputational model designed to show how SPA can be used to describe the neural mechanisms that generate emotional responses. We have not yet implemented this model computationally, but doing so should be straightforward using the NENGO (Neural Engineering Object) simulation software that Eliasmith and his colleagues have developed (*www.nengo.ca*). Once implemented in a running computer program, the model provides a way of testing the semantic pointer theory of emotions through simulations of neural and psychological experiments. This methodology is common in cognitive science: A theory is a proposal about structures and processes; a model is a computational specification of these structures and processes; and a program is a running instantiation whose performance can be directly compared with results of experiments (Thagard, 2012a, Chapter 1). We also discuss the relevance of the new theory and model of emotions for issues about psychological construction and variability.

Semantic Pointer Architecture

A cognitive architecture is a general proposal about the structures and processes that produce intelligent thought (Anderson, 1983, 2007; Newell, 1990; Thagard, 2012a). It hypothesizes the kinds of mental representations and computational procedures that constitute a mechanism for explaining a broad range of kinds of thinking, including perception, attention, memory, problem solving, reasoning, learning, decision making, motor control, language, emotion, and consciousness. The most influential cognitive architectures that have been developed are either rule-based, using if–then rules and procedures that operate on them to explain thinking, or connectionist, using artificial neural networks (Thagard, 2005). Eliasmith (2013; Eliasmith et al., 2012) has proposed a different kind of cognitive architecture that is tied much more closely to the operations of the brain but capable of many of the kinds of high-level reasoning that make rule-based explanations plausible. We now present a highly simplified and informal account of the key ideas in Eliasmith's SPA; please consult his book for a much more mathematically rigorous and neurologically detailed description.

SPA adopts a view of neural representation and processing that is much more biologically accurate than the connectionist (parallel distributed processing [PDP]) view of "brain-style" computing that has been highly influential in psychology since Rumelhart and McClelland (1986). SPA is based on the Neural Engineering Framework (NEF) developed by Eliasmith and Anderson (2003). Like connectionist views, SPA assumes that mental representations are distributed processes involving the firing of populations of neurons connected by excitatory and inhibitory links. But SPA differs from connectionist models in at least the following ways:

1. Neurons spike, so that firing patterns and not just activations (firing rates) contribute to representational capacity.
2. Neurons are heterogeneous, with different temporal patterns resulting from different neurotransmitters.
3. Neural networks are large, involving thousands or millions of neurons rather than the few dozens typical of connectionist models.
4. Neural networks are organized into functional subnetworks that may be mapped onto anatomical brain areas.

In summary, a mental representation according to SPA is a process involving the interaction of many thousands or millions of spiking neurons with varying dynamics.

Connectionism has been criticized as inadequate for explaining high-level cognitive phenomena such as reasoning and language use (e.g., Fodor

& Pylyshyn, 1988; Jackendoff, 2002). SPA meets this challenge by showing how neural processes can support the kinds of problem solving and linguistic understanding usually attributed to symbolic rules. The key bridge from biologically realistic neurons to cognitive symbols is the idea of a semantic pointer. We think that this idea is the best available candidate for solving the symbol–subsymbol problem, one of the most important in cognitive science, which concerns the relations between high-level symbols such as words and concepts and low-level distributed representations in neural networks. In the context of a psychological constructionist perspective on emotion, the semantic pointer idea is important, because it provides a detailed neural-level explanation of the conceptualization process thought to be central to the generation of specific emotions out of more blurry unspecific affective reactions (e.g., Barrett, 2006; Russell, 2009). More generally, we argue that understanding emotions as semantic pointers allows one to integrate biological, cognitive, and sociocultural constraints on emotional experience into a single framework.

Semantic pointers are neural processes that (1) provide *shallow meanings* through symbol-like relations to the world and other representations; (2) expand to provide *deeper meanings* with relations to perceptual, motor, and emotional information; (3) support complex syntactic operations; and (4) help to control the flow of information through a cognitive system to accomplish its goals. Thus, semantic pointers have semantic, syntactic, and pragmatic functions, just like the symbols in a rule-based system, but with a highly distributed, probabilistic operation. Below we show how emotions construed as semantic pointers have analogous semantic, syntactic, and pragmatic functions, while they are grounded in highly distributed representations of physiological states.

A semantic pointer comprises spiking patterns in a large population of neurons that provide a kind of compressed representation analogous to JPEG picture files or iTunes audio files. The term *pointer* comes from computer science, in which it refers to a kind of data structure that gets its value from a machine address to which it points. A semantic pointer is a neural process that compresses information in other neural processes to which it points and into which it can be expanded when needed. For example, the concept *car* can be understood as a semantic pointer that comprises spiking neurons that compress, point to, and expand into other populations of spiking neurons that contain a wide range of information in various modalities (e.g., verbal and visual).

Eliasmith (2013) shows how symbolic pointers provide a mechanistic elucidation of the physical symbol system hypothesis of Barsalou (1999), according to which symbols are higher-level representations of combined perceptual components extracted from sensorimotor experience. For example, full understanding of the concept *car* requires both semantic knowledge about related concepts, such as *machine* and *transportation*, and sensory and motor experiences, such as *color, sound,* and *movement,* which are semantic primitives cannot be defined linguistically (Johnson-Laird, 1983; Johnson-Laird & Quinn, 1976). The semantic pointer *car* includes a compressed mental model of that motor experience.

The SPA proposes a hierarchical organization of the cognitive system, in which higher-level symbol-like representations point to neural representations at lower levels more tied to sensorimotor experience. The semantic pointer theory of emotion is therefore compatible with the psychological constructionist approach, which also makes use of Barsalou's (1999) grounded cognition ideas (see Barrett, Wilson-Mendenhall, & Barsalou, Chapter 4, this volume). To some degree, SPA is also compatible with views of embodied affect, cognition, and conceptual metaphor (e.g., Crawford, 2009; Lakoff & Johnson, 2003; Niedenthal, Winkielman, Mondillon, Vermeulen, 2009), while avoiding some of the more radical views according to which the mind does not employ representation or computation (Thagard, 2010b). SPA holds that meaning is often grounded in bodily experience; but semantic pointers are sufficiently decoupled from lower-level deep meanings (which they only represent in compressed form) that they can operate with symbol-like properties.

Why is this important for emotion? As we describe in more detail below, such a hierarchical organization of the cognitive system allows for an integrative understanding of all the different facets of emotion, from the physiological components to socially constructed symbols. For example, the experience of *love* and *affection* that is ultimately grounded in the sensory experience of physical warmth that infants of all cultures feel in the arms of their mothers (Lakoff & Johnson, 2003) is also subject to considerable cultural symbolic construction and variation conveyed in the arts and literature over the centuries (Belli, Harré, & Íñiguez, 2010). Accordingly, Osgood and colleagues have shown that the semantic relations between culturally constructed symbols of language are constrained by the basic dimensions of emotion, evaluation–valence, potency–control, and activity–arousal (e.g., Fontaine, Scherer, Roesch, & Ellsworth, 2007; Heise, 2010; Osgood, May, & Miron, 1975; Osgood, Suci, & Tannenbaum, 1957; Rogers, Schröder, & von Scheve, 2014).

A major problem for connectionist cognitive architectures has been how to represent syntactically complex information such as relations (he loves her, which is different from she loves him) and rules (if she loves him, he is happy). The problem arose because early connectionist models were unable to represent such syntactic complexity, but various solutions have since been proposed. SPA adopts the solution proposed by Plate (2003) called *holographic reduced representations,* which shows how vectors can be bound together in ways capable of maintaining syntactic complexity. A *vector* is a mathematical structure that represents two or more quantities; a vector with *n* quantities is called *n-dimensional.* If *man, loves,* and *woman* are all represented by vectors, then *loves(man, woman)* can be represented by another vector that binds the original ones by various mathematical operations including convolution, which interweaves structures (for an introduction to holographic reduced representations and convolution, see Eliasmith & Thagard, 2001; Thagard & Stewart, 2011).

Representing symbolic concepts as vectors may sound technical, but it gains plausibility from a long tradition in the psychology of emotion. Specific emotions such as love or happiness have been represented as two-dimensional vectors in circumplex models of emotion (*pleasure* and *arousal*; Larsen & Diener, 1992; Russell, 1980) or as three-dimensional vectors in Osgood's affective space (*evaluation-valence, potency-control*, and *activity-arousal*; Osgood et al., 1957, 1975). More recently, Fontaine et al. (2007) mapped the Osgood space onto 144 single features of emotions (e.g., specific appraisals, physiological reactions, or muscle movements).

There is an analogy between these kinds of vectors and the SPA: Symbol-like three-dimensional representations of emotions (shallow meanings) can be viewed as compressed models of the underlying 144-dimensional representations of sensorimotor and appraisal correlates (deep meanings of emotion). Affect control theory (Heise, 2007), a mathematically formalized theory of social interaction and culturally shared emotional experience, represents social perception as vectors with nine or more dimensions, with the elements corresponding to Osgood's dimensions of affect (evaluation–valence, potency–control, and activity–arousal), as well as grammatical structure (agent, action, and recipient). The resulting mathematical model allows one to compute dynamic emotional states that occur during social interaction through combinations of vectors (Rogers et al., 2014).

Eliasmith has shown that these kinds of vector structures and operations can be accomplished by populations of spiking neurons. Hence, SPA networks are capable of all the syntactic complexity needed for many kinds of reasoning and language processing. Eliasmith et al. (2012) have used SPA to create a large-scale model of the functioning brain, whose 2.5 million artificial neurons that can perform tasks such as symbol recognition and reproduction, memory, and question answering. SPA can also be used to solve the famous Tower of Hanoi problem that has long been a benchmark of rule-based inference (Stewart & Eliasmith, 2011), to explain behavioral priming (Schröder & Thagard, 2013), and to model the interplay between intentional and impulsive action (Schröder, Stewart, & Thagard, 2014). In this chapter, we argue that SPA as a general cognitive architecture is also a candidate for understanding the neural mechanisms underlying the psychological construction of emotion, in line with the view that "affect is [also] a form of cognition" (Duncan & Barrett, 2007).

Ignoring the mathematics, we can say that a neural architecture can represent relations such as *loves(man, woman)* by producing a nested binding such as the following:

$$loves(man, woman) = BIND[BIND(loves, action),$$
$$BIND(man, agent), BIND(woman, recipient)]$$

That is, the relation *loves* is represented by a binding of three separate bindings of elements: the binding of loves as the action, the binding of the man as the agent, and the binding of the woman as the recipient. Each of the elements can be represented by a vector and can therefore be translated (using Eliasmith's method) into a pattern of activity in a population of neurons. The bindings themselves can be understood both as mathematical operations on the vectors and as neural processes that transform neural processes into more complex ones. Semantic pointers are important for this process, because they provide the high-level representation of concepts such as *love*.

In addition to semantics and syntax, a cognitive architecture must support *pragmatics*, the ability of a system to accomplish its goals by making decisions in particular contexts. Eliasmith (2013) describes the need for a system to manage the control of selection of which representations to employ, manipulation of current representations given current context, determination of what next course of action to pursue, and so on. SPA has various mechanisms for managing these kinds of control, correspondingto operations in the basal ganglia and other brain regions. Let us now see how SPA ideas about semantics, syntax, and pragmatics apply to emotions.

Emotions as Semantic Pointers

SPA is sufficiently broad that it can be used to provide neural mechanisms for any of the currently popular approaches to understanding emotions. The view that emotions are primarily perceptions of physiological states, espoused by Damasio (1994), Prinz (2004), and others, can be specified biologically by means of neural populations that respond to physiological variables such as heart rate, skin response, and hormone levels. This view is compatible with the claim that there are innate mechanisms for basic emotions such as happiness, fear, and anger (Ekman, 2003). Alternatively, the view that emotions are cognitive appraisals of the relevance of a situation to an agent's goals, espoused by Oatley (1992), Scherer, Schorr, and Johnstone (2001), and many others, can be specified biologically by means of neural populations that compute the goal relevance of a situation. The radical view of Harré (1989) and others that emotions are mere social constructions created by an individual's culture can be specified biologically by means of neural populations that respond to social communication. As mentioned before, the psychological constructionist view that emotional states emerge from a conceptualization process, in which linguistic categories are applied to make sense of inner representations of physiological states, can be specified through the compression and binding mechanisms of semantic pointers that connect deep, sensorimotor meanings with higher-level symbolic meanings.

Much more interesting is that SPA can be used to build a model that synthesizes physiological, appraisal, social, and psychological constructionist accounts of emotions, in line with the EMOCON account of emotional consciousness (Thagard & Aubie, 2008). In this account, physiological and appraisal theories of emotions are not alternatives, but can be unified by a neural model that shows how parallel processing in the brain can integrate both perception of physiological states and evaluation of the relevance of the current situation to the goals of the agent. Figure 6.1 shows some of the

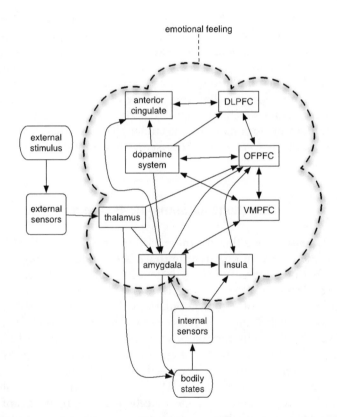

FIGURE 6.1. The EMOCON model of Thagard and Aubie (2008), which contains details and partial computational modeling. DLPFC, dorsolateral prefrontal cortex; OFPFC, orbitofrontal prefrontal cortex; VMPFC, ventromedial prefrontal cortex. The dashed line is intended to indicate that emotional consciousness emerges from activity in the whole system.

relevant brain areas; the amygdala and insula are most relevant to physiological perception, and the frontal areas are most relevant to cognitive appraisal.

EMOCON was too large and complex to be implemented computationally by the tools available when it was conceived in 2006, but SPA is supported by software that should make possible an enhanced model using new theoretical ideas such as semantic pointers. EMOCON is consistent with the view that there are social and cultural aspects of emotion, because appraisal is subject to social coordination through the interpersonal (often nonverbal) communication of affect (Manstead & Fischer, 2001; Parkinson & Simons, 2009). Furthermore, goals and beliefs that are relevant for the appraisal process are often culturally acquired. Let us examine how the general structure of EMOCON can be worked out in much more biological detail via the theoretical resources of SPA. Later we will sketch a new model, POEM, which includes the brain areas in Figure 6.1 plus additional ones identified as relevant to emotions by brain scanning experiments.

We need to spell out how the four main ideas of SPA—neural representation, semantic pointers, binding, and control—apply to emotions. To begin, we need to distinguish between *emotion tokens*, such as particular instances of happiness or fear, and *emotion types*, which are classes of emotional responses. For now, we are only concerned with emotion tokens, and we address the question of types below. We propose to identify instances of emotions with SPA-style neural representations that comprise spiking behavior in neural populations. This proposal assumes the contentious philosophical mind–brain identity theory, defended elsewhere (Thagard, 2010a).

It is crucial to note that a neural population need not be confined to a specific brain region, because there are extensive synaptic connections between neurons in different regions. We need to avoid the naive assumption that particular emotions reside in particular brain regions, for example, fear in the amygdala and happiness in the nucleus accumbens, because brain scans indicate that emotions are correlated with much more distributed brain activity (Lindquist, Wager, Kober, Bliss-Moreau, & Barrett, 2012). The EMOCON model in Figure 6.1 assumes that emotions are widely distributed across multiple brain areas, and a SPA account of emotions can similarly look at emotions as activity in populations of neurons not confined to a single region.

Now we get to the crucial contention of this chapter, that an emotion token is a semantic pointer. We need to show how emotions can possess shallow meanings through compressed representations that can be expanded into deeper representations, employing binding operations that support syntactic combinations and manage the control of the flow of information in a system capable of generating actions that accomplish goals.

What is going on in your brain when you feel an emotion such as being happy upon hearing that a paper has been accepted by a good journal? This occurrence of emotion comprises firing of interconnected neurons in a way that amounts to a compressed but expandable representation of the current situation. The compressed representation functions to produce verbal reports of the experience "I'm happy," as well as to link the incident to other occurrences of feeling happy. Moreover, this neural representation "points" to others that provide an expanded meaning, for it is based on *both* physiological perception and cognitive appraisal, in accord with the EMOCON model.

Binding operations of the sort that can be performed by convolution in SPA are crucial for the construction of the emotional response of being happy that your paper was accepted. In logical notation, we could represent the situation by this formula:

$$accept\ (journal,\ paper) \tag{P1}$$

Linguistically, the relevant proposition is actually more complicated, since it should also contain the information that the paper is yours, but we ignore the self until the next section. The neural processing of P1 requires a binding, something like

$$BIND[BIND(accept,\ action),\ BIND(journal,\ agent), \tag{P2}$$
$$BIND(paper,\ recipient)]$$

In SPA, this complex binding can be understood as mathematical operations on vectors that are performed by neural populations, producing a new vector that is also represented by a firing pattern in neurons. P2 is the proposition (vector, neural firing pattern) that results from accomplishing the bindings that unite the representations of *acceptance, journal*, and *paper* into a proposition representing an event.

Now we have to find a neural representation for the proposition that you are happy that the paper was accepted. Verbally, this is just something like

$$happy[accept(journal,\ paper)] \tag{P3}$$

But if happiness results from a combination of physiological perception and cognitive appraisal, then the binding is more complicated, something like

$$BIND\ (P2,\ physiology,\ appraisal) \tag{P4}$$

In P4, P2 is the firing pattern already produced by binding together *happy, journal,* and *paper,* and the other two ingredients need to be explained.

We can easily identify the physiological and appraisal aspects of the emotional response as firing patterns in neural populations. For physiology, the relevant process is detection by brain areas, including the amygdala and insula, of bodily changes such as heart rate, breathing rate, skin temperature, configuration of facial muscles, and hormone levels. For appraisal, the relevant process is a complex calculation of goal relevance that can perform constraint satisfaction, as in the EACO (Emotional Appraisal as Coherence) computational model in Thagard and Aubie (2008). The journal acceptance presumably satisfies a variety of personal goals, such as increasing your reputation and salary. Binding these three ingredients together—the situation representation P2, the representation of physiological changes, and the representation of appraisals—produces the semantic pointer that constitutes the neural representation of your emotional reaction. We are not using *bind* as a vague metaphor here, because SPA contains the required algorithms for using neural populations to perform such bindings. Some emotions may also involve a self-representation, discussed below.

To summarize, Figure 6.2 provides a rough picture of how an emotion token can be a semantic pointer through operations of compression and convolution. The groups of circles depict populations of thousands or millions of neurons. The semantic pointer is the result of binding of several key representations: the situation that the emotional response is about, the results of physiological perceptions, and the results of cognitive appraisal. Each of these three representations could be further decompressed into other representations. Usually, the situation representation is a pointer to a binding of an action with an agent. The physiological representation would be a compression of many kinds of changes in bodily states, such as breathing. The cognitive appraisal representation would be a compression of a complex parallel satisfaction process that determines the goal–significance of the situation. Hence the occurrence of emotions depends on a cascade of semantic pointers pointing to others, and emotion representations have rich meanings deriving from their relations to other representations and ultimately to perceptual inputs. Emotion representations in the form of semantic pointers are also able to contribute to complex syntactic structures via binding, making possible highly structured propositions such as "If you're happy and you know it, clap your hands."

Semantic pointers, as in Figure 6.2, can represent complex emotions, such as being happy about a journal acceptance, and can help to control the flow of information in your brain and form intentions, hence leading to action. The representation that you are happy will affect your behavior in various ways, including how you react to other people. Internally,

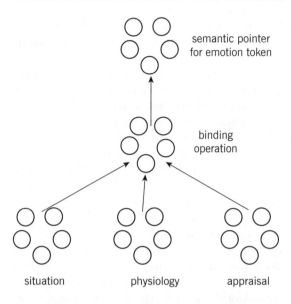

FIGURE 6.2. Schematic view of how a semantic pointer for an emotion occurrence compresses the binding of a situation, physiological reaction, and cognitive appraisal. The circles represent large and diverse neural populations, while the arrows represent transformations of neural activity in those populations through interactions with other populations.

the positive feelings associated with the journal, the paper, yourself, and the people with whom you collaborated will increase, leading to thoughts that may enhance your subsequent interactions with them. Elsewhere, we use the semantic pointer hypothesis to explain the influences of emotional states on automatic and intentional actions (Schröder et al., 2014; Schröder & Thagard, 2013). Moreover, the case can be made that all human cognition is controlled in part by emotion (Clore & Palmer, 2009), so the semantic pointer theory of emotions is potentially an important part of *any* cognitive theory (also see Duncan & Barrett, 2007). Because semantic pointers connect to control, and hence to action in particular contexts, they have important contributions to pragmatics, as well as to semantics and syntax.

Understanding emotions as semantic pointers has several theoretical advantages. First, it applies SPA, which provides a powerful synthesis of symbolic, connectionist, and embodiment approaches. Second, it shows how constructionist views of emotions can meld with biological accounts. Third, it provides a precise way to integrate physiological and appraisal views of emotion within a neural framework that is sufficiently rigorous to be amenable to computer simulation. In order to incorporate social construction accounts, we need to say more about self-representation.

Self-Representation and Social Construction

In the previous last section, P2 was used to represent your happiness that your paper was accepted by a journal but left out the "you." P2 needs to be expanded into something like

$$\text{happy[you, accept(journal, paper)]} \qquad \text{(P5)}$$

This indicates that you are happy that the journal accepted the paper, but how can we represent you? There is a voluminous literature in social psychology on the nature of the self, much of which is concerned with self-representations such as self-concepts (e.g., Thagard, 2014). Here we offer the novel view that a self-representation is a semantic pointer, that is, a neural representation that expands contextually into much richer multimodal representations of sensory experiences, bodily states, emotional memories, and social conceptions.

Once again, binding is the key idea for tying together diverse representations. Hume (1888) worried that the self was no more than a bundle of perceptions, whereas Kant (1965) and other dualistic philosophers sought the unity of the self in transcendental entities such as souls. Binding provides the clue to a semiunified, naturalistic view of self-representation as involving the integration of several factors by convolution and other neural transformations, along the following lines:

$$\text{self-representation} = \text{BIND(self-concepts, experiences,} \qquad \text{(P6)}$$
$$\text{memories)}$$

Here, self-concepts are themselves semantic pointers for general concepts that people apply to themselves, including roles such as *university professor, father,* and *colleague* and traits such as *tall, middle-aged, sociable,* and *conscientious.* Through making use of such concepts, people incorporate cultural knowledge and social structure into the current representation, since the meaning of roles and traits is culturally constructed and passed on across generations through language (Berger & Luckmann, 1966). MacKinnon and Heise (2010) have argued that language provides humans with an implicit cultural theory of people. Whenever one applies linguistic categories to make sense of oneself, one internalizes part of the institutional structure of society and its set of behavioral and emotion-related expectations that are crystallized in the language (Heise, 2007; MacKinnon & Heise, 2010).

The social constructionist interpretation of being happy upon acceptance of your journal article is that the emotion is a consequence of the culturally constructed meanings of the concepts included in that representation (cf. Rogers et al., 2014). With our semantic pointer theory of emotion, we intend to provide a detailed explanation of how such culturally constructed semantics are constrained by, and related to, the biological processes in the brain (for a more general discussion of social vs. psychological constructionist approaches, see Boiger & Mesquita, Chapter 15, this volume). All linguistic concepts include affective meanings (Osgood et al., 1975), which are widely shared among members of one culture (Ambrasat, von Scheve, Schauenburg, Conrad, & Schröder, 2014; Heise, 2010; Moore, Romney, Hsia, & Rusch, 1999). From our perspective, affective meanings are compressed representations of the corresponding appraisal patterns and physiological reactions that are bound into the complex representation of the emotion. Hence, the decompressing mechanisms of semantic pointers enable culturally shared symbolic concepts to activate and socially synchronize related cognitive and physiological processes in the generation of emotion and action (for details, see Schröder & Thagard, 2013).

In accord with the SPA operating within the NEF, both the process of binding and the structures bound are patterns of spiking activity in populations of neurons. Then, the complex proposition P5 that you are happy that the journal accepted your paper becomes the kind of nested, compressed structure shown in Figure 6.3.

Not all emotional experiences require a self-representation. The journal acceptance case does; it is important that it was *your* paper that was accepted for publication, and the emotional response is immediately identifiable as yours. But there are many species that seem to have emotional reactions similar to those of humans but have no detectable sense of self. Members of only eight species are currently known to be able to recognize

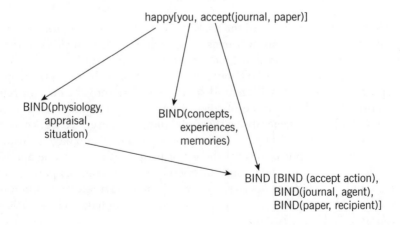

FIGURE 6.3. Representation of the proposition that you are happy that your paper was accepted as the semantic pointer to representations that bind emotion, self, and situation. The representation of you (the self) is the binding of concepts, experiences, and memories.

themselves in mirrors: humans, gorillas, chimpanzees, orangutans, elephants, dolphins, pigs, and magpies (Prior, Schwarz, & Güntürkün, 2008; Broom, Sena, & Moynihan, 2009). Yet behaviorally and neurologically, emotions such as fear seem to operate in very similar ways in a variety of mammals, such as rats (LeDoux, 1996). We conclude, therefore, that self-representations and their linguistic expressions are not essential to emotions, even though they are an important part of human emotions.

Self-representations are particularly important to social emotions such as pride, guilt, shame, and envy, which require an appreciation of one's location in a social situation. Pride, for example, usually involves a positive feeling of accomplishment as a result of feeling appreciated by a social group one cares about, such as family or members of one's profession. Such emotions clearly have a large cultural component, because different societies attach wildly different values to behaviors such as work, education, and gender roles. Depending on the broad values accepted in a society, substantially different behaviors can generate different social emotions. In this sense, emotions are socially constructed, but only partially, because underlying them are the same biological mechanisms, common to all people: representation, binding, and control operating in brain areas that collectively accomplish physiological perception and cognitive appraisal. The neuroanatomy is common to all humans, but the results of appraisal vary dramatically depending on what are viewed by individuals in a particular culture to be the appropriate goals.

Wierzbicka (1999) surveyed both the commonalities of emotions and their extensive diversity across many cultures. Our semantic pointer account of emotions can account for such findings: Whereas the neural mechanisms akin to all humans are the source of cross-cultural commonality, more complex semantic pointers such as those in our example of article acceptance are sufficiently decoupled from underlying bodily representations that they are influenced by culturally bound patterns of social interpretation.

Cultural influences on emotion are clearly not confined to high-level social emotions such as pride. Anger, fear, disgust, happiness, sadness, and surprise occur broadly (Ekman, 2003), but the evaluation of particular objects as scary, disgusting, and so on, varies with a culture's beliefs and attitudes about the objects. Hence, all human emotions have important social dimensions, but they are not mere social constructions because of their substantial underlying biological commonalities.

Building and Testing a Model

The ideas we sketched out about how the SPA can generate an integrative theory of emotions still need to be fleshed out by a much more fully developed computational model. We now present the design of such a model, called "POEM," for "POinters EMotions," to be implemented using the software platform NENGO, which incorporates the theoretical ideas of Eliasmith's NEF and SPA.

First, POEM will specify not only neural populations corresponding to the relevant brain areas, which will include all the ones in the EMOCON model (Figure 6.1) but also additional ones, such as the anterior temporal lobe, identified as important for emotions by various researchers (Lindquist et al., 2012). We will need to decide what dynamics are appropriate for the different brain areas. For example, areas that are part of the dopamine pathway, such as the nucleus accumbens and the orbitofrontal cortex, may have different temporal characteristics than other areas that employ different neurotransmitters. We will need to determine whether these temporal differences matter for the modeling of psychological phenomena.

Second, we will use neuroanatomical information to determine the interconnectivity of the brain areas selected, establishing links between the neurons in them.

Third, we will ensure that the resulting network can perform the following functions: input from external perception of information about a situation; input and interpretation of perceptual information from internal, bodily sources; appraisal of the situation information with respect to goals; and integration of all these kinds of information in an overall interpretation of the significance of the situation to generate a broadly distributed network whose firing patterns will be identifiable as corresponding to particular emotional responses.

Fourth, we will test the POEM model by seeing whether it is capable of simulating the results of important psychological experiments. The previous EMOCON model was never tested in this way, because available technology did not support a computational implementation and the main explanatory target of the model was emotional consciousness, about which little experimentation has taken place. In contrast, earlier neuro-computational models of emotion were strenuously tested for the ability to duplicate experimental results. The GAGE model (named after Phineas Gage) of Wagar and Thagard (2004) was used to simulate the behavior of participants in the Iowa gambling task experiments of Bechara, Damasio, Tranel, and Damasio (1997) and in the famous attribution experiments of Schacter and Singer (1962). The ANDREA (Affective Neuroscience of Decision through Reward-Based Evaluation of Alternatives) model (Litt, Eliasmith, & Thagard, 2008) was used to simulate the behavior of participants in experiments based on decision affect theory (Mellers, Schwartz, & Ritov, 1999) and prospect theory (Kahneman, & Tversky, 1979). Both of these models were used to duplicate not only the qualitative behavior of human participants in the relevant experiments but also the quantitative behavior, generating results similar to those found by the experimenters.

The theoretical assumptions behind POEM are highly compatible with those behind GAGE and ANDREA, so it should be feasible to incorporate the structure of these models into a broader one that includes new ideas about binding, semantic pointers, and self-representation.

Ideally, POEM will be able not only to match the ability of GAGE and ANDREA to simulate important experimental results about emotions but also to simulate quantitatively the results of additional key experiments from different paradigms such as embodiment (e.g., Niedenthal et al., 2009), appraisal theory (e.g., Siemer & Reisenzein, 2007), and sociology of emotion (e.g., Heise & Weir, 1999). In addition, POEM should be able to incorporate the ability of EMOCON to provide a mechanistic explanation of how conscious experiences of emotions arise by incorporating *competition* among semantic pointers (Thagard, in press). Building POEM is a daunting task, but within the range of the convenient software tools of NENGO and the powerful theoretical ideas of NEF and SPA.

As usual in cognitive science, the proof is in the programming (Thagard, 2012b). Success in building POEM will demonstrate the feasibility of semantic pointers, binding, and control for providing a mechanistic account of emotions. Progress in simulating the results of a broad variety of psychological and neurological experiments will provide evidence that the set of mechanisms incorporated into POEM correspond approximately to those that produce emotions in human brains. In addition to applying POEM to psychological experiments, we will need to validate its neurological assumptions by comparing its structure and performance to neuroscientific evidence, including brains scans using functional magnetic resonance imaging (fMRI) and other techniques.

Discussion

Earlier we made the claim that emotion tokens (particular occurrences of emotions; e.g., a person feeling happy at a particular time) are semantic pointers, a special kind of compressed neural pointer that decompresses into a binding of information about physiological states, cognitive appraisals, and sometimes the self. It would probably be just as reasonable to claim that an emotion token is the *combined* process that includes both the semantic pointer and the neural processes to which it points. Given the imprecise nature of folk psychological categories such as *happy*, more specific identification is not supportable by evidence. What matters is that we now have a plausible candidate for a neural mechanism that can have the various psychological effects produced by specific occurrences of emotions.

Even more problematic is the identification of the whole category or type of happiness and other emotions with a class of neural processes. There is insufficient evidence about the neural correlates of kinds of emotions to specify an identity relation between a whole class of occurrences of kinds of emotions and a whole class of neural processes. Hence we support a token–token mind–brain identity theory of emotions, while remaining agnostic concerning the viability of a type–type identity theory for emotions. There are indeterminacies on both sides: Not only is there insufficient neurological evidence about kinds of emotions, such as happiness, there is still uncertainty about whether categories derived from folk psychology will have a legitimate role in a well-worked-out theory of emotions supported by experimental evidence from both psychology and neuroscience. As Patricia Churchland (1986) suggested, we should not take folk categories for granted, but should expect a coevolution of psychological and neural theories that may substantially modify ideas such as happiness.

Recent technological advances may prove to be useful for establishing type–type identities. One is a novel brain-mapping approach that combines text mining and meta-analysis to enable accurate and generalizable classification of cognitive states (Yarkoni, Poldrack, Nichols, Van Essen, & Wager, 2011). In lexical brain decoding, the text of a large corpus of articles is retrieved, and a search string for a psychological state such as "pain" serves to retrieve a subset of articles that report neural coordinates. An automatic meta-analysis of the coordinates produces a whole-brain map of the probability of the psychological state given activation at each brain location.

Another potentially promising technique is the application of machine learning algorithms that can detect specific distributed activation patterns in the brain which reliably correspond to the mental representation of specific concepts. This method has proven useful for identifying the neural correlates of intentions (Haynes et al., 2007), cognitive tasks (Poldrack, Halchenko, & Hanson 2010), and tool concepts (Shinkareva et al., 2008). The combination of brain imaging and machine learning has been used for diagnosing eating disorders (Weygandt, Schaefer, Schienle, & Haynes, 2012). In principle, the challenge is no different for associating emotions with neural activity. Recognition of the locations that correlate generally with psychological states such as pain or happiness, along with a theoretical account of the neural processes that connect activities in those locations, may lead to reasonable type–type identifications of kinds of emotions with kinds of neural processes. We leave open the possibility, however, that such studies will provide grounds for revising everyday concepts of emotions.

We avoid pursuing philosophical issues about emotions that are not addressable by empirical methods. For example, whether emotions supervene on physical states and whether emotions have essences (one common interpretation of the claim that emotions are natural kinds) presuppose a conception of necessity, which most philosophers understand as truth in all possible worlds. Minds supervene on brains if and only if *necessarily* a difference in mental properties requires a difference in neural properties. An essence of something is a property that it has necessarily. It is hard enough to collect evidence concerning what emotions are in *this* world, let alone to pursue the impossible task of collecting evidence that would address questions about what they are in all possible worlds. To modify Wittgenstein, whereof one cannot collect evidence, thereof one must be silent. See Thagard (2010a) for a more thorough defense of philosophical naturalism in discussions of mental states, including rejection of the metaphysical concept of necessity. Hence, the concepts of *supervenience, essence,* and *natural kind* are best ignored in science-oriented discussions of emotions. Whether the general category of emotions (and the myriad categories of different types of emotions) survive in scientific discourse will depend on the roles they play in neuropsychological theorizing.

We have tried to contribute to such theorizing by outlining a new, neurocomputational theory of the neural construction of emotions. This theory is broadly compatible with psychological constructionist views that do not tie emotions to localized, programmed neural operations. Instead, we propose that emotions as semantic pointers are compressed representations of bindings of physiological perceptions and cognitive appraisals, operating in many different brain areas. The plausibility of this theory will depend on the success of the planned model POEM in explaining, more effectively than alternative models, the full range of psychological and neural evidence about emotions.

ACKNOWLEDGMENTS

Paul Thagard's work is supported by the Natural Sciences and Engineering Research Council of Canada. Tobias Schröder was awarded a research fellowship by the Deutsche Forschungsgemeinschaft (No.SCHR 1282/1-1) to support this work.

REFERENCES

Ambrasat, J., von Scheve, C., Schauenburg, G., Conrad, M., & Schröder, T. (2014). Consensus and stratification in the affective meaning of human sociality. *Proceedings of the National Academy of Sciences of the United States of America, 111,* 8001–8006.

Anderson, J. R. (1983). *The architecture of cognition.* Cambridge, MA: Harvard University Press.

Anderson, J. R. (2007). *How can the mind occur in the physical universe?* Oxford, UK: Oxford University Press.

Barrett, L. F. (2006). Solving the emotion paradox: Categorization and the experience of emotion. *Personality and Social Psychology Review, 10,* 20–46.

Barrett, L. F. (2009). The future of psychology: Connecting mind to brain. *Perspectives on Psychological Science, 4,* 326–339.

Barsalou, L. W. (1999). Perceptual symbol systems. *Behavioral and Brain Sciences, 22*, 577–660.

Bechara, A., Damasio, H., Tranel, D., & Damasio, A. R. (1997). Deciding advantageously before knowing the advantageous strategy. *Science, 275*, 1293–1295.

Belli, S., Harré, R., & Íñiguez, L. (2010). What is love?: Discourse about emotions in social sciences. *Human Affairs: A Postdisciplinary Journal for Humanities and Social Sciences, 20*, 240–270.

Berger, P. L., & Luckmann, T. (1966). *The social construction of reality: A treatise in the sociology of knowledge*, Garden City, NY: Anchor Books.

Broom, D. M., Sena, H., & Moynihan, K. L. (2009). Pigs learn what a mirror image represents and use it to obtain information. *Animal Behavior, 78*, 1037–1041.

Churchland, P. S. (1986). *Neurophilosophy*. Cambridge, MA: MIT Press.

Clore, G. L., & Palmer, J. E. (2009). Affective guidance of intelligent agents: How emotion controls cognition. *Cognitive Systems Research, 10*, 22–30

Crawford, L. E. (2009). Conceptual metaphors of affect. *Emotion Review, 1*, 129–139.

Damasio, A. R. (1994). *Descartes' error: Emotion, reason, and the human brain*. New York: Putnam.

Duncan, S., & Barrett, L. F. (2007). Affect is a form of cognition: A neurobiological analysis. *Cognition and Emotion, 21*, 1184–1211.

Ekman, P. (2003). *Emotions revealed: Recognizing faces and feelings to improve communication and emotional life*. New York: Holt.

Eliasmith, C. (2013). *How to build a brain*. Oxford, UK: Oxford University Press.

Eliasmith, C., & Anderson, C. H. (2003). *Neural engineering: Computation, representation and dynamics in neurobiological systems*. Cambridge, MA: MIT Press.

Eliasmith, C., Stewart, T. C., Choo, X., Bekolay, T., DeWolf, T., Tang, Y., et al. (2012). A large-scale model of the functioning brain. *Science, 338*, 1202–1205.

Eliasmith, C., & Thagard, P. (2001). Integrating structure and meaning: A distributed model of analogical mapping. *Cognitive Science, 25*, 245–286.

Fodor, J., & Pylyshyn, Z. (1988). Connectionism and cognitive architecture: A critical analysis. *Cognition, 28*, 3–81.

Fontaine, J. R. J., Scherer, K. R., Roesch, E. B., & Ellsworth, P. C. (2007). The world of emotions is not two-dimensional. *Psychological Science, 18*, 1050–1057.

Gross, J. J., & Barrett, L. F. (2011). Emotion generation and emotion regulation: One or two depends on your point of view. *Emotion Review, 3*, 8–16.

Harré, R. (Ed.). (1989). *The social construction of emotions*. Oxford, UK: Blackwell.

Haynes, J.-D., Sakai, K., Rees, G., Gilbert, S., Frith, C., & Passingham, R. E. (2007). Reading hidden intentions in the brain. *Current Biology, 17*, 323–328.

Heise, D. R. (2007). *Expressive order: Confirming sentiments in social action*. New York: Springer.

Heise, D. R. (2010). *Surveying cultures. Discovering shared conceptions and sentiments*. New York: Wiley.

Heise, D. R., & Weir, B. (1999). A test of symbolic interactionist predictions about emotions in imagined situations. *Symbolic Interaction, 22*, 139–161.

Hume, D. (1888). *A treatise of human nature*. Oxford, UK: Clarendon Press.

Jackendoff, R. (2002). *Foundations of language: Brain, meaning, grammar, evolution*. Oxford, UK: Oxford University Press.

Johnson-Laird, P. N. (1983). *Mental models: Towards a cognitive science of language, inference, and consciousness*. Cambridge, MA: Harvard University Press.

Johnson-Laird, P. N., & Quinn, J. G. (1976). To define true meaning. *Nature, 264*, 635–636.

Kahneman, D., & Tversky, A. (1979). Prospect theory: An analysis of decision under risk. *Econometrica, 47*, 263–291.

Kant, I. (1965). *Critique of pure reason* (N. K. Smith, Trans., 2nd ed.). London: MacMillan.

Lakoff, G., & Johnson, M. (2003). *Metaphors we live by* (2nd ed., with a new Afterword). Chicago: University of Chicago Press.

Larsen, R. J., & Diener, E. (1992). Promises and problems with the circumplex model of emotion. In M. S. Clark (Ed.), *Review of personality and social psychology* (Vol. 13, pp. 25–59). Thousand Oaks, CA: Sage.

LeDoux, J. (1996). *The emotional brain*. New York: Simon & Schuster.

Lindquist, K. A., & Gendron, M. (2013). What's in a word?: Language constructs emotion perception. *Emotion Review, 5*, 66–71.

Lindquist, K. A., Wager, T. D., Kober, H., Bliss-Moreau, E., & Barrett, L. F. (2012). The brain basis of emotion: A meta-analytic review. *Behavioral and Brain Sciences, 35*, 121–143.

Litt, A., Eliasmith, C., & Thagard, P. (2008). Neural affective decision theory: Choices, brains, and emotions. *Cognitive Systems Research, 9*, 252–273.

MacKinnon, N. J., & Heise, D. R. (2010). *Self, identity, and social institutions*. New York: Palgrave Macmillan.

Manstead, A. S. R., & Fischer, A. H. (2001). Social appraisal: The social world as object of and influence on appraisal processes. In K. R. Scherer, A. Schorr, & T. Johnstone (Eds.), *Appraisal processes in emotion: Theory, research, application* (pp. 221–232). New York: Oxford University Press.

Mellers, B., Schwartz, A., & Ritov, I. (1999). Emotion-based choice. *Journal of Experimental Psychology: General, 128*, 332–345.

Moore, C. C., Romney, A. K., Hsia, T.-L., & Rusch, C. D. (1999). The universality of the semantic structure of emotion terms: Methods for the study of inter- and intra-cultural variability. *American Anthropologist, 101*, 529–546.

Newell, A. (1990). *Unified theories of cognition*. Cambridge, MA: Harvard University Press.

Niedenthal, P. M., Winkielman, P., Mondillon, L., & Vermeulen, N. (2009). Embodiment of emotion concepts. *Journal of Personality and Social Psychology, 96*(6), 1120–1136.

Oatley, K. (1992). *Best laid schemes: The psychology of emotions*. Cambridge, UK: Cambridge University Press.

Osgood, C. E., May, W. H., & Miron, M. S. (1975). *Cross-cultural universals of affective meaning*. Urbana: University of Illinois Press.

Osgood, C. E., Suci, G. J., & Tannenbaum, P. H. (1957). *The measurement of meaning*. Urbana: University of Illinois Press.

Parkinson, B., & Simons, G. (2009). Affecting others: Social appraisal and emotion contagion in everyday decision making. *Personality and Social Psychology Bulletin, 35*, 1071–1084.

Plate, T. (2003). *Holographic reduced representations*. Stanford, CA: Center for the Study of Language and Information.

Poldrack, R. A., Halchenko, Y., & Hanson, S. J. (2010). Decoding the large-scale structure of brain function by classifying mental states across individuals. *Psychological Science, 20*, 1364–1372.

Prinz, J. (2004). *Gut reactions: A perceptual theory of emotion*. Oxford, UK: Oxford University Press.

Prior, H., Schwarz, A., & Güntürkün, O. (2008). Mirror-induced representation in magpies: Evidence of self-recognition. *PLoS Biology, 6*(8), e202.

Rogers, K. B., Schröder, T., & von Scheve, C. (2014). Dissecting the sociality of emotion: A multi-level approach. *Emotion Review, 6*, 124–133.

Russell, J. A. (1980). A circumplex model of affect. *Journal of Personality and Social Psychology, 39*, 1161–1178.

Russell, J. A. (2009). Emotion, core affect, and psychological construction. *Cognition and Emotion, 23*, 1259–1283.

Schacter, S., & Singer, J. (1962). Cognitive, social, and physiological determinants of emotional state. *Psychological Review, 69*, 379–399.

Scherer, K. R., Schorr, A., & Johnstone, T. (2001). *Appraisal processes in emotion: Theory, methods, research*. New York: Oxford University Press.

Schröder, T., Stewart, T. C., & Thagard, P. (2014). Intention, emotion, and action: A neural theory based on semantic pointers. *Cognitive Science, 38*, 851–880.

Schröder, T., & Thagard, P. (2013). The affective meanings of automatic social behaviors: Three mechanisms that explain priming. *Psychological Review, 120*, 255–280.

Shinkareva, S. V., Mason, R. A., Malave, V. L., Wang, W., Mitchell, T. M., & Just, M. A. (2008). Using fMRI brain activation to identify cognitive states associated with perception of tools and dwellings. *PLoS ONE, 3*, e1394.

Siemer, M., & Reisenzein, R. (2007). The process of emotion inference. *Emotion, 7*, 1–20.

Stewart, T. C., & Eliasmith, C. (2011). *Neural cognitive modelling: A biologically constrained spiking neuron model of the Tower of Hanoi task*. Presented at the 33rd Annual Conference of the Cognitive Science Society, Austin, TX.

Thagard, P. (1988). *Computational philosophy of science*. Cambridge, MA: MIT Press.

Thagard, P. (2005). *Mind: Introduction to cognitive science* (2nd ed.). Cambridge, MA: MIT Press.

Thagard, P. (2010a). *The brain and the meaning of life*. Princeton, NJ: Princeton University Press.

Thagard, P. (2010b). How brains make mental models. In L. Magnani, W. Carnielli, & C. Pizzi (Eds.), *Model-based reasoning in science and technology. Abduction, logic, and computational discovery* (pp. 447–461). Berlin: Springer.

Thagard, P. (2012a). Cognitive architectures. In K. Frankish & W. Ramsay (Eds.),

The Cambridge handbook of cognitive science (pp. 50–70). Cambridge, UK: Cambridge University Press.

Thagard, P. (2012b). *The cognitive science of science: Explanation, discovery, and conceptual change.* Cambridge, MA: MIT Press.

Thagard, P. (2014) The self as a system of multilevel interacting mechanisms. *Philosophical Psychology, 27,* 145–163.

Thagard, P. (in press). Creative intuition: How EUREKA results from three neural mechanisms. In L. M. Osbeck & B. S. Held (Eds.), *Rational intuition: Philosophical roots, scientific investigations.* Cambridge, UK: Cambridge University Press.

Thagard, P., & Aubie, B. (2008). Emotional consciousness: A neural model of how cognitive appraisal and somatic perception interact to produce qualitative experience. *Consciousness and Cognition, 17,* 811–834.

Thagard, P., & Stewart, T. C. (2011). The Aha! experience: Creativity through emergent binding in neural networks. *Cognitive Science, 35,* 1–33.

Wagar, B. M., & Thagard, P. (2004). Spiking Phineas Gage: A neurocomputational theory of cognitive-affective integration in decision making. *Psychological Review, 111,* 67–79.

Weygandt, M., Schaefer, A., Schienle, A., & Haynes, J.-D. (2012). Diagnosing different binge-eating disorders based on reward-related brain activation patterns. *Human Brain Mapping, 33,* 2135–2146.

Wierzbicka, A. (1999). *Emotions across languages and cultures: Diversity and universals.* Cambridge, UK: Cambridge University Press.

Yarkoni, T., Poldrack, R. A., Nichols, T. E., Van Essen, D. C., & Wager, T. D. (2011). Large-scale automated synthesis of human functional neuroimaging data. *Nature Methods, 8,* 665–670.

CHAPTER 7

Affect Dynamics

Iterative Reprocessing in the Production of Emotional Responses

WILLIAM A. CUNNINGHAM
KRISTEN DUNFIELD
PAUL E. STILLMAN

For thousands of years, categories such as cognition, emotion, and attitude have been used to simplify the challenge of understanding behavior and thought. Yet however useful these categories have been as starting points or heuristics, it is common practice in the psychological and neuroscience literature to treat these simplifying devices as if they are "natural kind" categories with dissociable causal properties, and unique localizable neural substrates. We argue in this chapter that this approach may not be ideal for understanding how nature is carved at its joints, and suggest that greater attention should be directed toward the more elemental and computational aspects of psychological process. More specifically with regard to emotion, the processes that underlie and build complex affective states are likely to be multifaceted, and when more fully articulated, may not even be amenable to description at the observable level of analysis (Barrett, 2009; Barrett & Satpute, 2013). By refocusing on the elemental level of analysis, with an eye toward linking levels of analysis (how the elements combine is as important as knowing what the elements are), we believe that it will be possible to understand not only the homogeneity of emotional experiences (there are likely similarities among instances of anger), but also the heterogeneity of emotional experience (not all instances of anger are the same). For our purposes in this chapter, we focus our discussion of the elements

168

1. *If emotions are psychological events constructed from more basic ingredients, then what are the key ingredients from which emotions are constructed? Are they specific to emotion or are they general ingredients of the mind? Which, if any, are specific to humans?*

According to our model, emotions are events that are constructed from more basic ingredients. Specifically, we propose that what we label as "emotions" arise from the processing of changes in affective trajectories across time. For example, noticing that one's fortunes are improving, or that they may in the near future, is an initial ingredient of emotion. Yet what one does to cope with, or benefit from, this change is also part of the emotion. These changes can be cognitive (appraising or labeling the event) or behavioral in nature. Altering ones thoughts or actions themselves alters the system and subsequently the affect (i.e., emotion) changes with it. Because of this, it is difficult to determine what aspects, if any, of emotion are separable from cognition. We suggest a gradient of processes that may differentiate humans from other animals, in that humans have a greater capacity for reflective thought and linguistic abilities to construe events in more abstract terms.

2. *What brings these ingredients together in the construction of an emotion? Which combinations are emotions and which are not (and how do we know)?*

According to our perspective, the sum total of processes attached to a particular affective change can be considered the emotion. In this sense, the differentiation between a combination that is labeled "emotion" and a combination that is labeled "cognition" is somewhat arbitrary.

3. *How important is variability (across instances within an emotion category, and in the categories that exist across cultures)? Is this variance epiphenomenal or a thing to be explained? To the extent that it makes sense, it would be desirable to address issues such as universality and evolution.*

Because different cultures can describe their experiences in different ways, it is likely there will also be differences in emotions. That is, the affective changes that underlie emotion may be consistent, but the appropriate ways of categorizing these changes, as well as the socially appropriate ways of using the affective information, may be radically different. As such, some aspects of the processes should be invariant (prediction errors in judgment), whereas others should be shaped (the appropriate way to deal with anger in public). The ingredients seem to be evolutionarily derived, whereas the social shaping of these ingredients seems more varied.

(continued)

> **4.** *What constitutes strong evidence to support a psychological construction to emotion? Point to or summarize empirical evidence that supports your model or outline what a key experiment would look like. What would falsify your model?*
>
> At the moment, the work on dynamical systems and computational cognitive neuroscience has shaped our understanding of the building blocks of mind. In the future, computational models of emotion from affective computing should provide new hypotheses that can be tested on neuropsychological populations and with neuroimaging methods.

of affect to the iterative reprocessing (IR) model (Cunningham & Zelazo, 2007; Zelazo & Cunningham, 2007), which proposes that affect and emotion result from dynamic and emergent information processing represented in **heterarchically** organized brain systems.

The IR Model

The IR model is a dynamical systems account of human information processing that is informed by the **heterarchical** organization of brain function. Instead of drawing strict distinctions along the lines traditional dichotomies, IR views information processing as an emergent property of a dynamic system that is rooted in the hierarchical organization of the brain (see also Barrett, Ochsner, & Gross, 2007). Importantly, IR seeks to understand human behavior as the output of a system that attempts to balance two competing goals: (1) achieving a veridical representation of the world, while (2) minimizing processing demands. At its base, the IR model is grounded in the observation that brain systems have reciprocal influences, such that relatively more automatic processes influence and are influenced by relatively more reflective processes. As people are aroused by events from the environment or by internal changes in cognitive processing (e.g., imagery or reconstrual), they automatically reprocess active information to determine its meaning, with evaluative meaning being particularly important (Clore & Ortony, 2008; Ortony & Clore, Chapter 13, this volume). Yet this initial processing that follows a perceived change does not necessarily provide a final affective state (or even affect for more than a few milliseconds). Rather, the information is continuously reprocessed through iterative cycles, potentially creating more reflective evaluations of the information and thereby more nuanced affect.

When an affective state is based on few iterations, it is traditionally labeled *automatic*. These initial states are obligatory and can occur without conscious monitoring (Fazio & Olsen, 2003; Bargh & Williams, 2006). In contrast, when affect is the result of multiple additional iterations, it occurs more slowly, allowing for additional computations, and is often labeled *conscious reflection*. Importantly, these traditionally dissociable states do not require separate independent evaluative systems for more automatic and more reflective evaluations. Rather, the processes operate on information within the system in order to generate dynamic evaluations that over time and processing incorporate prior experience into current information (e.g., context and goals) to achieve an optimal affective state in a given situation. As an event is reprocessed, it can be understood in a more nuanced manner by situating it in an ever-broadening array of considerations. The process of reappraisal continues until a solution is reached, which minimizes both errors and processing demands. That said, it is important to note that just because more time is spent processing an event, it is not always the case that multiple iterations lead to more nuanced levels of processing. For example, in the case of rumination, it is possible that a thought can be reprocessed repeatedly at a low level, without ever recruiting more high-level brain areas.

Representations Are Distributed

IR draws on current models from computational cognitive neuroscience that typically take a more or less connectionist approach to information processes (e.g., O'Reilly, Munakata, Frank, Hazy, & Contributors, 2012) to understand how different processes and representations are organized. An important component of these models is that what is often considered higher order mental activity (e.g., an evaluation or an affective state) can be considered an emergent property of the patterns and interactions of interconnected networks (e.g., units of neurons). Moreover, these frameworks have several properties to explain how the dynamics of information can be used to generate affective states, and how affect emerges in time.

A fundamental premise of connectionist models is that meaningful information resides across patterns of units rather than being encoded within the units per se (for in-depth reviews of connectionist models in social psychology, see Smith, 1996, 2009). As opposed to localist models, which propose that information is contained in a single "node" for each concept (e.g., one's grandmother), connectionist models posit that information is distributed across multiple units that together constitute the representation. Importantly, the same units are used in multiple distinct representations, allowing for a near limitless number of representations with relatively fewer units.

A second crucial component of connectionist models is that "memory" is the stored connection weights between units. Specifically, units are heavily interconnected, and the activation of Unit 1 carries a certain probability of activating Unit 2, and this probability is represented by the weight between the units. As the neurons coactivate more frequently, the weights between them get stronger (via Hebbian learning), and the activation of one is more and more likely to activate the other. If the connection weights are strong enough, a representation can be built with very sparse inputs. Importantly, these recreations are often imperfect and may lead to altered representations (McClelland, Rumelhart, & Hinton, 1986). In cognitive processing, the units of networks tend to gravitate toward stable patterns of activation called *attractor states*. An attractor state is a state of activation that is probable given a diverse array of neuronal activations. In other words, given different inputs, the network will settle on a single internal representation. For example, if you were playing catch, many different neuronal activation patterns would settle into the stable representation of "ball."

The strength of these attractor states is that they allow us quickly to reach a stable internal representation given inputs that are ambiguous, uncertain, or novel. This is particularly important in light of the processing goal to build a stable representation of the environment. The process of settling into a given pattern of activation (often referred to as *categorization*) allows us to predict how the event or stimulus will interact with the environment, thus giving our representations greater nuance (e.g., Barrett, Chapter 3, this volume; Barrett, Wilson-Mendenhall, & Barsalou, 2014). So when a roundish object comes flying at you and you categorize it as a "ball," you know that it will travel with certain physical properties, and that you can likely throw it back. Most of the time, the settling process is quick and accurate. However, the network can settle into an incorrect attractor state, resulting in inaccurate predictions. For example, if a small, green, roundish object came flying at you and you settled on "ball" instead of "grenade," it would most likely result in your death, because with the "ball" categorization there is no prediction of impending doom and impetus to rapidly throw it away and run.

A Distributed and Dynamic Mind

Because the recognition of any given stimulus is the function of the probabilistic sum of activation from multiple independent neurons, distributed representations allows for both stability and flexibility. The active representation of any given piece of information, be it an attitude, emotion, or self-perception, is the function of *both* the preexisting connection weights (that are relatively stable and stored in memory) and the current state of activation (which is a function of factors such as goals, context, and current hedonic experiences). Indeed, stronger connection weights (which are a function of previous experience/reinforcement) make it more likely that similar patterns of activation will be generated, whereas top-down foregrounding can change stimulus construals by reflectively creating distinct patterns of activation.

According to the IR model, when a stimulus is encountered, it initiates an iterative sequence of evaluative processes in which the stimuli are interpreted and reinterpreted in iterative cycles. Sometimes the processing and reprocessing are accomplished in a more automatic way, and other times, more meaningful and complex representations are recruited. By reprocessing the stimuli at multiple levels of resolution and reflective process it is possible to retain both stable representations and affective flexibility. For example, the interactive unfolding of process over time as a function of distributed representations can help us understand the complexities of the human experience, such as the relationship between attitudes and evaluations, the construction of emotions over time, and how we develop a working sense of self from the relevant autobiographical memories. In each of these examples, the IR model relies on the reciprocal interaction of multiple levels of neural hierarchy in order to achieve the optimal balance of accuracy and effort. Moreover, in each of these distinct domains, initial experiences and automatic impressions are transformed in light of relevant context in order to achieve a useful mental model that can appropriately guide behavior.

The iterative and distributed view of information processing proposed by the IR model utilizes a single set of representations to account for the typical "fast" and "slow" dimensions proposed in much of social cognition (see Chaiken & Trope, 1999). Connection weights, which update slowly, represent statistically reliable information that has been extracted from the environment, providing the basis for stable representations. Current activations are more malleable and shift rapidly as a function of context, goals, and presently active representations. A direct result of these interactive distributed representations is the idea that no two mental states are ever identical, and that at any given time current construals are being changed and updated in light of additional considerations.

One of the crucial factors differentiating IR from dual-process models is that greater "thought" (i.e., more iterations) need not necessarily lead to more advanced or more nuanced representations. For example, although rumination involves further iterations, active representations remain fairly static. Similarly, if relatively more top-down processes have already set the weights for the attractor sets, more iterations may not be necessary for the system to settle into a certain representation. In this way, greater "thought" is neither necessary nor sufficient for richer representations, though it often does make it more likely.

Change, Time, and Entropy

The goal of the mind is to settle into a stable, predictive internal representation of the environment. A useful description of this process is that of a system going from a high entropy state to a low entropy state. Here, what we mean by *entropy* is the degree of organization of active representations. Unorganized (or "unsettled") representations have a possibility of settling into a number of different stable internal representations; thus, there is greater uncertainty about how they will settle. Put another way, unstable, uncategorized representations have many possible configurations; that is, the same (unstable) representation can be generated by many different patterns of activation. As the stimulus or event settles into a stable pattern of activation, the number of probable forms the representation may take decreases, thereby reducing entropy. Successive iterations allow for more nuanced representations and therefore less entropy and greater prescriptive predictions.

Entropy, from an information theory perspective, is the number of possible microstates that can account for a given observable macrostate (Boltzmann, 1877; Shannon, 1948; also see Hirsh, Mar, & Peterson, 2012). For a given representation (i.e., a stable representation into which that the network has settled), entropy may be thought of as the number of possible arrangements of the neuronal network that can produce that representation. In other words, entropy is the number of possible inputs (microstates) that can create the observed representation (macrostate). A stimulus that has just been encountered and has not settled into a stable internal representation creates the highest entropy. Entropy is reduced by engaging in pattern extraction, which reduces the number of possible network states that could give rise to the given representation. With each successive iteration, the macrostate (representation) is further refined and narrows the number of possible arrangements that can give rise to that representation, thus (1) increasing predictive power and (2) reducing network entropy. An equivalent way of saying this is that each iteration reduces the number of potential ways the mind can solve the given inputs, that is, the number of potential stable representations that may result from a given input. The number of possible arrangements of the neuronal network, and therefore entropy, that give rise to a given representation is reduced when the representation goes from "bad" to "bad, furry, and charging." In other words, the neuronal network is always working to reduce entropy, which simultaneously increases predictive power.

This conceptualization has several implications. First and foremost is that any change creates entropy—be it small changes, such as encountering a new stimulus, or big changes, such as a friend punching one in the face. The increase in entropy is proportional to the degree to which one's internal representations shift based on the event (and will usually correspond to how novel the event is or how much it violates expectation). It also suggests that whereas some sources of entropy (e.g., basic perception and seeing changes) are easily reducible because the network can easily settle into a stable representation, other sources may create entropy that is much more difficult to reduce. Entropy can be difficult to reduce for a number of reasons, but two important sources of persistent entropy are either novel stimuli that do not settle easily into a preset attractor state, or violations of expectation that not only fundamentally alter one's current representation but also disrupt other representations in the network (or at other layers of the network). Since the brain is trying to reduce entropy, these persistent entropy sources will warrant further iterations in order to reduce the entropy by arriving at a stable internal representation for that event.

Another important source of network entropy is incompatible representations. If a dog bites its owner, this creates entropy, because the representation at one layer (i.e., dog bite = bad) is inconsistent with the "higher-order" representation (i.e., dog = loyal). Between-representation entropy more generally occurs not just between different levels of representation but also laterally, between representations at the same level. Simultaneous incompatible representations lead to unstable representations, and as such require more iterations to resolve. With subsequent iterations, the network ideally will settle on one of the two representations, or re-solve the data entirely to arrive at a solution that allows for stability across all representations. However, some events do not lend themselves to easily reducible entropy. We label events that cause persistent, not-immediately-reducible entropy "anomalies," and they are critical for the understanding of how IR relates to emotions. According to the IR model, an emotional experience is the process of reducing (or trying to reduce) entropy created by anomalies.

One of the crucial implications of a dynamic iterative system is that the prior state of the system is extremely important. Because the system is constantly updating its representations through rerepresentation, and because these rerepresentations are at least in part dependent on the previous representation, taking into account the state of the system at time $n - 1$ is necessary to understand and predict the state of the system at the time of interest. In this way, the previous states of the system act as powerful biasing factors for the further processing of information. Put another way, from an IR perspective, there is no such thing as time 0; the previous states of the system are always influencing the representation process in principled and important ways, for example, by altering the attractor state weights for subsequent processing. This is true regardless of whether state $n - 1$ has begun to iterate on the event or stimulus. Even "new" stimuli that are encountered will be impacted by the previous states of the system, including both how previous states bias processing of new information and whether or how often a particular stimulus has been encountered. In this way, all cognitive processing is occurring across time.

The Construction of (More) Specific Emotions

From a psychological constructivist perspective, we take as a starting point the premise that the wide variety of emotional experiences can be generated through the interactions of a more limited number of basic mental ingredients (Barrett, 2006, 2009, Chapter 3, this volume; Russell, Chapter 8, this volume). In our view, however, the affective ingredients typically proposed are not sufficient to capture the processes of affect, because they, too, are constructed from more elemental processing units. That is, although affect experientially may comprise a circumplex structure of two axes capturing some degree of valence and arousal (Russell, 1980, 2003; Plutchik, 1962; Watson & Tellegen, 1985; Yik, Russell, & Barrett, 1999), the processing of valence occurs dynamically in time, with separable representations of valence for the present, past, and future (Cunningham & Van Bavel, 2009; Kirkland & Cunningham, 2012). As described earlier, evaluative states are constructed dynamically through a series of iterative neural loops occurring multiple times per second. These multiple mental systems serve as a way to track our affective trajectories through time. Incoming information can inform the system as it is compared to previous information and the discrepancy between these two states is computed. This in turn informs interpretation of future updates. Thus, we are constantly situated at a time point in affective space that comprises of our past, our present, and what we predict for our future. Construction of the current affective state is based on the newest incoming information (what just happened, including comparisons to previous predictions) and the information that existed before (past events or feeling states), as well as any predictions about what may occur next (see also Carver & Scheier, 1990, for a similar argument about goal pursuit). Our emotion categories are therefore a way to label and differentiate the various affective trajectories we experience as we move continuously through time.

To the extent that affect is dynamic and reprocessed from moment to moment, it is likely that the affective states labeled as "emotional" also reflect the ongoing dynamics of affective experience within a temporally sensitive framework. *Previous* affective states comprise memory representations of an individual's immediate affective past. The *current* affective state is an evaluation of one's present state based on outcomes. *Predicted* affective states are evaluations of what is likely to happen next. Critically, comparisons can be made between these time points through communication among the relevant neural circuits, allowing us to map out our particular affective place in time (Cunningham & Van Bavel, 2009; Kirkland & Cunningham, 2012). Focusing on affective dynamics as a starting point for emotional processing suggests that emotional states result primarily from changes in the representation of affect within or between systems. That is, just as our perceptual systems are sensitive to changes in sensory input, our affective system is sensitive to various *changes* in valence (Kirkland & Cunningham, 2012). This change or discrepancy, especially if it cannot be resolved quickly, leads to changes in the overall entropy state of the system and a motivation to reduce the entropy either through behavioral or cognitive change. According to this view, a predicted negative state may be labeled "fear," whereas a current negative state may be labeled "sadness." Differentiating between these categories is important, because they provide information as to where in the system the change has occurred. A negative event that can still be avoided may lead to a different set of behavioral options than one that has already occurred (Lazarus, 1982).

As an emotional experience unfolds, these processes contentiously interact to generate an emotion episode. Because the episode lasts until entropy is reduced, different emotions can last quite different periods of time, from an instant of joy quickly resolved to a weeklong bout of anxiety regarding a long past-due chapter deadline. Thus, although emotions are generated through a dynamic cycle of processing, some emotions may result from attention to only parts of the system. For example, the emotion category "fear" may simply require labeling the feeling state generated by a negative prediction signal. Others, such as "joy" or "sadness," may require more comparison; for these examples, this comparison might reveal an upward or downward affective trajectory, respectively. In contrast to models that tacitly begin emotional processing after stimulus presentation (at a figurative "time 0"), this perspective suggests that emotional states are rarely separate from the affective and motivational context in which they arise and may, in fact, necessarily require changes in affective processing from previous to current states. Within this frame, the hard distinction among *cognition, motivation*, and *emotion* falls away; each of these terms refers to a different aspect of a unified dynamic system.

To the extent that these changes in dynamic affect, at least in part, underlie the construction of emotional experience, we should expect that the linguistic categories we use should mirror our predictions. To test this hypothesis, Kirkland and Cunningham (2012) presented participants with information about affective trajectories and recorded which emotion they thought best fit the scenario. To eliminate any semantic information that could be used to determine emotional categories, participants were simply provided with information about past, present, and predicted valence. For example, "You are feeling good, and you predict that something bad will happen. Which emotional label best characterizes this situation?" or "You expect something good to happen, but something worse than expected happens. Which emotional label best characterizes this situation?" Importantly, participants were given the option of reporting that they would not experience any emotion. As expected, each of the "basic emotions" fit into particular quadrants of the affective space. For example, when a worse-than-expected outcome follows the prediction that something good will happen, that situation is labeled as causing anger, but when a worse-than-expected outcome follows the prediction that something bad will happen, that situation is labeled as causing sadness. Additionally, emotion categories are differentiated to a greater extent when participants are required to think categorically than when they have the option to consider the possibility of multiple emotions and degrees of emotions. This work indicates that information about affective movement through time and changes in affective trajectory may be a fundamental aspect of emotion categories.

It is important to note that these relatively automatic comparisons among valence representations alone are likely insufficient to account for the full heterogeneity of emotional experience. Automatic feedback is a key feature of emotional experience; sometimes it is even the essence of emotion itself. For example, Barrett and Bliss-Moreau (2009) suggest that sensory information from the world is represented in somatovisceral, kinesthetic, proprioceptive, and neurochemical fluctuations, and that these bodily representations form a "core" affective state. This body state, which is cortically rerepresented in the somatosensory cortex, particularly the insula, can then be integrated into subsequent steps of affective processing through connections to the amygdala and orbitofrontal cortex (OFC). Cortical interpretations of these body states provide information about the state of the individual and, following some cognitive interpretation, lead to the development of more nuanced emotional experiences. In addition to using information from the body to inform brain states, changes in affectively related brain states often lead to changes in body states. For example, once a potential threat has been detected, the body may need to organize in preparation for an immediate fight-or-flight response. This organization of body into action provides an important cue for future iterative reprocessing of valenced information.

Furthermore, although automatic comparisons can provide movement toward the construction of a particular emotional experience, iterative reprocessing allows for processing to become more refined with time. That is, although affective responses begin with some combination of physiological activation and neural evaluations, emotional episodes also appear to involve some degree of cognitive interpretation. Our appraisals about affect—such as who or what is causing it, how much control we have, whether the state is consistent with our goals, and so forth—help us to understand and even define our emotional experience. The particular emotion that is experienced may be largely dependent on aspects of the situation or object to which one is attending. Indeed, the final outcome will reflect the perceiver's unique interpretation of his or her surroundings in terms of personal relevance.

We propose a topography of emotion, in which emotion categories represent different combinations of expected events and actual outcomes. For example, we predict that simply anticipating a negative event is sufficient for people to use the "fear" label, whereas "anger" typically requires a discrepancy between an anticipated and an experienced state. Furthermore, although we may label our emotion as "joy" or "happiness" when a positive event occurs, this is especially the case when the positive event occurs after a negative one. In other words, people amplify their sense of happiness by comparison to what once was. Thus, we suggest that whereas some emotions are highly related to predictions, others are outcome-dependent, and still others require comparisons between prediction and outcome, reflecting a particular affective trajectory through time (Kirkland & Cunningham, 2012). Additional affective states, such as moods, may be reliant only on current information, without necessitating comparisons. Importantly, these comparisons do not require any contextual details or semantic appraisals and, as such, may be a basic ingredient that can be elaborated by other processes. Whereas a cognitive appraisal- focused approach (e.g., Arnold, 1960; Lazarus, 1982; Scherer, 1993) predicts that emotion requires some degree of evaluation regarding the situation, likelihood of a particular outcome, goal consistency, and so forth, our model suggests that emotion labels (indeed, perhaps emotions themselves) can begin to arise using only information about affective states in time. Although we do not mean to imply that these are the *only* processes that may inform emotion (see next section), we propose, critically, that affective trajectories may be among the fundamental building blocks of emotional experience, and that trajectory-related information alone may help to differentiate emotion categories.

Adding Additional Ingredients to Affective Trajectories

In this chapter, we highlight the role that affective trajectories play in the development of emotional episodes. Although we believe that changes in affective processes are required for an emotional episode, we do not believe that these changes are sufficient to generate the large heterogeneity of emotions that people experience. Although outside the scope of this chapter, we believe that this trajectory information is combined with appraisals (Ortony & Clore, Chapter 13, this volume), conceptualizations (Barrett, Chapter 3, this volume), and behavioral options and choices to create more nuanced emotional life. Indeed, a primary goal of appraisal theorists has been to understand which cognitive interpretations are necessary and/or sufficient for an emotional response. The particular emotion that is experienced may be largely dependent on the aspects of the situation or object to which one attends (Ortonty & Clore, Chapter 13, this volume). The situation reflects the perceiver's unique interpretation of his or her surroundings in terms of personal relevance. Given the computational nature of these appraisals, current models propose an iterative sequence of appraisal checks that begins with a basic sense of relevance and valence, and builds in complexity toward a differentiated emotional experience (Scherer, 2009).

As with the conceptual act model (Barrett, 2006), our model of emotion requires the integration of affective changes with cognitive categories to understand the heterogeneity of emotions. Thus, we propose that affective trajectories are among the ingredients used in combination with other processes. Based on this view, a pattern of valence information regarding the past, the present, and the anticipated future prime our cognitive systems toward a particular emotional state. If one is predicting that something bad will happen, emotional responses typically associated with fear are more likely. If one also experiences a change toward negative valence, but this is a downward trajectory, then emotional responses typically associated with sadness are more likely. Yet the increased probability that the state will be labeled as "sadness" is not the same as saying that the particular pattern of valence representations is sadness. Rather, this information needs to be combined with our interpretations of the environment (appraisals) and the different behavioral options that are available at the moment. A predicted bad event in which one potentially can escape is likely experienced quite differently than an event in which one is trapped. Thus, the trajectory model can be thought of as providing a "preappraisal" of dynamic valence.

Conclusion

Neuroscience methodologies and perspectives have been useful tools in the continuing process of understanding how affect manifests in the human brain, and the implications of these findings for models of emotion. Much that is now known about the systems involved in affective processing was relatively inaccessible even 20 years ago. These include the generation of affective predictions for the future, the representation of current affective states, the integration of information from the body, and the engagement of reflective processing to integrate appraisals, interpretation, categorization, and meaning. When taken together, these aspects of affective processing may result in the experience of discrete emotional states.

REFERENCES

Arnold, M. B. (1960). *Emotion and personality*. New York: Columbia University Press.

Bargh, J. A., & Williams, E. L. (2006). The automaticity of social life. *Current Directions in Psychological Science, 15*, 1–4.

Barrett, L. F. (2006). Emotions as natural kinds? *Perspectives on Psychological Science, 1*, 28–58.

Barrett, L. F. (2009). The future of psychology: Connecting mind to brain. *Perspectives in Psychological Science, 4*, 326–339.

Barrett, L. F., & Bliss-Moreau, E. (2009). Affect as a psychological primitive. *Advances in Experimental Social Psychology, 41*, 167–218.

Barrett, L. F., Ochsner, K. N., & Gross, J. J. (2007). On the automaticity of emotion. In J. Bargh (Ed.), *Social psychology and the unconscious: The automaticity of higher mental processes* (pp. 173–217). New York: Psychology Press

Barrett, L. F., & Satpute, A. B. (2013). Large-scale brain networks in affective and social neuroscience: Towards an integrative architecture of the human brain. *Current Opinion in Neurobiology, 23*(3), 361–372.

Barrett, L. F., Wilson-Mendenhall, C. D., & Barsalou, L. W. (2014). A psychological construction account of emotion regulation and dysregulation: The role of situated conceptualizations. In J. J. Gross (Ed.), *Handbook of emotion regulation* (2nd ed., pp. 447–468). New York: Guilford Press.

Boltzmann, L. (1877). Uber die beziehung zwischen dem zweiten hauptsatz der mechanischen warmetheorie und der wahrscheinlichkeitsrechnung respektive den satzen uber das wrmegleichgewicht [On the relationship between the second law of the mechanical theory of heat and the probability calculus]. *Wiener Berichte, 76*, 373–435.

Carver, C. S., & Scheier, M. F. (1990). Origins and functions of positive and negative affect: A control-process view. *Psychological Review, 97*, 19–35.

Chaiken, S., & Trope, Y. (1999). *Dual-process theories in social psychology*. New York: Guilford Press.

Clore, G. L., & Ortony, A. (2008). Appraisal theories: How cognition shapes affect into emotion. In M. Lewis, J. M. Haviland-Jones, & L. F. Barrett (Eds.), *Handbook of emotions* (3rd ed., pp. 628–642). New York: Guilford Press.

Cunningham, W. A., & Van Bavel, J. J. (2009). Varieties of emotional experience: Differences in object or computation? *Emotion Review, 1*, 56–57.

Cunningham, W. A., & Zelazo, P. D. (2007). Attitudes and evaluations: A social cognitive neuroscience perspective. *Trends in Cognitive Sciences, 11*, 97–104.

Fazio, R. H., & Olson, M. A. (2003). Attitudes: Foundations, functions, and consequences. In M. A. Hogg & J. Cooper (Eds.), *The handbook of social psychology* (pp. 139–160). London: Sage.

Hirsh, J. B., Mar, R. A., & Peterson, J. B. (2012). Psychological entropy: A framework for understanding uncertainty-related anxiety. *Psychological Review, 119*, 304–320.

Kirkland, T., & Cunningham, W. A. (2012). Mapping emotions through time: How affective trajectories inform the language of emotion. *Emotion, 12*(2), 268–282.

Lazarus, R. S. (1982). Thoughts on the relations between emotions and cognition. *American Physiologist, 37*(10), 1019–1024.

McClelland, J. L., Rumelhart, D. E., & Hinton, G. E. (1986). The appeal of parallel distributed processing. In J. L. McClelland & D. E. Rumelhard (Eds.), *Parallel distributed processing: Explorations in the microstructure of cognition* (Vol. 2, pp. 3–44). Cambridge, MA: MIT Press.

Öhman, A., & Mineka, S. (2001). Fear, phobias and preparedness: Toward an evolved module of fear and fear learning. *Psychological Review, 108*, 483–522.

O'Reilly, R. C., Munakata, Y., Frank, M. J., Hazy, T. E., & Contributors. (2012). *Computational cognitive neuroscience*. Available online at *http://ccnbook. colorado.edu*.

Plutchik, R. (1962). *The emotions: Facts, theories, and a new model*. New York: Random House.

Russell, J. A. (1980). A circumplex model of affect. *Journal of Personality and Social Psychology, 39*, 1161–1178.

Russell, J. A. (2003). Core affect and the psychological construction of emotion. *Psychological Review, 110*, 145–172.

Scherer, K. R. (1993). Studying the emotion–antecedent appraisal process. *Cognition and Emotion, 7*, 325–355.

Scherer, K. R. (2009). Emotions are emergent processes: They require a dynamic computational architecture. *Philisophical Transactions of the Royal Society B: Biological Sciences, 1535*, 3459–3474.

Shannon, C. E. (1948). A mathematical theory of communication. *Bell System Technical Journal 27*(3), 379–423.

Smith, E. R. (1996). What do connectionism and social psychology offer each other? *Journal of Personality and Social Psychology, 70*, 893–912.

Smith, E. R. (2009). Distributed connectionist models in social psychology. *Social and Personality Psychology Compass, 3*, 64–76.

Watson, D., & Tellegen, A. (1985). Toward a consensual structure of mood. *Psychological Bulletin, 98*, 219–235.

Yik, M. S. M., Russell, J. A., & Barrett, L. F. (1999). Integrating four structures of current mood into a circumplex: Integration and beyond. *Journal of Personality and Social Psychology, 77*, 600–619.

Zelazo, P. D., & Cunningham, W. (2007). Executive function: Mechanisms underlying emotion regulation. In J. J. Gross (Ed.), *Handbook of emotion regulation* (pp. 135–158). New York: Guilford Press.

CHAPTER 8

My Psychological Constructionist Perspective, with a Focus on Conscious Affective Experience

JAMES A. RUSSELL

Much psychological theorizing and research on emotion rest on ancient prescientific assumptions that we all hold as intuition and common sense. As Gross pointed out, everyday concepts and assumptions have a gravitational pull: Even when an assumption is found wanting, it continuously reappears. The words we use to ask questions and formulate answers—words such as *emotion, feeling, anger, fear,* and *joy*—rest on an implicit understanding that is part of our cultural heritage, an understanding that rests on principles of cognitive economy. For example, much writing in science simply presupposes that emotions are the cause of the observable components of the episode: fear makes us tremble, makes us frown, makes us want to flee, and so on. Thus, questions are asked about the functions and other effects of different emotions; correlations between emotion and another outcome are interpreted as showing causality. Even writers who explicitly define emotion as the set of observable components slip into writing of the emotion as their cause.

Psychological construction is a family of accounts—in Lakatos's (1970) terms, a research program—that offers an alternative to the ancient prescientific assumptions that underlie much of the thinking found in affective science to this day. Constructionist accounts have a family history (Gendron & Barrett, 2009). The family is growing, as demonstrated in the chapters of this book. Here, I first state some of my assumptions, which I

1. *If emotions are psychological events constructed from more basic ingredients, then what are the key ingredients from which emotions are constructed? Are they specific to emotion or are they general ingredients of the mind? Which, if any, are specific to humans?*

As occurrent events, emotional episodes are indeed constructed at the time of occurrence from simpler ingredients that are general ingredients of the mind (and body). In principle, any ingredient could play a role, but the usually named "components"—peripheral physiological changes, attributions and appraisals, subjective experiences, plans and goals and behaviors—are certainly important. What is true for emotional episodes may also be said for the construction of what I call attributed affect, perception of affective quality, and emotional meta-experience. Core affect provides the pleasant or unpleasant and the energized or enervated feeling to an emotional episode, but core affect is always present, including times when no emotional episode is occurring. I doubt that any of these processes are unique to humans, although perhaps emotional meta-experience is.

2. *What brings these ingredients together in the construction of an emotion? Which combinations are emotions and which are not (and how do we know)?*

The rejection of essentialism implies that no emotion, affect program, neural module, appraisal, act of labeling, conceptual act, bolt of lightning, or the like, brings the ingredients together in all and only emotional episodes (or fear episodes, anger episodes, etc.). Of course, each ingredient (component) is produced by a causal mechanism. And human episodes, emotional or otherwise, are coordinated. Ingredients co-occur for a variety of reasons. Some are ongoing and therefore necessarily co-occur. Some ingredients influence others (appraisals influence goals and plans, which influence behavior). Others are influenced by the same central mechanisms (attention influences both appraisal and peripheral ANS). External events influence many ingredients, and external events have a correlational structure, which influences the correlational structure of the ingredients. All events we call, say, *fear* typically have a similar pattern of ingredients in common, because they have to in order to count as *fear*. Emotional episodes are coordinated, just as are all human episodes, because a primitive function of the brain is to coordinate the various subsystems of the body, but no subsection of the brain is dedicated to coordinating all and only emotions or all and only specific types of emotional episode.

Which combinations are emotions? *Emotion* is an English word, so one interpretation of this question is that it is about the semantics of English, which is interesting but only a small part of affective science. The question then is what events do native speakers of English call *emotion*, and research has provided a good start to answering this question. For example, membership is graded with no clear boundary between emotions and not-emotions. We do not need to answer this question when explaining emotional episodes. Emotional

(continued)

episodes require explanation because all human episodes require explanation, whether they are or are not classified as emotional. Scientists who use *emotion* as a scientific concept need to specify its boundaries: which events are and which are not emotions in their account. But a sharp boundary can be created only by stipulation. The sharply bounded category cannot be equivalent to the vaguely bounded category named in everyday language.

3. *How important is variability (across instances within an emotion category, and in the categories that exist across cultures)? Is this variance epiphenomenal or a thing to be explained? To the extent that it makes sense, it would be desirable to address issues such as universality and evolution.*

Variability of instances within a category and of categories across cultures is a fact. Affective science requires a good account of this variability; it must be explained. Variability has consequences; it is not epiphenomenal. Universality is also a fact. There are levels of description in which most or all human activity is universal, but other levels of description bring out cultural and individual variability. So eating is universal, but eating sushi, beef, insects, or pork varies with group membership. Unconditioned reflexes are universal; conditioned ones vary. We can find levels of description of human psychology that state what is universal and what is culture-specific. Starting with a Western concept, then using dubious methods and statistics to prove it universal is not a useful enterprise. I hypothesize that core affect, attributed affect, perception of affective quality, and emotional meta-experience are universal processes, but that specific categories of emotional episode and emotional meta-experience (shame vs. *verguenza*; Hurtado de Mendoza, Fernandez Dols, Parrott, & Carrera, 2010) are culture-specific. Evolution is a fact; we are products of evolution, but we evolved mechanisms whereby we adapt and learn and create culture.

4. *What constitutes strong evidence to support a psychological construction to emotion? Point to or summarize empirical evidence that supports your model or outline what a key experiment would look like. What would falsify your model?*

My specific account includes many hypotheses, evidence concerning which is reviewed elsewhere (Russell, 2003a). Falsifiable? Each specific hypothesis would be easily falsified. For example, my claim that core affect is a universal psychological mechanism would be falsified by the existence of a group of normal human beings lacking core affect. Or finding that primitive feelings lack the properties I hypothesized for core affect. For example, the claim that core affect includes one bipolar pleasure–displeasure dimension is currently being seriously questioned (Larsen et al., 2001). My hypothesis that the categories into which humans divide emotions is not universal would be falsified by finding that the categories are invariant with culture, language, and so on. I have offered an analysis of emotion concepts (Fehr & Russell, 1984), of the development of those concepts (Widen & Russell, 2013), of the perception

(continued)

of emotion from facial expression (Carroll & Russell, 1996, 1997; Russell, 1994, 1997), of the psychometrics of affect measurement (Russell & Carroll, 1999), and of neurophysiological correlates of core affect (Posner et al., 2005). The pattern of available evidence is consistent with these analyses and therefore with my version of psychological construction, but it will undoubtedly need to be modified as more evidence comes in.

As a family of accounts, psychological construction is a research program in Lakatos's sense. Such a program includes but is not limited to any one analysis or model. Evaluation of a full research program is not as simple as verifying or falsifying a single hypothesis. A research program is a set of assumptions, methods, theories, and historical antecedents that ideally spawns scientific progress and that, when it can no longer do so, withers.

share with (perhaps most) other family members. I then summarize, elaborate, and develop my specific account as it bears on the first two questions that are the focus of this book.

Assumptions Shared

Here are some of my assumptions shared with most, but perhaps not all, other psychological constructionist accounts.

1. Intuition, common sense, and folk psychology are important topics to study, but we cannot take them as truth, as the "gold standard" for knowledge about emotion. Theories of quantum mechanics, relativity, plate tectonics, and evolution through natural selection illustrate how far science can move beyond its roots in the everyday way of thinking. Scientists typically use the concepts of folk understanding to begin their investigation, but prescientific concepts and the assumptions underlying them are typically found to be approximations at best and often are simply wrong. In the study of emotion, the situation is more complicated, because the folk concepts are part of (but not all) the subject matter of that study. The problem in affective science is captured by something Will Rogers once said: "The problem is not so much what we don't know as it is what we know that ain't so."

2. The everyday, ordinary words *emotion, fear, anger, love,* and the like name categories that have proven to be vague and heterogeneous. Instances that fall within each of these categories share a family resemblance rather than a common core. Instances are more or less emotional (or more or less fear, etc.), with no clear border to be found between emotion and not-emotion (or fear and not-fear, etc.). Ortony and Turner (1990)

pointed to the vagueness of everyday language as a problem for theories that use everyday terms as scientific terms. We have an intuition that if we have a word for something, that word must name a clearly definable category. Yet this intuition has been undermined for words in general and for emotion words in particular. The instances within the category named *emotion* are qualitatively different: occurrent events and dispositions, intentional and nonintentional states, automatic and controlled processes, motives and lack of motivation, reflexes and cognitive states, and so forth. The implications of this heterogeneity are vast. Heterogeneity undermines the seemingly endless search for a precise definition of emotion. It undermines categorical statements purporting to be laws of emotion. It underscores the need to take seriously the variability within our commonly used emotion categories and the variability of categories across individuals and groups. We can limit this heterogeneity a bit, but cannot eliminate it, by using subcategories. In the remainder of this chapter, I typically limit the discussion to *emotional episodes*, which are stipulated to be occurrent events. Of course, there is more to emotion than just emotional episodes: moods, sentiments, emotional dispositions, and many more categories that need to be considered.

3. The everyday, ordinary words *emotion, fear, anger, love*, and the like name important folk concepts that must be studied and understood. In psychological construction, these concepts are treated as topics of study because they are part of the human understanding of emotional life. Of course, *emotion, fear*, and so on, are words in modern English. Other languages and the same language at different times (Barfield, 1954) name different concepts, equally worthy of study. Language provides an invaluable tool with which we can examine the conceptual world of different people in different cultures and eras. Language evolved because it served a function, namely, transferring information about one person's mental state to someone else. Language serves to transfer one's conception of the emotional world to another person; thus, language enables an adult to transfer a conception of emotion to a child.

4. Emotional episodes and cognitive episodes are closer and more intertwined than common sense would have it. Both involve information processing and reactions based on that information. More generally, the old black-and-white dichotomies that pervaded thinking about human beings—nature–nurture, biology–culture, mind–body—are all being replaced. Thus, traditional distinctions such as emotion versus reason or feeling versus thought are viewed with skepticism. Both involve the body, both involve the brain. Thinking is affectively charged, feeling is a form of thinking.

5. Not all emotional episodes are predetermined reaction patterns that are simply triggered, although a few are. A type of emotional episode

(anger, fear, etc.) is not a set of simple repeatable units that recur under specifiable circumstances. Thus, not all emotional episodes are products of emotion-specific brain modules or neural affect programs. Of course, the brain is doing all the work, but the appropriate neural account is not so simple (LeDoux, 2012).

6. An emotional episode is multicomponential. It comprises various components (ingredients, manifestations), no single one of which is itself an emotion. Furthermore, no single component is given a privileged scientific status. The conscious feeling of the emotion (feeling scared, feeling sad, etc.) is not a single, irreducible primitive unit of consciousness. An emotional episode is not well described in a simple stimulus–response framework. Instead, an emotional episode comprises various component processes, each unfolding over time, changing moment to moment as the components interact with each other, with other processes, and with the surrounding world. A token emotional episode is put together at the time of its occurrence.

7. The traditional measurement model for an emotional episode—in which emotion (or fear, anger, etc.) is an inferred latent variable that causes its observable components—is inappropriate. There is no "unseen entity" (Clore & Ortony, 2008, p. 630) causing all and only emotional episodes. As Coan and Gonzalez (Chapter 9, this volume) outlined, an alternative measurement model resonant with psychological construction has emotion emerging from its indicators (now a misnomer).

Assumptions Rejected

One side of my research program is an investigation of the common assumptions made about emotion. One early project concerned the assumption that everyday concepts of emotion, fear, and so on, are each definable in the classical way, through individually necessary and collectively sufficient features. A series of empirical studies showed that this assumption is unwarranted (Fehr, Russell, & Ward, 1982; Fehr & Russell, 1984). There are no necessary and sufficient features to be found, no border separating emotion from not-emotion. This analysis was later extended to types of emotion, such as anger and love (Fehr & Russell, 1991; Russell & Fehr, 1994).

The received folk psychological account of emotion has been most clearly articulated as basic emotion theory, which has served an invaluable historical function. It has been the dominant guide to research for at least a generation. Although some evidence is consistent with basic emotion theory, much is not. Table 8.1 lists a set of core assumptions of basic emotion theory and evidence on those assumptions.

TABLE 8.1. Problems Uncovered in Studies of Basic Emotions

Presupposition	Problem
Specific emotions are universal aspects of human nature.	There are cultural differences in all known aspects of emotion.
Words such *fear, anger,* and *disgust* provide scientific terms for the emotions of all human beings.	Different languages lack a one-to-one correspondence between emotion terms.
Emotion and other terms can be precisely defined.	Theories based on traditional assumptions have not led to increased precision of terms. Each term lacks inclusion and exclusion rules.
Basic emotions are the building blocks of all emotions.	Basic emotions rarely occur alone, and yet no accepted theory of how they co-occur or blend has been developed.
Certain facial expressions are automatically produced by an emotion and automatically recognized by onlookers.	Failure to find convincing evidence that emotions produce "facial expressions of emotion." Failure to find convincing evidence that observers recognize the specific emotion from the purported facial expression.
Each basic emotion has a signature pattern in the autonomic nervous system.	Failure to find convincing evidence of a unique pattern for each emotion in the autonomic nervous system.
The conscious feeling of fear, anger, disgust, and the rest are primitive irreducible qualia common to human beings, akin to sensations.	Failure to find separate factors corresponding to basic emotions in studies of self-reported emotional experience.
Each emotion includes (or causes) a specific instrumental behavior; thus, flight is explained by fear.	Failure to find a class of behaviour common to instances of a given emotion.
The various components produced by the emotion, because they have a common cause, are highly associated.	Dissociation rather than predicted associations among manifest components.

The evidence for basic emotion theory that researchers have found most compelling concerns facial expressions. That facial expressions express something, presumably emotions, is embedded in our everyday way of speaking, but is it true? Research from my laboratory joins that from others in challenging the widely cited claim of universal recognition of seven basic emotions from people's facial expression. That claim is undermined by four lines of evidence. First, rather than being universal, observers' ability to match a specific face to its predicted emotion varies significantly with language and culture (Russell, 1994; Nelson & Russell, 2013). Similarly, the specific expected expression associated with a given emotion varies with culture (Jack, Blais, Scheepers, Schyns, & Caldara, 2009).

The evidence widely cited as demonstrating universal recognition is largely, although not completely, an artifact of method. In the most commonly used method, an observer is shown a series of highly exaggerated posed facial expressions, without being given information about the situation encountered or the expresser's bodily movements and behavior. The observer is asked to select one and only one emotion term from a short list. None of these method factors is a fatal flaw, but each has been shown to nudge the results in the predicted direction. Cumulatively, these method factors are largely responsible for the widely cited results. The results are then held to an inappropriate statistical standard (Nelson & Russell, 2013).

Second, the emotion seen in a face varies with context to a degree that is inconsistent with basic emotion theory. In basic emotion theory, the facial movement is *part of* the emotional response itself. If this is so, the facial movement provides direct information about the emotion; this information should supersede information provided by less direct sources, such as the situation the expresser has encountered or the expresser's behavior as seen in bodily movements—events that are probabilistically associated with the emotion rather than part of it. In contrast to this theory, when the observer has information about both the face and context, the face fails to dominate in the way predicted (Aviezer, Trope, & Todorov, 2012; Hassin, Aviezer, & Bentin, 2013; Carroll & Russell, 1996). Furthermore, the observer's context (e.g., other facial expressions the observers happens to have seen) also influences the observer's judgment (Russell & Fehr, 1987; Yik, Widen, & Russell, 2013).

Third, basic emotion theory relies on an evolutionary story to account for the alleged universal recognition. For example, Izard (1994) noted the improved chance of survival of the preverbal child who avoids the dangers of poisons and pathogens by recognizing disgust in the faces of others. Empirically, however, until age 9 years, the majority of children interpret the standard face purported to express disgust as a display of anger rather than disgust. More generally, children's matching of a facial expression with the emotion it allegedly expresses is poor and improves only gradually with age (Widen, 2013; Widen & Russell, 2013). Conceptually, an evolutionary account of emotion need not predict facial signaling of the emotion (Buss, in press).

Fourth, one prediction from basic emotion theory was so much a part of common sense that it was rarely tested. An emotion results in the corresponding facial expression: happy people smile, and so on. So, it has been a surprise that this prediction has repeatedly failed to be supported (Aviezer et al., 2012; Fernandez Dols & Ruiz Belda, 1995; Fernandez Dols & Crivelli, 2013; Reisenzein, Studmann, & Horstmann, 2013).

Scarantino's New Basic Emotion Theory: A New Hope?

My critique of basic emotion theory is based on previously published versions. In another chapter in this book, Scarantino faults psychological construction and proposes a new basic emotion theory. However, much of what he writes is consistent with psychological construction. His proposed version of basic emotion theory is so different from current versions that it raises the question of how much a research program can be changed and still be the same program. I do not believe that the new version can save that program.

Correlation ≠ Coordination

Earlier I pointed to low correlations between the predicted components of basic emotions (the frown of fear, the peripheral physiological signature of fear, the subjective experience of fear, appraisal of danger, etc.). Traditional basic emotion theory makes a strong prediction about these correlations, namely, because they all stem from activation of the same neural program (or at least some emotion-specific mechanism), the same or a highly similar pattern of these specific components recurs in all or most episodes of fear or any other basic emotion. Therefore, across individuals, or across time for one individual, occurrence and intensity of each specified fear component was predicted to be highly correlated with the occurrence and intensity of each of the other fear components. One of the most surprising empirical findings of affective science is how low these correlations are in fact. I offered an explanation for why the correlations are low but not zero. Scarantino does not challenge the empirical findings and, indeed, seems to reject traditional basic emotion theory on this basis. He speculates that there are new categories of events in which the correlations will be found to be larger, categories such as "core ingestive basic disgust." This is likely so, but it is irrelevant to the prediction of traditional basic emotion theory; to my explanation of the empirical findings about events ordinarily described as fear, anger, disgust, and so forth; and to much of human emotional life.

Scarantino wrote that psychological construction claims "low coordination between neurobiological, physiological, expressive, behavioral, or phenomenological responses" (Chapter 14, this volume, p. 343). Not so. For any token human episode, including any token emotional episode (Sally's encounter with the bear last Saturday morning), all the neurobiological, physiological, expressive, cognitive, behavioral, and phenomenological subevents within the episode are highly coordinated. Coordination is simply a feature of biological systems, and it is a primary function of the brain. Even if the correlations among basic emotion theory's *predicted* components of an emotion were zero, that correlation would not challenge the coordination among subevents (many of which are often not the ones predicted by basic emotion theory) within the token episode. Emotional episodes are coordinated, just not in the way predicted by basic emotion theory.

Analysis of Psychological Construction

Scarantino offers no criticisms of most versions of psychological construction seen in this book or elsewhere. Relative to my account, he mentions correlation and coordination, discussed earlier. Relative to Barrett's conceptual act theory, Scarantino relies on an implicit definition of *emotion* as a behavioral response pattern. When Barrett uses *emotion* (as did James) to mean what I call "emotional meta-experience" and what is commonly called the conscious feeling of emotion (or fear or anger, etc.), then Scarantino's criticisms dissolve. When Barrett writes of emotion as perceived by others (witness or scientist), Scarantino's criticisms similarly dissolve. I see no reason to accept Scarantino's assumption that the components of an emotional episode cannot occur without an emotion. His assumptions seem to rule out acquisition of a new concept.

Scarantino offers no criticisms of the major premises of psychological construction. Indeed, he explicitly accepts much of psychological construction—including the problems entailed in using folk concepts as technical concepts in a scientific theory; the concept of core affect; the way in which an emotional episode is dependent on context, prior history, a myriad of psychological processes, and so on; and the heterogeneity of emotion and types of emotion. Scarantino's rejection of our natural language emotion categories as scientific concepts is extremely important, not simply because every current basic emotion theory relies on them, but because researchers outside of basic emotion theory simply assume that if we have a word for a type of emotion, there must be a corresponding distinct entity that causes that emotion's manifestations in all cases.

Analysis of Basic Emotion Theory

Scarantino echoes my criticisms of traditional basic emotion theory to the degree that he calls for a new basic emotion theory. Yet his new basic emotion theory is so vague that it is difficult to evaluate. He assumes that emotional episodes can be divided into categories, but not the categories currently used in basic emotion theory. In his new basic emotion theory, fear is replaced with multiple fear categories. (He provides no defense for his apparent assumption—and may not even accept it—that the new fear categories are all subsets of fear, and that they collectively coincide with fear and only fear. Indeed, he does not address the question.) Left to be determined in the future is how many categories there are, what defines them, and what scientifically interesting explanatory and predictive generalizations are true of them. In his new basic emotion theory, the categories and the relations among them remain completely unspecified, and so only the vaguest of predictions are made. No amount of evidence can rule out the possibility that, in the future, some new category will be found that possesses the properties Scarantino specifies. In this regard, his new basic emotion theory cannot be falsified. Traditional basic emotion theory, in contrast, was a highly productive theory because it made specific predictions, which turned out to be largely false, but it was the predictions that led to research.

What Scarantino preserves from basic emotion theory are "basic emotion programs" (Chapter 14, this volume, p. 363): unspecified emotion-specific neural mechanisms. This claim is especially problematic because, as Scarantino acknowledges, the concept of emotion is undefined, culture-specific, and too heterogeneous to be useful in science. Some of the supposed programs are output-rigid (i.e., reflexes). We gag at certain things, blink at this, startle at that, and so forth. Of course, I agree that reflexes exist, although I speculate that reflexes are a tiny part of human emotional life. Scarantino's more important claim is that emotion-specific output-flexible programs exist, but he offers no evidence or other reason to think that the neural circuitry corresponding to such programs is specific to emotion. LeDoux (2012) recently argued against thinking in terms of emotion-specific circuits, and thinking instead in terms of survival circuits—another way of stating psychological construction's project. Furthermore, Scarantino provides a "protective belt" for his hypothesis: The observable components produced as output of his output-flexible basic emotion programs cannot be predicted, because the actual components depend on other information processing, other concurrent states, prior history, context, and so on—in other words, according to psychological construction, all the things on which observable components depend. Thus, given LeDoux's framework at the neural level and psychological construction's framework at the psychological level, we have no need of the undefined "basic emotion programs."

Scarantino seems to think that the neural mechanisms underlying emotional episodes must be specific just to emotion. Indeed, he offers an implausible interpretation of William James as a basic emotion theorist by presupposing that James, too, must have presupposed just emotion-specific mechanisms despite his explicit statements to the contrary. Scarantino's seventh footnote (Chapter 14, this volume, p. 369) points to one of the obvious problems with this interpretation of James.

In summary, Scarantino says that he offers a theory (a new basic emotion theory), but it is not so much a theory as a hope. The hope is that someday someone will discover that human emotional life divides into a limited number of natural kinds, each resulting from a dedicated neural circuit unique to that kind. James (1890/1950) was skeptical of these assumptions: "There is no limit to the number of possible different emotions. . . . Any classification of the emotions is seen to be as true and as 'natural' as any other." Still, this hope is a logical possibility, and it will remain so no matter how often we fail to find those natural categories.

Reconciliation

I join with Scarantino in the theme he strikes in his conclusion. All of us are working to build a science of emotion. Both psychological construction and basic emotion theory are research programs, as defined by Lakatos (1970); each includes a family of related assumptions, theories, hypotheses, methods, and so on. Each is progressing. We will progress faster by working together.

My Positive Account of Affective Experience

The second part of my research program has been an attempt to articulate an alternative account by proposing a set of concepts and hypotheses for the analysis of emotional episodes. My account is aimed at the psychological level. Of course, other levels of analysis—evolutionary, neuroscientific, developmental, and sociocultural—need to be added, but that task remains for another day. Emotional episodes include various components, such as peripheral physiological changes, expressive signs, instrumental actions, and conscious experiences. By *component*, I mean an event that by itself, an observer (the self, a witness, a scientist) would take to be a sign of an emotion. Of course, such components in turn depend on many processes, often difficult to observe, some of which are fast, automatic, and nonconscious. I next elaborate on my account of one component: conscious affective experience.

Most accounts of emotional episodes, especially historically, have focused on conscious experience. Indeed, many writers have simply presupposed that emotion *is* a conscious experience. Still, conscious experiences within an emotional episode are a heterogeneous lot. Without claiming to be exhaustive, I distinguish four kinds of conscious experiences that are components of an emotional episode: emotional meta-experience, perception of affective quality, core affect, and attributed affect.

Emotional Meta-Experience

I begin with my version of what has been the focus of much writing on emotion, indeed, what has often been synonymous with *emotion*: the conscious experience of having a specific emotion such as anger, jealousy, fear, love, and so on. My term for this experience, *emotional meta-experience*, emphasizes that the experience of anger, for example, is not the recurrence of the same, simple, irreducible mental quale. Instead, emotional meta-experience is a form of self-perception. It is a meta-experience in that it depends on other aspects of experience, some of which are themselves consciously accessible. Emotional meta-experience presupposes concepts—in these examples, concepts of anger, jealousy, fear, and love. Like all perceptions, emotional meta-experiences are intentional mental states; that is, they include a representation of something: what one is angry about, jealous of, afraid of, or in love with. Like all perceptions, emotional meta-experiences are interpretations. The raw data on which the interpretation is based are both top-down (e.g., concepts, stored knowledge, expectations, attributions, appraisals, and memories) and bottom-up (from both the internal world via somatosensory feedback and the external world).

A person typically has a fair amount of such information on which the perception—the emotional meta-experience—is based, but, all the same, no one is infallible. The perception can be mistaken in the sense that unbiased observers would give a different interpretation. An emotional episode or individual components within that episode can also occur with no emotional meta-experience.

The hypothesis of emotional meta-experience contrasts with any account in which the conscious experiences of anger, fear, and so on, are irreducible and universal qualia (Oatley & Johnson-Laird, 1987). Referring to such experiences as *sensations* seems to imply the same. When Barrett (Chapter 3, this volume) uses *emotion* to mean what I call emotional meta-experience, then my account resonates with hers, although we rely on different accounts of the categorization process involved.

Perception of Affective Quality

The objects and events that we perceive in the world or remember or imagine are affectively coded as pleasant, distressing, calming, and so on (i.e., they are coded by their ability to alter core affect, which is described below). Perception of affective qualities is not limited to emotional episodes but is a routine aspect of perceiving the world. In some cases, the dominant aspect of an emotional episode is its intentional object. People sometimes report that in extreme cases of fear they had no time to experience fear, that their attention was focused on the coiled snake, the car out of control, or the gun pointed at them. That is, in my terms, they did not form the emotional meta-experience of being afraid, but, rather, the dominant aspect of consciousness was the terrifying object—the snake, or car, or gun perceived largely in terms of its affective quality.

Core Affect

My concept of core affect has surprisingly often been misunderstood. Core affect is a part of what are commonly called emotions, feelings, and moods, but it is not synonymous with any of these. Thus, core affect is not a substitute term for *emotion*, nor is it the essence of emotion or an additional discrete emotion. For example, whereas emotional episodes are said to begin and then, after a short time, end, one is always in some state of core affect, which simply varies over time (sometimes slowly, sometimes rapidly) without beginning or end. Emotional episodes are typically directed at something (one is angry with, afraid of, or sad about something). In contrast, core affect is not necessarily directed at anything. Like mood, core affect per se can be free-floating (as in feeling down but not about anything and without knowing why), but it can come to be directed at something. Still, the everyday concept of mood typically implies a long lasting and mild state, whereas core affect has neither implication.

Core affect is "a neurophysiological state that is consciously accessible as a simple, non-reflective feeling that is an integral blend of hedonic (pleasure–displeasure) and arousal (sleepy–activated) values" (Russell, 2003a, p. 147). This seemingly simple definition contains a series of empirical proposals. First, calling core affect a neurophysiological state is a promissory note that so far has been left unfulfilled. The neural basis of core affect is an active research concern (Gerber et al., 2008; Posner, Russell, & Peterson, 2005; Barrett, Wilson-Mendenhall, & Barsalou, Chapter 4, this volume). There are some attractive leads (Kringelbach, 2010; Leknes & Tracey, 2008; Pfaff, 2006; Smith, Mahler, Peciña, & Berridge, 2010).

Second, this neurophysiological state has important functions. Core affect is a continuous assessment of one's current state, and it influences other psychological processes accordingly. A change in core affect evokes a search for its cause and therefore facilitates attention to and accessibility of like-valenced material. Core affect guides cognitive processing according to the principle of mood congruency. When core affect is positive, then events encountered, remembered, or envisioned tend to seem more positive— provided that the core affect is not attributed elsewhere (Schwarz & Clore, 1983). Core affect is part of the information used to estimate affective quality and is therefore implicated in incidental acquisition of preferences and attitudes. Core affect influences behavior, from reflexes to complex decision making. Core affect is a background state that continuously changes in response to a host of events, most beyond conscious monitoring. Core affect in turn provides a powerful bias in processing of new information. In this way, core affect is involved in one's current state, including what are conventionally distinguished as cognitive state, motivational state, mood state, and so on, including the past, the present, and forecasts of the future.

One can seek to alter or maintain core affect directly—*affect regulation*—from one's morning coffee to the evening brandy. People generally (but not always) seek behavioral options that maximize pleasure and minimize displeasure. Decisions therefore involve predictions of future core affect (March, 1978). Core affect is involved in motivation, reward, and reinforcement. An intriguing question is which of these functions requires conscious attention and which do not.

Third is the proposal that core affect is a state to which all humans have conscious access, although people do not always attend to it. When core affect is accessed, it is experienced as a simple, nonreflective feeling that is an integral blend of hedonic (pleasure–displeasure) and arousal (sleepy–activated) values. At the level of consciousness, core affect is simple in the sense that it cannot be decomposed at that level (although, of course, it can at a neurological level); that is, feeling good cannot be analyzed into simpler constituents. Rather, core affect is an elemental building block of other psychological events, such as feeling good about having an article accepted for publication. Core affect is therefore one ingredient of an emotional episode: It is the hedonic tone and subjective sense of energy or mobilization in the episode.

Concepts for types of emotional episode can be thought of as scripts, with actual instances varying in degree of prototypicality. Some instances are prototypical, which means that they resemble the script closely, but other instances resemble the script less, and some events may or may not be instances. The script often specifies core affect. Fear includes the anticipation of displeasure. Hope includes the anticipation of pleasure. Anger includes displeasure attributed to someone's blameworthy action. And so on.

Core affect is, at a psychological level, a preconceptual primitive process. Indeed, I tentatively hypothesized that core affect has many of the features of modularity (Faucher & Tappolet, 2008): fast, mandatory, unique output, an evolutionary explanation, dedicated brain circuitry, and encapsulation (Russell, 2006). This unitary view of core affect contrasts with some alternative views. For example, some have theorized many qualitatively different types of pleasure (multiplicity view; see Russell 2003b). Similarly, for the vertical dimension of arousal, others have theorized qualitatively different types of arousal. That core affect is encapsulated from general beliefs and desires is consistent with the common-sense idea that affect is involuntary. Core affect does not change simply because we desire it to change, or because we believe it will change. Instead, we must create conditions that then influence core affect.

At any point in time, people can answer the question, how do you feel? Studies of their answers have led to the concept of core affect. At a psychological level, core affect is the most elementary, simple, primitive affective feeling. A map of core affect is seen in Figure 8.1, which shows a circumplex representation of self-reported moods and feelings. A person's core affect at any one moment in time is represented by one point somewhere inside the space. Therefore, the person has only one core affect at a time. The center can be thought of as an adaptation level (a neutral point midway between pleasure and displeasure, and midway between low and high arousal), with distance from the center representing intensity or extremity of feeling. Core affect can be extremely intense at times, milder at other times.

Let me caution the reader against certain misinterpretations of Figure 8.1. Core affect is defined by bipolar dimensions, but it also can be broken into categories. For example, it includes feeling states that might be categorized as excitement (feels good + highly energized), serenity (feels good + low in energy), tension (feels bad + highly energized), and depression (feels bad + low in energy). In the previous sentence, the words *excitement, serenity, tension,* and *depression* are not used in their full senses, but only as shorthand for the specified combinations of pleasure and arousal. In the same way, the terms shown on the periphery of many empirical versions of the circumplex are not used in their full sense. More generally, core affect is part of, but not the whole of, the states labeled in the circumplex. Put differently, core affect is not the set of all states listed in a figure; rather, it is a feature of all those states. Furthermore, all token events called *fear,* for example, do not fall at the same point in core affect space.

Searle (1992) suggested thinking of consciousness as a single field that is modified. If so, core affect is one property of the field, a property that changes from time to time. Like sensations and perceptions, core affect is experienced as involuntary: It is given rather than chosen, but can be changed indirectly by creating conditions that alter it. A person is always in some state of core affect, just as a particular color falls at some point in the color space. That is, although its structural description requires two dimensions, core affect is a single feeling. This feature parallels the way a description of a particular color requires three dimensions (hue, saturation, and brightness), but the sensation of a particular color is a single sensation. In both cases, dimensions combine in an integral fashion to form the experience. The conscious side of core affect is primary consciousness (Farthing, 1992).

Core affect, when assessed through verbal report of conscious experience, has also been shown to be related to changes in the autonomic nervous

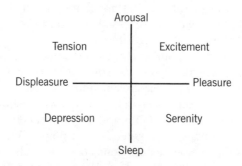

FIGURE 8.1. A circumplex representation of core affect.

system (ANS), facial and vocal behavior, instrumental behavior, cognitive processes, reflexes, and a host of other things (Russell, 2003a). Core affect is clearly related to stimulants, depressants, and euphoric and dysphoric drugs. These relations are all empirical discoveries rather than part of the definition of core affect.

The account of core affect I have just outlined is an empirically testable proposal currently under scrutiny. First is the hypothesis that core affect at the level of conscious experience can be represented by two dimensions. Others have proposed more or other dimensions such as power (Fontaine, Scherer, & Soriano, 2013).

Second, in the hypothesis of core affect, the dimensions of pleasure–displeasure and activation–deactivation are represented as independent of one another. Alternative representations are that pleasure is maximized at intermediate values of activation; that activation is equal to the intensity of pleasure or displeasure (activation is a V-shaped function of pleasure–displeasure); or that pleasure is equal to low activation, displeasure to high. An analysis of eight datasets found that (1) there is a weak but consistent V-shaped relationship of activation as a function of pleasure–displeasure at the nomothetic level, yet (2) there is large variation at the idiographic level, so that (3) activation and pleasure–displeasure can in principle show a variety of relationships depending on person or circumstances (Kuppens, Tuerlinckx, Russell, & Barrett, 2013).

Third, the hypothesis about core affect represents pleasure–displeasure as a single bipolar dimension. Correlational data from various sources had seemed to challenge the assumption of bipolarity; the alternative offered was independent dimensions of positive affect and negative affect. A more careful analysis of how bipolar dimensions are manifest in correlational data showed that the data were fully consistent with a single bipolar dimension (Russell & Carroll, 1999). A more recent challenge to bipolarity comes from experimental data (Larsen, McGraw, & Cacioppo, 2001), and the jury is still out on this issue.

Attributed Affect

When core affect is attributed to a cause, I name the resultant event *attributed affect*. Core affect is caused by both bottom-up and top-down processes (Ochsner et al., 2009). Sometimes a change in core affect results from a single salient event, but more typically core affect is multidetermined; it is a bottom-line assessment of one's current situation. The pleasure and arousal elicited by the event are not intrinsic properties of the event but experiences of a person. A mechanism is needed to bind the change in core affect to the event that elicited it. Although we often have a good idea of why we feel as we do, we sometimes do not, as shown by free-floating emotions and moods, and everyday feelings. Because there are usually too many influences on core affect for a person to track, and because some of those influences are beyond our ability to detect (e.g., infrasound), we can make mistakes about the cause of our core affect. Noting that people do not have conscious access to the origin of hedonic processes, Kringelbach (2010) suggested that people are "happy to confabulate about the causes" (p. 203). We attribute our core affect to a specific cause (Weiner, 1985), but we can get the cause wrong; indeed, the sheer number of influences on core affect suggests that we consistently oversimplify. That is, in philosophers' terms, attributed affect is not incorrigible. An interesting consequence of its corrigibility is that we can be wrong on just what emotion we perceive in ourselves (Neumann, 2000).

Emotion's Ingredients

The word *emotion* covers so many kinds of things that I earlier changed the book's first question to begin, "Emotional episodes are . . . " An emotional episode is any short-term episode that we call *emotional*. Because emotion includes dispositions, attitudes, occurrent events, and so on, the category of *emotional episode* is narrower and more tractable than the category of *emotion*. Still, emotional episode remains defined by an everyday word and therefore suffers from problems similar to those plaguing emotion. I therefore do not believe that we can formulate a theory for all and only emotional episodes: The psychology of emotional episodes is all of psychology. All the same, the set of emotional episodes includes all the cases of occurrent emotions that we think of as typical and that inspire emotion researchers. Emotional episodes must be explained.

Emotional episodes are real and important. They do not just happen; each is caused and organized. An emotional episode—even the clearest case—is a one-time event built on the fly. Each emotional episode is constructed out of simpler components (constituents or ingredients), which, in turn, are constructed out of even simpler components, and so on, down to the most minute level. Each emotional episode is a unique, complicated event in which the components change rapidly while interacting with each other, with other psychological processes, and with the surrounding environment in a way that is dependent on the history of the person undergoing that episode. Humans do not always passively undergo emotional episodes; they can actively seek them and steer them (Tamir, 2009).

By *component*, I mean an event that by itself an observer might take to be a sign of emotion: the core affect, emotional meta-experience, attributed affect, and perception of affective quality mentioned earlier plus appraisal, attribution, expression, and instrumental action. Each component in turn is the tip of the iceberg of a set of processes that often are nonconscious. I do not offer accounts of the components here but instead make five points. First, no one component defines or is essential to the emotional episode; rather the more components that resemble the script of a specific emotion, the more likely that episode will be categorized as that emotion. Second, the components do not necessarily occur in a fixed order. Third, none of these components is itself an emotion. Instead, components are processes, many of which are continuous, unfolding over time at their own pace while interacting collaboratively with each other, with other psychological processes, and with the external world, and dependent on prior conditions, both moment to moment and longer term. And fifth, the components must themselves be explained, as must relations among the components. A constructionist critique might well apply to the components I have posited: appraisal, attribution, and so forth. Perhaps these, too, fail to cut nature at the joints and need to be reconceptualized in terms of more basic processes. This is a project not just for affective psychology but for all of psychology, indeed for various sciences.

What do all and only emotional episodes have in common? They bear a family resemblance to one another, but what they and only they have in common is that our language community calls them *emotional*. (Thus, categorizing an event as *emotional* is based on its family resemblance to other events.) That is not to say that the person undergoing the emotional episode necessarily calls it emotional—just that someone would. Categorizing an episode as emotional is itself an important event.

What are the processes involved? I see no psychological process that can be excluded. (Of course, some events carry more weight than others in categorizing an event as emotional or as a specific type of emotion.) Accounting for these processes is surely a question for all of psychology. There is no necessary ingredient in an emotional episode, no single process that is or produces the episode in all cases, no fixed order of events. Even the list of ingredients that make up an emotional episode is not fixed. As persons move through their day, various interacting psychological processes continuously occur—sensation, perception, cognition, planning, and behaving. (Thus, psychological construction cannot be well represented by a flowchart of a few boxes connected by arrows.) Each ingredient in an emotional episode has its underlying physiological process that similarly occurs continuously. Emotion researchers have pointed to some of these processes as ingredients in emotional episodes, but I suspect that all psychological processes and their underlying physiology need to be included, with nothing excluded. Of course, a theory of "psychological processes" is no easy feat; indeed, it is a central quest for all of psychology. One implication of this line of reasoning is that scientific work on fear or any other type of emotion is replaced by questions about the episode's components and relations among them. Evidence of, for example, a subcortical circuit for fear raises the question of just which component(s) of a fear episode that circuit innervates. Similarly, evidence that fear has a certain effect raises the question of which component(s) is doing the work.

Emotions in Nonhuman Animals

The question of which species exhibit emotional episodes requires that we begin by asking about the function of each component in the episode, for different components serve different functions and likely appear in different species. Most of the components serve primitive functions— emotional behavior, perception of the external world, monitoring of the internal world, preparing for and executing actions. Thus, simple reflexes fall under the term *emotional behavior* (Panksepp, 2012) and are ancient. Appraisal processes typically serve to characterize the current situation, especially with respect to dimensions important to the organism. Appraisal defined abstractly occurs in any species with capacity to process information, although the specific aspects of appraisal vary with the species. Core affect serves to characterize one's own current self (core self) with respect to valence and arousal. This information is needed in the planning of behavior. Thus, I expect to find core affect in any species in which reflexes have been replaced with a more flexible behavioral repertoire. Attribution serves to link a change in core affect to its cause. Facial movements serve to enhance perception and to communicate behavioral intentions to an audience. Changes in the peripheral nervous system serve to prepare for action.

On the other hand, emotional meta-experience serves to categorize oneself with respect to important social norms and roles attached to culture-specific categories of emotion and to internalized standards of self. It might also require language and be limited to humans. In this regard, emotional meta-experience is similar to categorizing another as having an emotion.

Coordinating Emotional Episodes

There is no "common agent behind" emotional episodes: No emotion, faculty of mind, psychic entity, affect program, neural module, appraisal, act of labeling, conceptual act, bolt of lightning, or the like brings the components together and orchestrates them in all and only emotional episodes. Part of rejecting essentialism is rejecting a single cause to all and only emotional episodes. Thus, the components are not signs, indicators, or manifestations of an inferred agent, the emotion.

What coordinates the components? There is no orchestra leader for emotional episodes that does not coordinate nonemotional episodes. Like all human episodes, emotional episodes are coordinated by the brain, but there is no neural circuitry dedicated exclusively to all and only emotional episodes. LeDoux (2012) noted that it has long been known that the body is a highly integrated system that comprises multiple subsystems working in concert to sustain life, both moment to moment and over longer time periods. A major function of the brain is to coordinate the activity of all the body's various subsystems. Indeed, a neuroscientific account of each of the component processes and their coordination is a much needed complement to the psychological account. Gazzaniga (1995) noted that although the brain produces a unified, coordinated pattern, there is no single coordinating mechanism: no orchestra leader.

This question illustrates the gravitational pull of intuition on our assumptions about emotion. In the folk psychology of emotion, an emotion is a psychic entity that triggers a pattern of manifestations. For example, fear triggers activation of a fear-specific pattern in the ANS, a facial expression, flight, and so on. This assumption of an orchestra leader—a common cause to fear-specific components—implies high correlations among those components. Empirical evidence has consistently found just the opposite, low correlations. What correlations exist can be explained without assuming a common cause. The external world has a correlational structure that influences the correlation among components. Components influence one another. Multiple components are influenced by the same nonemotional mechanisms, such as attention. We must also take into account the observer: To be categorized as an instance of fear, the instance must at least some extent resemble the fear script, in which all the prototypical components co-occur.

Defining Emotion

Each author was asked which combinations of ingredients are emotion. We can also ask which combinations are anger? Which are fear? And so on. These seemingly simple questions have yet to achieve consensual answers. Indeed, they are a perpetual thorn in the side of emotion researchers. The questions may be perplexing because the terms *emotion, anger, fear*, and so on, are used in two distinct ways: in everyday discourse by everyday folk, and as technical terms by scientists to express scientific concepts (Russell, 1991b). The different uses yield different answers to the question. I consider each use in turn.

Descriptive Definitions

Because all these questions are framed in terms of English words, such as *emotion, anger, fear*, and so on, the questions concern the semantics of English. Emphasizing that *emotion* and the rest are English words is not simply being pedantic. The nearest equivalent terms in other languages have somewhat different meanings (Wierzbicka, 1999; Russell & Sato, 1995; Russell, 1991a). As everyday terms, they (or something like them) have been in common use for centuries by everyone, and scientists need to understand them.

For descriptive definitions, we need to discover their meaning in every-day natural language, because the everyday concepts named *emotion, fear*, and so on—like those named *water, witch, weatherman, wallet*, or *wizard*—play a role in everyday thinking and other psychological processes, including emotional episodes. As everyday concepts, *emotion, fear*, and so on, look much like other concepts studied by Rosch (1975) that do not fit the classical mold but instead show blurry borders and degrees of membership. Thus, although some episodes are prototypical cases of emotion, many are mediocre or borderline examples. Similarly, although some episodes are prototypical cases of fear, love, jealousy, and the rest, many episodes are mediocre or borderline examples. Many episodes fit no single emotion category well. All the same, a person's perception that he or she is afraid, in love, or jealous (or *amae, song, fago*, or *liget*) is an important and influential event, fully worthy of study. *Emotion* and other concepts thus remain in my account but only as everyday concepts, because, as concepts, they play an actual role as in, for example, emotional meta-experience and the perception of emotion in others, which in turn play a role in social interactions.

Because everyday concepts of emotion are open ended, with no sharp boundaries, we can offer various approximations rather than precise descriptive definitions. As a first approximation, earlier I pointed to some terms that can be defined as a first approximation by core affect, as illustrated in Figure 8.1. Other terms require a more elaborate first approximation, which can be achieved by specifying both core affect and its cause. *Triumph* is excitement caused by success; *fear* is tension caused by anticipation of displeasure. *Relief* is serenity caused by nonoccurrence of an anticipated displeasure; *sorrow* is depression caused by a loss. Other terms require core affect plus cause plus behavior or motive to behave. *Anger* is distress caused by some blameworthy action plus a motive to aggress (for more elaborate characterizations of individual emotion concepts, see Ortony, Clore & Collins, 1990; Wierzbicka, 1999).

Prescriptive Definitions

For scientific purposes, researchers have borrowed *emotion, anger, fear*, and so forth, for use as technical terms in their theories, a role often played by everyday concepts in the early stages of science. Having done so, researchers then ask how to define these terms, but it is often unclear whether the definitions typically offered are meant to be descriptive or prescriptive. As a scientific term, *emotion* is separated from *not-emotion* (or *fear* from *not-fear*, etc.) in a precise way only by stipulation. I therefore suggest that we begin to move away from these everyday words as technical terms. If we do so, we would not need to define *emotion* prescriptively; that is, we would not need to stipulate a scientific definition that states the boundaries of the set of events to be explained, because *emotion* is given no scientific work to do. For example, my concept of core affect is not defined in terms of emotion. On the other hand, *emotional episode* does contain the word *emotional*. Emotional episodes must be explained, because all human episodes must be explained, and not because emotional episodes are qualitatively different from nonemotional episodes, whatever those might be. In other words, the goal of psychological construction is an account that includes, but is not exclusive to, all events labeled as *emotional*. So, in my account of emotional episodes, *emotion* functions something like a chapter heading and does not function as a technical term.

To illustrate, consider the scientific status of the concept of a *house*. All houses (whether palace, mansion, shack, toy house, birdhouse, or houseboat) conform to the laws of physics, and the builder of houses does well to take those laws into account. Houses are real, but, all the same, *house* is not a technical term in physics. Similarly, speaking colloquially, we say that Jack was angry; Jill was afraid. All the phenomena remain in my account, and what is at issue are the technical terms in affective science. Bickle (2012) termed this philosophical stance *eliminative materialism with a small e*. Emotional episodes are simply an especially interesting and important subset of human episodes, much as houses are an interesting and important subset of physical systems.

ACKNOWLEDGMENTS

I thank Sherri Widen, Joe Pochedly, Erin Heitzman, Nicole Trauffer, Joshua Rottman, James Dungan, Cecilea Mun, and Jordan Theriault for their comments on a draft of this chapter. This study was funded by a grant from the National Science Foundation (No. 1025563).

REFERENCES

Aviezer, H., Trope, Y., & Todorov, A. (2012). Body cues, not facial expressions, discriminate basic emotion theoryween intense positive and negative emotions. *Science, 338,* 1225–1229.

Barfield, O. (1954). *History in English words.* London: Methuen.

Bickle, J. (2012). Lessons for affective science from a metascience of "molecular and cellular cognition." In P. Zachar & R. D. Ellis (Eds.), *Categorical versus dimensional models of affect: A seminar on the theories of Panksepp and Russell* (pp. 175–188). Amsterdam: Benjamins.

Buss, D. M. (in press). Evolutionary criteria for considering an emotion "basic": Jealousy as an illustration. *Emotion Review.*

Carroll, J. M., & Russell, J. A. (1996). Do facial expressions express specific emotions?: Judging emotion from the face in context. *Journal of Personality and Social Psychology, 70,* 205–218.

Carroll, J. M., & Russell, J. A. (1997). Facial expressions in Hollywood's portrayal of emotion. *Journal of Personality and Social Psychology, 72,* 164–176.

Clore, G. L., & Ortony, A. (2008) Appraisal theories: How cognition shapes affect into emotion. In M. Lewis, J. M. Haviland-Jones, & L. F. Barrett (Eds.), *Handbook of emotions* (pp. 628–642). New York: Guilford Press.

Farthing, G. W. (1992). *The psychology of consciousness.* Englewood Cliffs, NJ: Prentice-Hall.

Faucher, L., & Tappolet, C. (Eds.). (2008). *The modularity of emotions.* Calgary, Canada: University of Calgary Press.

Fehr, B., & Russell, J. A. (1984). Concept of emotion viewed from a prototype perspective. *Journal of Experimental Psychology: General, 113,* 464–486.

Fehr, B., & Russell, J. A. (1991). The concept of love viewed from a prototype perspective. *Journal of Personality and Social Psychology, 60,* 425–438.

Fehr, B., Russell, J. A., & Ward, L. M. (1982). Prototypicality of emotions: A reaction time study. *Bulletin of the Psychonomic Society, 20,* 253–254.

Fernandez-Dols, J. M., & Crivelli, C. (2013). Emotion and expression: Naturalistic studies. *Emotion Review, 5,* 24–29.

Fernandez-Dols, J. M., & Ruiz-Belda, M. A. (1995). Are smiles a sign of happiness?: Gold medal winners at the Olympic Games. *Journal of Personality and Social Psychology, 69,* 1113–1119.

Fontaine, J. R. J., Scherer, K. R., & Soriano, C. (2013). *Components of emotional meaning: A sourcebook.* Oxford, UK: Oxford University Press.

Gazzaniga, M. S. (1995). Principles of human brain organization derived from split-brain studies. *Neuron, 14*(2), 217–228.

Gendron, M., & Barrett, L. F. (2009). Reconstructing the past: A century of ideas about emotion in psychology. *Emotion Review, 1,* 316–339.

Gerber, A. J., Posner, J., Gorman, D., Colibazzi, T., Yu, S., Wang, Z., et al. (2008). An affective circumplex model of neural systems subserving valence, arousal, and cognitive overlay during the appraisal of emotional faces. *Neuropsychologia, 46,* 2129–2139.

Hassin, R. R., Aviezer, H., & Bentin, S. (2013). Inherently ambiguous: Facial expressions of emotions, in context. *Emotion Review, 5,* 60–65.

Hurtado de Mendoza, A., Fernandez Dols, J. M., Parrott, W. G., & Carrera, P. (2010). Emotion terms, category structure, and the problem of translation: The case of *shame* and *verguenza. Cognition and Emotion, 24*(4), 661–680.

Izard, C. E. (1994). Innate and universal facial expressions: Evidence from developmental and cross-cultural research. *Psychological Bulletin, 115,* 288–299

Jack, R. E., Blais, C., Scheepers, C., Schyns, P. G., & Caldara, R. (2009). Cultural confusions show that facial expressions are not universal. *Current Biology, 19*(18), 1543–1548.

James, W. (1950). *The principles of psychology.* New York: Dover. (Original work published 1890)

Kringelbach, M. L. (2010). The hedonic brain: A functional neuroanatomy of human pleasure. In M. L. Kringelbach & K. C. Berridge (Eds.), *Pleasures of the brain* (pp. 202–221). Oxford, UK: Oxford University Press.

Kuppens, P., Tuerlinckx, F., Russell, J. A., & Barrett, L. F. (2013). The relationship between valence and arousal in subjective experience. *Psychological Bulletin, 139,* 917–940.

Lakatos, I. (1970). Falsification and the methodology of scientific research programs. In I. Lakatos & A. Musgrave (Eds.), *Criticism and the growth of knowledge* (pp. 91–195). Cambridge, UK: Cambridge University Press.

Larsen, J., McGraw, A. P., & Cacioppo, J. (2001). Can people feel happy and sad at the same time? *Journal of Personality and Social Psychology, 81*(4), 684–696.

LeDoux, J. (2012). Rethinking the emotional brain. *Neuron, 73*(4), 653–676.

Leknes, S., & Tracey, I. (2008). A common neurobiology for pain and pleasure. *Nature Reviews Neuroscience, 9,* 313–320.

March, J. (1978). Bounded rationality, ambiguity and the engineering of choice. *Bell Journal of Economics, 9,* 587–608.

Nelson, N., & Russell, J. A. (2013). Universality revisited. *Emotion Review, 5*(1), 8–15.

Neumann, R. (2000). The causal influences of attributions on emotions: A procedural priming approach. *Psychological Science, 11,* 179–182.

Oatley, K., & Johnson-Laird, P. N. (1987). Towards a cognitive theory of emotions. *Cognition and Emotion, 1,* 29–50.

Ochsner, K. N., Ray, R. R., Hughes, B., McRae, K., Cooper, J. C., Weber, J., et al. (2009). Bottom-up and top-down processes in emotion generation common and distinct neural mechanisms. *Psychological Science, 20*(11), 1322–1331.

Ortony, A., Clore, G. L., & Collins, A. (1990). *The cognitive structure of emotions.* Cambridge, UK: Cambridge University Press.

Ortony, A., & Turner, T. J. (1990). What's basic about basic emotions? *Psychological Review, 97*(3), 315.

Panksepp, J. (2012). In defense of multiple core affects. In P. Zachar & R. Ellis (Eds.), *Categorical versus dimensional models of affect: A seminar on the theories of Panksepp and Russell* (pp. 31–78). Amsterdam: Benjamins.

Pfaff, D. (2006). *Brain arousal and information theory: Neural and genetic mechanisms.* Cambridge, MA: Harvard University Press.

Posner, J., Russell, J. A., & Peterson, B. S. (2005). A circumplex model of affect: An integrative approach to affective neuroscience, cognitive development, and psychopathology. *Development and Psychopathology, 17,* 715–734.

Reisenzein, R., Studmann, M., & Horstmann, G. (2013). Coherence between emotion and facial expression: Evidence from laboratory experiments. *Emotion Review, 5,* 16–23.

Rosch, E. (1975). Cognitive representations of semantic categories. *Journal of Experimental Psychology: General, 104*(3), 192–233.

Russell, J. A. (1991a). Culture and the categorization of emotion. *Psychological Bulletin, 110,* 426–450.

Russell, J. A. (1991b). Natural language concepts of emotion. In D. J. Ozer, J. M.

Healy, Jr., & A. J. Stewart (Eds.), *Perspectives in personality: Self and emotion* (pp. 119–137). London: Jessica Kingsley.

Russell, J. A. (1994). Is there universal recognition of emotion from facial expression?: A review of the cross-cultural studies. *Psychological Bulletin, 115,* 102–141.

Russell, J. A. (1997) Reading emotion from and into faces: Resurrecting a dimensional-contextual perspective. In J. A. Russell & J. M. Fernandez-Dols (Eds.), *The psychology of facial expression* (pp. 295–320). New York: Cambridge University Press.

Russell, J. A. (2003a). Core affect and the psychological construction of emotion. *Psychological Review, 110,* 145–172.

Russell, J. A. (2003b). Introduction: The return of pleasure. *Cognition and Emotion, 17,* 161–165.

Russell, J. A. (2006). Emotions are not modules. *Canadian Journal of Philosophy, 36,* 53–71.

Russell, J. A., & Carroll, J. M. (1999). On the bipolarity of positive and negative affect. *Psychological Bulletin, 125,* 3–30.

Russell, J. A., & Fehr, B. (1987). Relativity in the perception of emotion in facial expressions. *Journal of Experimental Psychology: General, 116,* 223–237.

Russell, J. A., & Fehr, B. (1994). Fuzzy concepts in a fuzzy hierarchy: Varieties of anger. *Journal of Personality and Social Psychology, 67,* 186–205.

Russell, J. A., & Sato, K. (1995). Comparing emotion words between languages. *Journal of Cross-Cultural Psychology, 26,* 384–391.

Schwarz, N., & Clore, G. L. (1983). Mood, misattribution, and judgments of well-being: Informative and directive functions of affective states. *Journal of Personality and Social Psychology, 45,* 513–523.

Searle, J. R. (1992). *The rediscovery of the mind.* Cambridge, MA: MIT Press.

Smith, K. S., Mahler, S. V., Peciña, S., & Berridge, K. (2010). Hedonic hotspots: Generating Sensory pleasure in the brain. In M. L. Kringelbach & K. C. Berridge (Eds.), *Pleasures in the brain* (pp. 27–49). Oxford, UK: Oxford University Press.

Tamir, M. (2009). What do people want to feel and why?: Pleasure and utility in emotion regulation. *Current Directions in Psychological Science, 18(2),* 101–105.

Weiner, B. (1985). An attributional theory of achievement, motivation, and emotion. *Psychological Review, 92,* 548–573.

Widen, S. C. (2013). Children's interpretation of facial expressions: The long path from valence-based to specific discrete categories. *Emotion Review, 5,* 72–77.

Widen, S. C., & Russell, J. A. (2013). Children's recognition of disgust in others. *Psychological Bulletin, 139(2),* 271–299.

Wierzbicka, A. (1999). *Emotions across languages and cultures: Diversity and universals.* Cambridge, UK: Cambridge University Press.

Yik, M., Widen, S. C., & Russell, J. A. (2013). The within-subject design in the study of facial expressions. *Cognition and Emotion, 27,* 1062–1072.

CHAPTER 9

Emotions as Emergent Variables

JAMES A. COAN
MARLEN Z. GONZALEZ

> In order to find the real artichoke, we have divested it of its leaves.
> —WITTGENSTEIN (2010, p. 164)

Few scientific puzzles are as emotionally charged as the question of what emotions *are*. To some, emotions are subjectively experienced by-products of contextually controlled bodily responses (James, 1884), or useful labels to describe the interaction between gross physiological responses and prevailing circumstances (Schachter & Singer, 1962; Barret 2006a). Others regard the wide variety of emotions as deriving from a small set of human universals (Ekman, Rolls, Perrett, & Ellis, 1992) that might be reducible to discrete, phylogenetically determined circuits in the brain (Panksepp, 1998). The duration and intensity of arguments about what constitutes a "real emotion" reveal an important psychological perspective on the question itself: emotions, it seems, *matter*. And they should. Once seen as the unwanted by-products of otherwise rational creatures, contemporary psychology now suggests that emotional processes are integral to both our psychological well-being and physiological health (Diener, Sapyta, & Suh, 1998; Salovey, Rothman, Detweiler, & Steward, 2000). They are central to the dynamics of our interpersonal relationships (Coan & Gottman, 2007), and likely play a critical role in the success of traditionally "cold" cognitive acts such as decision making (Bechara, Damasio,

1. *If emotions are psychological events constructed from more basic ingredients, then what are the key ingredients from which emotions are constructed? Are they specific to emotion or are they general ingredients of the mind? Which, if any, are specific to humans?*

Emotions are likely built from basic units of the mind that are not unique to emotions per se. Although we cannot measure the contents of the mind directly, we generally accept self-reports, physiological markers, overt behaviors, and, increasingly, patterns of neural activity as reasonably good *indicators* of an emotion response. We say "reasonably good" because, in isolation, each indicator is compromised by errors of measurement that place limits on reliability and, therefore, validity, but the impact of measurement error can be tempered when multiple indicators are combined in a single model. For example, self-reports can be highly unreliable as measures of emotional experience. But even more "objective" measurements, such as physiological arousal and neural activation, introduce other risks, most notably errors of causal inference (Cacioppo, Tassinary, & Berntson, 2007). Highly similar patterns of central and autonomic activity can result from highly *dis*similar stimulus conditions (Cacioppo et al., 2003), as can be seen when many neuroimaging studies implicate the anterior cingulate and insular cortices in a diverse range of regulatory, behavioral, physiological, and experiential phenomena beyond just emotion (Allman, Hakeem, Erwin, Nimchinsky, & Hof, 2001; Craig, 2009). The evolving story of the amygdala may offer the quintessential illustration of this problem. Once thought to be "the seat of fear" in the brain, it turns out that the amygdala (1) becomes active for many reasons, and (2) is in any case better understood as a bundle of dissociable nuclei dedicated to a diverse array of activity (Hariri & Whalen, 2011). Similarly, electromyographic (EMG) data on emotional facial expressions reveal no muscular patterns for specific emotional states other than broad dimensions of valence and arousal (Cacioppo, Berntson, Larsen, Poehlmann, & Ito, 2000).

2. *What brings these ingredients together in the construction of an emotion? Which combinations are emotions and which are not (and how do we know)?*

If emotions do not occupy well-defined origins in the brain or body, then we must look elsewhere for sources of organization among emotion indicators. A strong candidate for this is the constellation of demands in a specific context (Barrett, 2006a). For example, encountering a bear in the woods may require high levels of vigilance, the mobilization of physiological resources, and a strong behavioral tendency to run, but viewing a bear at the zoo poses fewer risks and commensurably fewer demands—at most, one might become more vigilant for potential trouble. However, if the ultimate emotion that occurs is yoked to the demands of a situation, then perhaps there would be as many emotions as there are situations. Seeing a bear in an obvious plexiglass enclosure may have a totally different set of demands—hence, a different emotion—than

(continued)

seeing a bear in an open enclosure where there appears to be no barrier between oneself and the bear. The problem of locating "fear" in affective space is then compounded, for which bear-related situation results in fear per se, and which does not? Are life or death situations the only *real* fear-evoking situations? Can a quickening heartbeat and a subjective report of fear be said not to represent *real* fear? One resolution to this problem may be to talk about "fuzzy sets" of emotional categories that share some situational, behavioral, physiological, and experiential properties—that the gradient between levels of fear is not strictly binary. Conceptually, this view is similar to Ekman's (1992) notion of "emotion families" and Scherer's (1994) idea of "modal emotions"—those more common emotions that arise because some human situations are themselves more common than others. Ultimately, it is difficult to say whether any psychological state is absolutely devoid of emotional content given that all stimuli seem to be initially evaluated for their harmfulness or helpfulness (Cunningham & Zelazo, 2007). And if emotion experience is the conscious awareness of our response to situational demands, then we may again be back to William James's pragmatism, in which an experience is encoded as emotional because it is important to our goals, our learning, and our language (Barrett, 2006a; Scherer, 2009).

3. *How important is variability (across instances within an emotion category, and in the categories that exist across cultures)? Is this variance epiphenomenal or a thing to be explained? To the extent that it makes sense, it would be desirable to address issues such as universality and evolution.*

In considering evidence for or against either the latent or emergent variable models, it is vitally important to consider—and measure—key sources of variability. At a minimum, these sources likely include the specifics of given situations, cultural background, specific and putatively emotional behavior, the emotion category, and individual differences. From the perspective of the latent variable model, most of the variability in emotional responding should lie with the emotion categories. That is, there should be tremendous variability across emotions (e.g., fear should be very different from anger), but relatively little variability *within* emotions across cultures and individuals. It could be that variability across situations would covary strongly with variability in emotions, especially if we view the phylogeny of emotional states as stereotypical responses to key situations (e.g., threats, opportunities, loss). But, according to this view, even variability across situations could in theory be limited if it were possible to stimulate the neural systems supporting specific, stereotyped emotions directly. Presumably, this would result, again, in highly differentiated emotional states regardless of the situation. By contrast, the emergent variable perspective suggests that most of the variability in emotional responses would derive from differences in situational demands, with relatively little variation within cultures and individuals. Moreover, because situations and not specific neural circuits organize emotional responses, it would not make sense to think

(continued)

of variability across emotions per se. This suggests further that emotional invariance across situations, given direct neural stimulation, would be extremely difficult and potentially impossible. That said, the emergent variable model can accommodate a wider range of cultural influences, because culture can have a marked impact on the construal of situational demands. Importantly, the research to date has not strongly evaluated either the latent or emergent variable model. It is true that the latent variable model makes stronger claims and is beholden to more restrictive parameters than the emergent variable model. However, it would be a mistake to view the relative lack of supporting evidence for the latent variable model as evidence in itself supporting the emergent variable model, or vice versa.

4. *What constitutes strong evidence to support a psychological construction to emotion? Point to or summarize empirical evidence that supports your model or outline what a key experiment would look like. What would falsify your model?*

Importantly, strong support for the emergent variable model of emotion *necessarily* involves predicting important outcomes. This is why we have framed our discussion of the latent and emergent models in terms of SEM and MANOVA. From either statistical perspective, it is only actually possible to model—hence, *measure*—an emergent variable if we can assign *weights* to the emergent variable's indicators, and this will only be possible if there is some criterion against which those weights are being estimated that is extrinsic to the emergent variable itself. Indeed, we prefer the SEM approach, because it is more stringent in its measurement demands. Specifically, if we are going to use SEM to estimate an emergent variable model of emotion, then the structural model into which the emergent variable is embedded must be *identified* (MacCallum & Browne, 1993), which requires in turn that it predict at least two important outcomes. Here, *identification* refers to a computational requirement of the overall model, which is that a unique solution exists for each of the model's parameters. At a minimum, this usually requires that the number of estimable parameters not exceed the number of observations in the variance–covariance matrix. If this requirement is not met, the model is essentially unsolvable. Thus far, we have expressed some basic requirements of a kind of "existence proof" for emergent variables in purely statistical terms, but Figueredo (1998) has described an ontological analogue to the statistics, which he calls "emergent entitivity." At bottom, emergent entitivity requires the same evidence as the SEM restrictions described earlier. That is, it suggests that an emergent variable must *matter*, which is to say that it must have consequences that are important to us. On the one hand, if our emergent variable does not predict important outcomes, then we have no criteria against which to estimate the model's parameters. On the other hand, if there are no obvious consequences to the estimation of our emergent variable, then there is little (or no) logical justification for estimating it in the first place.

& Damasio, 2000), individual economic behavior (Sanfey, Rilling, Aronson, Nystrom, & Cohen, 2003), and even the activity of markets (Ackert, Church, & Deaves, 2003).

Recent years have seen a modern iteration of debates on the question of what emotions are. Although belief in basic affective programs has long held sway, psychological constructionist points of views have posed real challenges at both the theoretical and methodological levels (e.g., Barrett 2006b; Barrett et al., 2007; Lindquist, Wager, Kober, Bliss-Moreau, & Barrett, 2012). The constructionist view suggests that emotions are not in any lawful sense located in specific neural circuits or predictable physiological responses; rather, they *emerge* from the confluence of core affect, other basic nonspecific processes, and our categorization of the holistic experience as an instance of an emotion (Barrett, 2012; Russell, 2003). For example, Barrett (2006b) has argued that anger is not an absolute entity but an "emergent phenomenon" that exists as an interaction between context and perception.

As a practical matter, most emotion research has assumed measurement models that preclude the study of constructionist models. The best example of this is what we call the *latent variable model* of emotion, which assumes a central emotion circuit whose variation precedes variation in its various measured indicators. As reviewed in more detail below, moderate to high covariation between measured indicators is assumed in these models, but it is rarely tested. By contrast, what we call the *emergent variable model* posits that emotions do not cause, but rather *are caused by*, their measured indicators. In the emergent variable model, variation in measured indicators is assumed to precede rather than follow variation in the emotion itself, requiring no assumption of covariation among those indicators, and no need for some central neural circuit. We argue that the emergent variable model can incorporate the contextual flexibility in emotion that is predicted by psychological constructionist views (Barrett, 2011), while accommodating results supporting latent variable views. Importantly, the emergent variable model of emotion does not exclude the possibility of high covariation between elements, which would support theories of emotion circuits or networks.

Below, we argue that emergent measurement models offer the opportunity to move from philosophical debates about the nature of emotion to empirical tests of competing measurement models of emotion. We first discuss the study of emotion as a measurement problem, using "fear" as an example. Next, we discuss what we mean when we say that emotions might be "emergent phenomena," and apply our discussions of measurement and emergence to the emergent measurement model. From there, we review the qualities and limitations of the traditional latent variable model, as applied to emotion. Finally, we discuss how emergent models may be more accommodating of observed emotional phenomena than latent variable models.

Measuring Emotion

As with many psychological concepts, we measure "emotions" through proxies or *indicators* in order to determine the presence and/or intensity of the psychological experience. Although emotion theorists may not agree on much, there is at least implicit agreement that emotional states or processes can be inferred through measuring physiological changes, behavioral action tendencies or expressive behavior, and subjective experience. Although it will seem (and indeed *is*) overly simplistic (Kievet et al., 2011; Barrett, 2011), we use these four domains to construct the models of emotion discussed below. For example, *fear*, whether seen as a "natural kind" or a useful social category, depending on the study and the laboratory (and often enough the a priori assumptions about what constitutes a likely fear stimulus), has often corresponded with changes in the amygdala, autonomic arousal, avoidance behavior, and the subjective experience of being afraid. This is not to say that there are no other potential indicators of fear, or that the indicators just mentioned necessarily suggest an instance of fear. Indeed, in our simplified model, it is possible that subjective experience is the only unique factor when comparing "fear" to, say, "anger." Nevertheless, most researchers would agree that amygdala activation, autonomic arousal, avoidance behavior, and subjective fear experiences are each at least *plausibly* (though not necessarily) linked to fear as a construct, so we use these imperfect indicators to ground the forthcoming discussion.

Emergence

Emergent properties arise from the interactions or co-instances of a collection of concrete, directly measureable constituent elements (Coan, 2010; McClelland, 2010; Barrett, 2011); the colloquial equivalent is to say that something is "more than the sum of its parts"(Laughlin, 2005). Another way to describe emergence is to say that the properties of the whole—of the components in interaction—are not observed in any of its components per se. For example, water is made of hydrogen and oxygen, yet water's property of wetness can be found neither in oxygen nor in hydrogen.

Philosophers have distinguished between *weak* and *strong* emergence, and the distinction serves as a useful point of entry into the view of emergence we endorse. In weak emergence, a combination of elements may yield surprising or unexpected results, but the path from the emergent whole back to its elements can be more or less understood. Weak forms of emergence can be nothing more complex than a linear combination of causes (Bollen, 2002; Bollen & Davis, 2009)—the main criterion being that variation in the emergent variable follows variation in its measured indicators. The construct of *socioeconomic status* (SES) is a good example of this.

In SES, variation in parental education levels and personal income self-evidently precede variation in SES itself (Bollen & Davis, 2009). And SES is *useful* to us, because it predicts important outcomes that are relatively independent of each of its indicators in isolation. For example, individuals with high SES have substantially increased access to important people and institutions, while individuals with low SES are at risk for a number of social, psychological, and medical problems. It is possible to construe weakly emergent variables as little more than categories that are useful for organizing or classifying clusters of phenomena—that exist in our lexicon mainly for their usefulness and are "real" only to the extent that people agree to regard them as such (Hacking, 1999). For example, the concept of *city* eases communication about the size, structure, and number of people living in one geographical location. By contrast, strong emergence suggests that emergent phenomena are qualitative shifts that are at once irreducible to and "nondeducible" from the properties of their constituent elements (e.g., Chalmers, 2006). This is to say that even if one can find the constituent elements, the path from constituent elements to the emergent properties is either unknown or unknowable. An example of this might be consciousness, which has no obvious single substrate in the brain but nevertheless seems to be a property of the brain.

These views may strike readers as more philosophical than empirical. But measurement models are beholden to logical as well as statistical imperatives, and are often grounded in philosophical arguments (Coan, 2010; Barrett, 2011). Our own philosophical perspective is that emergent emotional phenomena are (1) *relatively* irreducible (e.g., not merely simple linear combinations of causes or conceptual conveniences); (2) entities whose variation is preceded by variation in their measured indicators; and (3) entities that are practically as well as theoretically *useful*. It may seem counterintuitive to construe a construct as being caused by rather than causing variation in its features. Still, the emergent variable model presented below may provide a step toward better measurement of emotional phenomena.

The Emergent Variable Model

Figure 9.1 depicts an emergent variable model of "fear" using the language of structural equation modeling (SEM). For illustration purposes, we have chosen two physiological measurements, autonomic arousal and amygdala activation, a measure of behavioral action tendencies (fleeing or freezing) and a measure of subjective experience through self-report. Each of these indicators has been implicated in the study of fear, as well as many other putative emotional states (e.g., Collet, Vernet-Maury, Delhomme, & Dittmar, 1997; Costafreda, Brammer, David, & Fu, 2008; Adolphs, 2013).

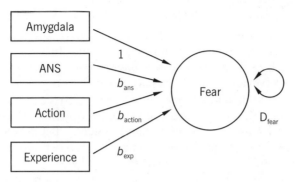

Fear = Amygdala + b_{ans}ANS + b_{action}Action + b_{exp}Experience + D_{fear}

FIGURE 9.1. A proposed emergent variable model of fear.

This list does not constitute an argument that there are no other—or no better—potential indicators of fear, or that they *necessarily* suggest an instance of fear. Rather, it is simply safe to say that, for this discussion, most would agree that amygdala activation, autonomic arousal, avoidance behavior, and subjective fear experiences are each at least plausibly linked to fear as a construct, regardless of one's theoretical perspective.

In this emergent variable model, "fear" is depicted using a circle, which in the graphical language of SEM indicates that it is a hypothetical construct that cannot be measured directly. Instead, it is detected through the measurement of its indicators—depicted in graphical SEM language using rectangles. The direction of the arrows from indicators to latent construct suggests causal direction and, hence, that variation in indicators precedes variation in fear. From this perspective, we can derive the following assumptions:

1. Fear is a relatively irreducible property of the co-occurrence of, and interaction among, amygdala activation, autonomic nervous system (ANS) arousal, withdrawal/freezing behavior, and subjective experience, as well as other unmeasured or immeasurable indicators.
2. There are no fear-specific neural circuits or networks.
3. The goal of affective neuroscience is to identify the neural, contextual, and experiential variables that give rise to an instance of fear.

The emergent variable model of emotion is roughly compatible with the component process and conceptual act models of Scherer (1984) and Barrett (2006a), respectively. In the component process model, an emotion experience is contingent on the appraisals of prevailing contextual demands. That is, variation in fairly dissociable indicators precedes the emotion experience. The level of coactivation or coherence among emotion indicators is determined by ongoing evaluations of stimuli in the environment, particularly the degree to which stimuli are novel, pleasant, aligned with current goals, manageable within the limits of current resources, and compatible with normative expectations (Scherer, 1982, 1984). The component process model is not, strictly speaking, a psychological constructionist theory of emotion even if it is consistent with an emergent variable view. Instead, the component process model suggests a lawful sequence in individual appraisal processes, that the synchrony between processes *is* what determines the presence or absence of an emotion, and that emotions are only mildly constructed, in that the categorization of nonverbal appraisal processes allows for situation-dependent meaning (Scherer, 2004, 2009).

Barrett's conceptual act model (see Barrett, Wilson-Mendenhall, & Barsalou, Chapter 4, this volume) is a true psychological constructionist view of emotions. In the conceptual act model, emotions are emergent phenomena comprised of discreet mental events that themselves are not specific to any emotion (Barrett, 2006a). Such mental events can include core affect (the goodness or badness of things), language, higher-order conceptualizations of social and situational context (schemas), and executive control. These elements are always combining to create mental states, only some of which are emotions (Barrett, 2006a; Barrett, 2012; Barrett, Mesquita, Ochsner, & Gross, 2007). Because variation in these elements always precedes variation in the emotion category, it is consistent with an emergent variable model.

These theoretical stances strongly emphasize the organizing properties of context—how the components of any emotional response are recruited to solve perceived contextual problems. It is the patterning of these problem–solution pairings, as well as the subjective experience of them, that combine to determine a given emotional state (Barrett 2006a; Scherer, 2001). Within this broad view, there has been some debate about whether the number of emotions is relatively fixed (Lazarus, 1991) or at least potentially infinite (Scherer, 1984, 2000). But Scherer has argued that any point of view permits a relatively small number of *modal emotions*—those that are more common not because of phylogenetically determined neural circuitry but because of the high frequency of certain situations in human experience (Scherer, 1994). In this way, modal emotions, such as fear, occupy imprecisely defined classes or "fuzzy sets" (e.g., Zadeh, 1965).

Following the causal direction of the arrows in Figure 9.1, the emergent variable model posits just this point of view. Here, the variability in the indicators is not caused by the hypothetical construct; rather, it *causes* variability in the construct. In this way, emergent variable models of emotion can be considered *formative*. The direction of causality dismisses the classical assumption that indicators must be positively correlated, although, critically in our view, it is flexible enough to permit the possibility (Bollen, 1984). Finally, error variance estimates are not assigned to the indicators themselves. Instead, model error is captured by what is called a *disturbance* term, or D_{fear}. In the emergent variable model, all indicator variances and covariances are treated as model parameters, and all measurement errors are manifest in the disturbance, which represents the remaining, unmeasured causes integral to the construct (Diamantopoulos, Riefler, & Roth, 2008). A large disturbance term constitutes poor score reliability among indicators. This is similar to multivariate analysis of variance (MANOVA), which makes use of possibly uncorrelated but individually reliable indicators to create a mathematically derived linear composite (Hancock & Mueller, 2006).

B weights are assigned to each indicator (strictly speaking, *causal* variables). In our example, the *b* weight of amygdala activity is fixed to 1 to create a scale for the emergent fear variable. There is no expectation that an increase in amygdala activity should coincide with an increase in other indicators. If amygdala activity increases it may be responding to a large portion of visible sclera above the iris (Whalen et al., 2004), for example. However, if the exposure of sclera from another human does not also come with the presence of some threatening force—say, an intruder, rather than one observed in a movie—it may not necessarily correspond with a rise in ANS activity, an increased probability of fleeing or freezing behavior, or a subjective experience of fear.

Again, in understanding the probabilistic organization—or lack thereof—among the indicators of fear in an emergent variable, context is key. One may view, for example, a bear in or out of a zoo. In the case of encountering a bear in the woods, the brain perceives possibly life-threatening danger and very quickly engages in parallel problem solving. Problem–solution pairs may include running to avoid real danger (behavior action plan), autonomic arousal to meet the metabolic challenge of running, or, possibly, fighting for one's life, and amygdala activity may intensify for the purpose of tagging the situation as highly salient in order to facilitate memory consolidation, learning, and, ultimately, future avoidance. Most controversially (in terms of the precise problem the brain is solving), all of these will be consciously experienced and very likely labeled an instance of fear. By contrast, encountering a bear (from a credibly safe distance) at a zoo entails a very different set of problem–solution pairs. For example, because real personal danger is likely to be low, a behavioral avoidance plan may be unnecessary. For similar reasons, ANS activity may be limited due to a minimal change in predicted metabolic demands. Amygdala activity may be relatively high, however, indicating that the novelty of the situation will be tagged as salient in memory, and the subjective experience associated with all of these may be highly variable from person to person, with some regarding themselves to be "afraid," others "excited," and still others merely "interested." Ultimately, context becomes the primary organizing principle in determining the degree to which the putative indicators of fear cohere, and, perhaps, whether fear actually occurs.

Limitations of the Latent Variable Model

If the emergent model sounds sensible, it is otherwise uncommon in emotion research. Traditionally, research on emotion has either explicitly or implicitly followed a latent rather than emergent variable model. Figure 9.2 summarizes the logical framework of the latent variable model of emotion, once more using fear. In this model, fear is assumed to be some module or neural circuit (Ekman, 1992; Izard, 2007) that, when activated, necessarily activates all of its indicators. This brings an assumption of strong covariation among indicators. It follows, if one believes a priori that indicators will cohere based on activation of the fear module, that there is relatively little need to measure multiple indicators. The latent variable model, therefore, privileges basic emotion models above constructionist views both theoretically and practically, because constructionist approaches may necessitate multiple measures.

Though latent variable models have dominated emotion research, much criticism has surfaced (Barrett 2006a; Barrett et al., 2007; Murphy, Nimmo-Smith, & Lawrence, 2003; Phan, Wager, Taylor, & Liberzon, 2002), and few studies have tested or resulted in covariation among indicators (for an exception, however, see Mauss, Levenson, McCarter, Wilhelm,

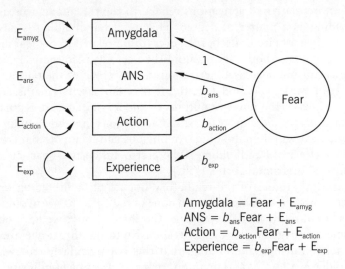

$$\text{Amygdala} = \text{Fear} + E_{amyg}$$
$$\text{ANS} = b_{ans}\text{Fear} + E_{ans}$$
$$\text{Action} = b_{action}\text{Fear} + E_{action}$$
$$\text{Experience} = b_{exp}\text{Fear} + E_{exp}$$

FIGURE 9.2. A proposed latent variable model of fear.

& Gross, 2005). Unlike latent variable models, the emergent variable model can accommodate lack of coherence in indicators and therefore explain a larger proportion of empirical findings in emotion research (Barrett et al., 2007; Clore & Ortony, 2008). For example, in our model of watching a bear in a zoo, only amygdala activity and a subjective perception of "fear" are apparent. Was this fear? The latent variable model cannot accommodate a "yes" answer, at least not without positing an additional qualification such as selective regulatory control imposed on some of the outputs of the fear circuit (more on this later). On the other hand, the emergent variable model posits that there were simply fewer problems to solve, so we may have a *fear-like* experience without having "fear" at its most coherent. The folk psychological term is not the construct itself (Barrett, 2011).

Our own work challenges the latent variable view of dedicated and reflexive emotion circuits. In a series of studies, we have observed that neural activity under threat of electric shock—activity attributable to the perception of the threat cue itself, increased awareness of internal states of the body, the regulation of threat-related processing, and so on—is diminished by the presence of a trusted friend or loved one (e.g., Coan, Beckes, & Allen, 2013; Coan, Shaefer, & Davidson, 2006; Conner et al., 2012). That is, many typically threat-activated structures are less active when one holds hands with someone than when alone. If the latent variable model is true, we might first expect that threat cues in these studies activate a stereotyped set of threat-related activations following from the activation of the fear circuit (e.g., amygdala and periaqueductal gray). Then, with the application of handholding, we might expect regulation either of the fear circuit per se, or its outputs. In the first instance, we would expect to see the entire matrix of activations related to the threat cue decrease with handholding as a matter of degree. That is, if handholding is having its effects on the fear circuit itself, then everything related to the fear circuit— all of its outputs—should show diminished activity. Alternatively, if handholding is causing decreased activation in only some of the outputs of the fear circuit, we should find that the fear circuit itself remains activated while portions of the putative outputs of the fear circuit are regulated. In either case, we would expect *increased* activations in some regulatory system associated with handholding. An obvious candidate mechanism of the regulatory effect of handholding is the prefrontal cortex—particularly the ventromedial prefrontal cortex (PFC).

In several studies of the regulatory impact of handholding or social presence, however, we have observed none of the outcomes we would expect if the latent variable model were true. On the contrary, we have observed that some neural regions typically responsive to the threat cue are simply not as active during handholding, that this is particularly true when the hand holder is a familiar companion, that the effect of familiarity is itself augmented by high-quality relationships, and that none of the previous situations is obviously mediated by inhibitory or regulatory processes in the PFC or elsewhere (Coan et al., 2006, 2013; Conner et al., 2012). This set of observations may be more compatible with an emergent perspective, which suggests that the critical variable in our experiment is the set of situational circumstances that demand more or less from the brain. Our interpretation of these results has indeed been that perceived access to social resources decreases the set of perceived demands occasioned by the threat cue, and that the brain is commensurably less active not because of inhibitory activity (as one often sees in self-regulation experiments) but because there is simply less work for the brain and body to do (Beckes & Coan, 2011).

Conclusion

Of course, evidence exists that is consistent with the latent variable model of emotion—some of which derives from our own work (e.g., Coan & Allen, 2003; Coan, Allen, & Harmon-Jones, 2001). Arguably, the most compelling evidence for neural circuits dedicated to basic emotional states is found in animal research, in which direct stimulation of such circuits is possible. Indeed, Panksepp (2007, 2008) has argued that it is only really possible to test what we refer to here as latent variable models in animal research. For example, Panksepp (1998) has suggested a fear circuit located in the bed nucleus of the stria terminalis and the central amygdala. Nevertheless, even in Panksepp's neural fear model there is a suggestion that effects and behaviors associated with fear are dissociable and contextually dependant. For example, fleeing behavior becomes more likely when the threatening stimulus is near. And variations in the intensity of direct neural stimulation can result in qualitatively different behaviors (Panksepp, 1998).

Still, even if emergent models are theoretically more capable of accounting for diversity of observations in the history of emotion research, direct empirical comparisons of the latent and emergent variable models do not exist. In this chapter we have presented a novel way of measuring emotions that may be more flexible and better suited to the measurement of emotion. The material we have presented here is covered in greater detail elsewhere, and we would like to remind our readers to view this chapter as a gentle introduction to the idea of emergent measurement models—not as a definitive statement of them. Moreover, it bears emphasizing that the emergent model we have presented does not constitute an argument that emotions— fear among them—are not real, a point that warrants additional reading on the existence of emotions from constructionist perspectives (Barrett, 2012; Barrett et al., Chapter 4, this volume). Ultimately, our perspective is primarily fueled by the conviction that framing theoretical positions in concrete and pragmatic measurement terms will add to our understanding of both psychological construction and emotion.

REFERENCES

Ackert, L., Church, B., & Deaves, R. (2003). Emotion and financial markets. *Economic Review–Federal Reserve Bank of Atlanta, 88*(2), 33–42.

Adolphs, R. (2013). The biology of fear. *Current Biology, 23*(2), R79–R93.

Allman, J. M., Hakeem, A., Erwin, J. M., Nimchinsky, E., & Hof, P. (2001). The anterior cingulate cortex. *Annals of the New York Academy of Sciences, 935*(1), 107–117.

Barrett, L. F. (2006a). Solving the emotion paradox: Categorization and the experience of emotion. *Personality and Social Psychology Review, 10*(1), 20–46.

Barrett, L. F. (2006b). Are emotions natural kinds? *Perspectives on Psychological Science, 1*(1), 28–58.

Barrett, L. F. (2011). Bridging token identity theory and supervenience theory through psychological construction. *Psychological Inquiry, 22*(2), 115–127.

Barrett, L. F. (2012). Emotions are real. *Emotion, 12*(3), 413–429.

Barrett, L. F., Lindquist, K. A., Bliss-Moreau, E., Duncan, S., Gendron, M., Mize, J., et al. (2007). Of mice and men: Natural kinds of emotions in the mammalian brain?: A response to Panksepp and Izard. *Perspectives on Psycholgical Science, 2*(3), 297–311.

Barrett, L. F., Mesquita, B., Ochsner, K. N., & Gross, J. J. (2007). The experience of emotion. *Annual Review of Psycholology, 58*, 373–403.

Bechara, A., Damasio, H., & Damasio, A. (2000). Emotion, decision making and the orbitofrontal cortex. *Cerebral Cortex, 10*(3), 295–307.

Beckes, L., & Coan, J. A. (2011). Social baseline theory: The role of social proximity in emotion and economy of action. *Social and Personality Psychology Compass, 5*(12), 976–988.

Bollen, K. A. (1984). Multiple indicators: Internal consistency or no necessary relationship? *Quality and Quantity, 18*(4), 377–385.

Bollen, K. A. (2002). Latent variables in psychology and the social sciences. *Annual Review of Psychology, 53*, 605–634.

Bollen, K. A., & Davis, W. R. (2009). Causal indicator models: Identification, estimation, and testing. *Structural Equation Modeling: A Multidisciplinary Journal, 16*(3), 498–522.

Cacioppo, J. T., Berntson, G. G., Larsen, J. T., Poehlmann, K. M., & Ito, T. A. (2000). The psychophysiology of emotion. In M. Lewis & J. M. Haviland-Jones (Eds.), *Handbook of emotions* (2nd ed., pp. 173–191). New York: Guilford Press.

Cacioppo, J. T., Berntson, G. G., Lorig, T. S., Norris, C. J., Rickett, E., & Nusbaum, H. (2003). Just because you're imaging the brain doesn't mean you can stop using your head: A primer and set of first principles. *Journal of Personality and Social Psychology, 85*(4), 650.

Cacioppo, J. T., Tassinary, L. G., & Berntson, G. G. (2007). Psychophysiological science. In J. T. Cacioppo, L. G. Tassinary, & G. G. Berntson (Eds.), *Handbook of psychophysiology* (3rd ed., pp. 3–23). New York: Cambridge University Press.

Chalmers, D. J. (2006). Strong and weak emergence. In P. Clayton & P. Davies (Eds.), *The re-emergence of emergence: The emergist hypothesis from science to religion* (pp. 244–256). New York: Oxford University Press.

Clore, G. L., & Ortony, A. (2008). Appraisal theories: How cognition shapes affect into emotion. In M. Lewis, J. M. Haviland-Jones, & L. F. Barrett (Eds.), *Handbook of emotions* (3rd ed., pp. 628–642). New York: Guilford Press.

Coan, J. A. (2010). Emergent ghosts of the emotion machine. *Emotion Review, 2,* 274–285.

Coan, J. A., & Allen, J. J. B. (2003). Frontal EEG asymmetry and the behavioral activation and inhibition systems. *Psychophysiology, 40,* 106–114.

Coan, J. A., Allen, J. J. B., & Harmon-Jones, E. (2001). Voluntary facial expression and hemispheric asymmetry over the frontal cortex. *Psychophysiology, 38*(6), 912–925.

Coan, J. A., Beckes, L., & Allen, J. P. (2013). Childhood maternal support and social capital moderate the regulatory impact of social relationships in adulthood. *International Journal of Psychophysiology, 88*(3), 224–231.

Coan, J. A., & Gottman, J. M. (2007). The specific affect coding system (SPAFF). In J. A. Coan & J. J. B. Allen (Eds.), *Handbook of emotion elicitation and assessment* (pp. 267–285). New York: Oxford University Press.

Coan, J. A., Schaefer, H. S., & Davidson, R. J. (2006). Lending a hand: Social regulation of the neural response to threat. *Psychological Science, 17,* 1032–1039.

Collet, C., Vernet-Maury, E., Delhomme, G., & Dittmar, A. (1997). Autonomic nervous system response patterns specificity to basic emotions. *Journal of the Autonomic Nervous System, 62*(1–2), 45–57.

Conner, O. L., Siegle, G. J., McFarland, A. M., Silk, J. S., Ladouceur, C. D., Dahl, R. E., et al. (2012). Mom—It helps when you're right here!: Attenuation of neural stress markers in anxious youths whose caregivers are present during fMRI. *PloS One, 7*(12), e50680.

Costafreda, S. G., Brammer, M. J., David, A. S., & Fu, C. H. (2008). Predictors of amygdala activation during the processing of emotional stimuli: A meta-analysis of 385 PET and fMRI studies. *Brain Research Reviews, 58*(1), 57–70.

Craig, A. D. (2009). How do you feel—now?: The anterior insula and human awareness. *Nature Reviews Neuroscience, 10*(1), 59–70.

Cunningham, W. A., & Zelazo, P. D. (2007). Attitudes and evaluations: A social cognitive neuroscience perspective. *Trends in Cognitive Sciences, 11*(3), 97–104.

Diamantopoulos, A., Riefler, P., & Roth, K. P. (2008). Advancing formative measurement models. *Journal of Business Research, 61*(12), 1203–1218.

Diener, E., Sapyta, J., & Suh, E. (1998). Subjective well-being is essential to well-being. *Psychological Inquiry, 9*(1), 33–37.

Ekman, P. (1992). Facial expressions of emotion: New findings, new questions. *Psychological Science, 3*(1), 34–38.

Ekman, P., Rolls, E., Perrett, D., & Ellis, H. (1992). Facial expressions of emotion: An old controversy and new findings [and discussion]. *Philosophical Transactions of the Royal Society B: Biological Sciences, 335*(1273), 63–69.

Figueredo, A. J. (1998, November). *The entitivity of emergent variables.* Paper presented at the annual meeting of the American Evaluation Association, Chicago, IL.

Hancock, G. R., & Mueller, R. O. (Eds.). (2006). *Structural equation modeling: A second course.* Greenwich, CT: Information Age.

Hariri, A. R., & Whalen, P. J. (2011). The amygdala: Inside and out. *F1000 Biology Reports, 3,* 2-2.

Izard, C. (2007). Basic emotions, natural kinds, emotion schemas, and a new paradigm. *Perspectives on Psychological Science, 2*(3), 260–280.

James, W. (1884). What is an emotion? *Mind, 9*(34), 188–205.

Kievit, R. A., Romeijn, J., Waldorp, L. J., Wicherts, J. M., Scholte, H. S., & Borsboom, D. (2011). Mind the gap: A psychometric approach to the reduction problem. *Psychological Inquiry, 22*(2), 67–87.

Laughlin, R. B. (2005). *A different universe: Reinventing physics from the bottom down.* New York: Basic Books.

Lazarus, R. S. (1991). *Emotion and adaptation.* New York: Oxford University Press.

Lindquist, K. A., Wager, T. D., Kober, H., Bliss-Moreau, E., & Barrett, L. F. (2012). The brain basis of emotion: A meta-analytic review. *Behavioral and Brain Sciences, 35*(3), 121–143.

MacCallum, R. C., & Browne, M. W. (1993). The use of causal indicators in covariance structure models: Some practical issues. *Psychological Bulletin, 114*(3), 533.

Mauss, I. B., Levenson, R. W., McCarter, L., Wilhelm, F. H., & Gross, J. J. (2005). The tie that binds?: Coherence among emotion experience, behavior, and physiology. *Emotion, 5*, 175–190.

McClelland, J. L. (2010). Emergence in cognitive science. *Topics in Cognitive Science, 2*(4), 751–770.

Murphy, F. C., Nimmo-Smith, I., & Lawrence, A. D. (2003). Functional neuroanatomy of emotions: A meta-analysis. *Cognitive Affective and Behavioral Neuroscience, 3*, 207–233.

Panksepp, J. (1998). *Affective neuroscience: The foundations of human and animal emotions.* New York: Oxford University Press.

Panksepp, J. (2007). Neurologizing the psychology of affects: How appraisal-based constructivism and basic emotion theory can coexist. *Perspectives on Psychological Science, 2*(3), 281–296.

Panksepp, J. (2008). Cognitive conceptualism—where have all the affects gone?: Additional corrections for Barrett et al.(2007). *Perspectives on Psychological Science, 3*(4), 305–308.

Phan, K., Wager, T., Taylor, S., & Liberzon, I. (2002). Functional neuroanatomy of emotion: A meta-analysis of emotion activation studies in PET and fMRI. *NeuroImage, 16*(2), 331–348.

Russell, J. (2003). Core affect and the psychological construction of emotion. *Psychological Review, 110*(1), 145–172.

Salovey, P., Rothman, A., Detweiler, J., & Steward, W. (2000). Emotional states and physical health. *American Psychologist, 55*(1), 110–121.

Sanfey, A., Rilling, J., Aronson, J., Nystrom, L., & Cohen, J. (2003). The neural basis of economic decision-making in the ultimatum game. *Science, 300*(5626), 1755–1758.

Schachter, S., & Singer, J. (1962). Cognitive, social and physiological determinants of emotional state. *Psychological Review, 69*, 379–399.

Scherer, K. R. (1982). Emotion as a process: Function, origin and regulation. *Social Science Information, 21*, 555–570.

Scherer, K. R. (1984). On the nature and function of emotion: A component process approach. In K. R. Scherer & P. Ekman (Eds.), *Approaches to emotion* (pp. 293–317). Hillsdale, NJ: Erlbaum.

Scherer, K. R. (1994). Toward a concept of modal emotions. In P. Ekman & R. J. Davidson (Eds.), *The nature of emotion: Fundamental questions* (pp. 25–31). New York: Oxford University Press.

Scherer, K. R. (2000). Psychological models of emotion. In J. C. Borod (Ed.), *The neuropsychology of emotions* (pp. 137–162). New York: Oxford University Press.

Scherer, K. R. (2001). On the nature and function of emotion: A component process approach. In K. R. Scherer, A. Schorr, & T. Johnstone (Eds.), *Appraisal processes in emotion: Theory, methods, research* (pp. 92–120). New York: Oxford University Press.

Scherer, K. R. (2004). Feelings integrate the central representation of appraisal-driven response organization in emotion. In A. S. R. Manstead (Ed.), *Feelings and emotions: The Amsterdam Symposium* (pp. 136–157). Cambridge, UK: Cambridge University Press.

Scherer, K. R. (2009). Emotions are emergent processes: They require a dynamic computational architecture. *Philosophical Transactions of the Royal Society B: Biological Sciences, 364*(1535), 3459–3474.

Whalen, P. J., Kagan, J., Cook, R. G., Davis, F. C., Kim, H., Polis, S., et al. (2004). Human amygdala responsivity to masked fearful eye whites. *Science, 306,* 2061.

Wittgenstein, L. (2010). *Philosophical investigations* [Philosophische Untersuchungen] (G. E. M. Anscombe, P. M. S. Hacker & J. Schulte, Trans.). (4th ed.). Singapore: Wiley-Blackwell.

Zadeh, L. A. (1965). Fuzzy sets. *Information and Control, 8*(3), 338–353.

PART III

CORE AFFECT

CHAPTER 10

Brain Mechanisms of Pleasure

The Core Affect Component of Emotion

MORTEN L. KRINGELBACH
KENT C. BERRIDGE

Emotion plays a central role for the brain, allowing adaptive function and ensuring survival. Pleasure and displeasure, as core affect components of emotion, determine the valence of emotional reactions. Pleasure contributes to emotional adaptiveness by optimizing decision making and balancing brain resource allocation. The cyclical time course of pleasure reactions often consists of wanting (incentive motivation and pleasure anticipation), liking (pleasure itself) and satiety (termination of wanting and liking), where rewards act as motivational magnets that facilitate the switching between different phases. Here, we examine the evidence for the nature of brain networks and mechanisms involved in these processes and in generating and registering the pleasure cycle. In particular, human neuroimaging has shown that remarkably similar underlying pleasure systems are engaged by fundamental and higher-order rewards. Other studies have helped pinpoint distinct brain networks for generating liking and wanting. This new understanding may help understand anhedonia, the lack of pleasure, which is a hallmark of many emotional disorders. In particular, this could lead to better ways of balancing reward networks through the development of new interventions which could in turn lead to more balanced states of positive well-being.

The previous decade has seen significant progress in the scientific study of pleasure. One strategy has been to define pleasure as a driving force for ensuring survival and procreation of both individuals and species

(Kringelbach, 2005; Kringelbach & Berridge, 2010). As such, pleasure may be seen as evolution's boldest trick, and substantial neural mechanisms for pleasure have been selected for and conserved if they ultimately serve a central role in fulfilling evolutionary imperatives of gene proliferation via improved survival and procreation. This view suggests that the capacity for pleasure must have been fundamentally important in evolutionary fitness (Berridge & Kringelbach, 2008; Darwin, 1872; Panksepp, 1999).

A main challenge for any brain is to balance resource allocation successfully for survival through maintaining appropriate energy levels and supporting procreation (Lou Joensson, & Kringelbach., 2011). In order to achieve this balance, different rewards compete for an individual's resources and therefore typically follow a cyclical time course (see Figure 10.1). Within this framework, pleasure helps to initiate, sustain, or terminate phases of *wanting, liking* and *satiety,* and as such plays a crucial role in guiding the survival-related decision making involved in optimizing resource allocation of brain resources.

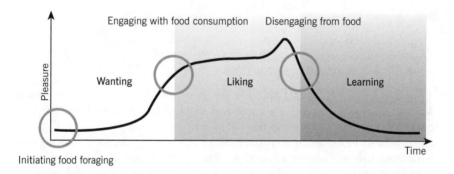

FIGURE 10.1. Pleasure cycles. Fundamental pleasures are associated with behaviors necessary for species survival and, together with higher order pleasures, are associated with a cyclical time course. Typically, rewarding moments go through a phase of expectation or wanting for a reward, which leads to initiating (e.g., food foraging). Given the right circumstances, this can lead to a phase of consummation or liking of the reward that can have a peak level of pleasure (e.g., encountering a loved one, a tasty meal, sexual orgasm, drug rush, winning a gambling bet). This can be followed by a satiety phase, in which one disengages from the reward, learns, and updates predictions for the reward. Note, however, that wanting, liking, and learning can take place throughout the cycle but that wanting is found mostly during expectation and likely mostly during the consummatory phase. These various phases have been identified at many levels of investigation, and the recent research on the computational mechanisms underlying prediction, evaluation, and prediction error are particularly interesting (Friston & Kiebel, 2009; Zhang et al., 2009). Very few rewards might possibly lack a satiety phase. Candidates for brief or missing satiety phase include money, some abstract rewards, and some drug and brain stimulation rewards that activate dopamine systems rather directly.

This chapter reviews the main findings from *hedonia* research; the term *hedonia* is derived from the ancient Greek word *hedone*, which in turn comes from *hedus*, the sweet taste of honey. This research has demonstrated that pleasure involves multiple brain networks and processes relating to incentive salience ('wanting'), hedonic valuation ('liking') and learning (Berridge, 1996; Berridge & Kringelbach, 2008; Kringelbach, 2005). Pleasure and displeasure have also been suggested to be primary core affects that may comprise many different socially constructed emotions (Lindquist, Wager, Kober, Bliss-Moreau, & Barrett., 2012; Posner, Russell, & Peterson, 2005; Russell & Barrett, 1999; also, in this volume, see Barrett, Wilson-Mendenhall, & Barsalou, Chapter 4, and Russell, Chapter 8. Please note the use of single quotation marks for 'wanting' and 'liking' which is meant to indicate the objective neural processing linked to overt behavioral changes rather than the subjective hedonic reactions (without quotation marks).

The discovery of specific brain mechanisms for generating pleasure and registering pleasure for further cognitive use or construction has primarily come from food research on the sensory pleasure of tastes (Berridge & Kringelbach, 2008; Kringelbach, Stein, & van Hartevelt, 2012). Due to the overlap in brain mechanisms among multiple diverse pleasures, that understanding in turn has informed the study of other fundamental and higher-order pleasures (Georgiadis & Kringelbach, 2012). As we demonstrate below, the evidence suggests that the underlying principles are shared across many different rewards, so the generation and encoding of quite different pleasures may also share a common substrate.

Pleasure also plays a role in more abstract states of human happiness. In our view, general pleasure mechanisms may contribute to balanced states of well-being, generating hedonic components of happiness and linking that hedonia to *eudaimonia*, the cognitive construals that let a life be experienced as engaging, valuable, and meaningful. In particular, the reward networks are integral parts of more general resting state networks in the brain. We review some of the evidence that balancing the reward networks may help more generally to rebalance the resting state networks that can become unbalanced in affective disorders.

A Science of Pleasure

As we mentioned earlier, pleasure is central to fulfilling the Darwinian imperatives of survival and procreation. In practice, this has meant that original pleasure mechanisms evolved first for the fundamental sensory pleasures related to survival, including food and sex (Berridge, 1996; Georgiadis & Kringelbach, 2012; Kringelbach, 2004). In social animals, the propagation of genes is linked to the social interactions with conspecifics that are important for both survival and procreation. Social pleasures are therefore part of the repertoire of fundamental pleasures for humans and for many animals (Kringelbach & Rolls, 2003). In particular, for the development of the social pleasures, the early attachment bonds between parents and infants are likely to be extremely important (Lorenz, 1943; Stein et al., 1991). In social species such as humans, it may well be that the social pleasures are at least as pleasurable as the sensory and the sexual pleasures (Aragona et al., 2006; Atzil, Hendler, & Feldman, 2011; Britton et al., 2006; Frith & Frith, 2010; King-Casas et al., 2005; Kringelbach et al., 2008; Leknes & Tracey, 2008; Parsons, Young, Murray, Stein, & Kringelbach, 2010).

In addition to these fundamental pleasures, there are a large number of higher-order pleasures, including monetary, artistic, musical, altruistic, and transcendent pleasures (Frijda, 2010; Kringelbach, 2005; Leknes & Tracey, 2010; Salimpoor, Benovoy, Larcher, Dagher, & Zatorre, 2011; Skov, 2010; Vuust & Kringelbach, 2010). Even rewarding drugs of abuse are widely viewed as hijacking the same hedonic brain systems that evolved to mediate food, sex, and other natural sensory pleasures (Everitt et al., 2008; Kelley & Berridge, 2002; Koob & Volkow, 2010). As such, brains may be viewed as having conserved and recycled some of the same neural mechanisms of hedonic generation for higher pleasures that originated early in evolution for simpler sensory pleasures.

Over the last century a large corpus of nonhuman animal experimentation has investigated reward processing in the brain. Many researchers have subsequently defined pleasure to be the conscious experience of reward, but it is questionable whether such a narrow definition is meaningful or indeed useful. Such as definition would rather limit pleasure to conscious organisms, which is problematic for a number of reasons, not least of which is that it is difficult to provide a good definition of consciousness. Plus there is also empirical evidence that in some cases human pleasures or displeasures might exist, yet not rise to consciousness.

Pleasure is never merely a sensation, even for sensory pleasures (Frijda, 2010; Kringelbach, 2010; Kringelbach & Berridge, 2010; Ryle, 1954). Instead pleasure always requires the active recruitment of specialized brain systems to paint an additional "hedonic gloss" onto a sensation. Active recruitment of brain pleasure-generating systems is what makes a pleasant experience 'liked.'

   The capacity of certain stimuli, such as a sweet taste or a loved one, reliably to elicit pleasure—to be painted nearly always with a hedonic gloss—reflects the privileged ability of such stimuli to activate these hedonic brain systems that are responsible for manufacturing and applying the gloss. Hedonic brain systems are well-developed in the brain, spanning subcortical and cortical levels, and are rather similar across humans and other animals. Pleasure reactions can be elicited by many stimuli and, in the normal brain, lead to activity in widespread brain networks, including deep in the brain (nucleus accumbens, ventral pallidum, brainstem; see Salamone, Correa, Randall, & Nunes, Chapter 11, this volume), while other candidates are found in the cortex (orbitofrontal, cingulate, and medial prefrontal and insular cortices; Amodio & Frith, 2006; Berridge, 1996; Cardinal, Parkinson, Hall, & Everitt, 2002; Everitt & Robbins, 2005; Kringelbach, 2010; Kringelbach, O'Doherty, Rolls, & Andrews, 2003; Kringelbach & Rolls, 2004; Watson, Shepherd, & Platt, 2010; see Figure 10.2).

In what follows we look at how different regions or nodes in this distributed pleasure network play different roles in terms of controlling the transition between the various phases of the pleasure cycle. One of the most important distinctions is between regions involved in the wanting and the liking phases, in which 'wanting' corresponds to the motivational salience, while 'liking' corresponds to the hedonic valence of stimuli. Regions involved in liking can be further subdivided into those regions involved in generating pleasure (hedonic hotspots) versus regions involved in decoding pleasure, although some regions are involved in both. Typically the former hedonic hotspots are inferred on the basis of a *change* in pleasure as a *consequence of a brain manipulation* such as a lesion or stimulation (Green, Pereira, & Aziz, 2010; Smith, Mahler, Peciña, & Berridge, 2010), while pleasure coding regions are inferred by measuring brain *activity correlated to a pleasant stimulus*, using human neuroimaging techniques (De Araujo, Kringelbach, Rolls, & Hobden, 2003a; De Araujo, Kringelbach, Rolls, & McGlone, 2003b; Kringelbach et al., 2003).

Generation and Decoding of Pleasure: 'Liking' Mechanisms

Only a few of the previously mentioned brain regions have been identified as involved in actually generating pleasure. Pleasure generation can be determined by identifying which brain systems can cause an increase in 'liking' reactions to a fundamental sensory pleasure, such as sweetness, consequent to brain manipulation. These hedonic hotspots have been found in subcortical structures in the rodent brain. They are typically only around one cubic-millimeter or so in volume in the rodent brain (Figure 10.2D). In humans, hedonic hotspots have yet to be identified, but if scaled to the size of the human brain they would measure around one cubic centimeter. Rodent hedonic hotspots have been identified in the nucleus accumbens shell, ventral pallidum, and in deep brainstem regions, including the parabrachial nucleus in the pons (Peciña, Smith, & Berridge, 2006). The pleasure-generating capacity of these hotspots has been revealed in part by studies in which microinjections of drugs stimulated neurochemical

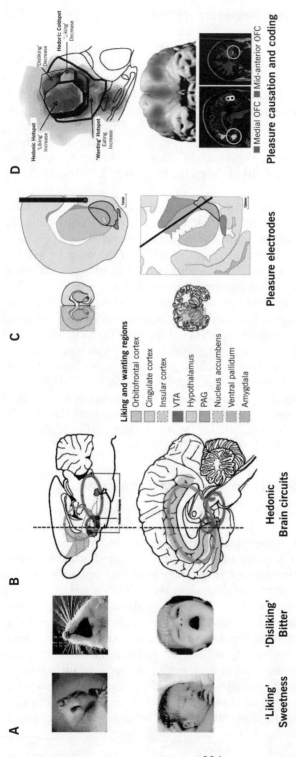

FIGURE 10.2. Hedonic brain circuitry. The schematic shows the brain regions for causing and coding fundamental pleasures in rodents and humans. (A) Facial 'liking' and 'disliking' expressions elicited by sweet and bitter taste are similar in rodents and human infants. (B, D) Pleasure causation has been identified in rodents as arising from interlinked subcortical hedonic hotspots, such as in nucleus accumbens and ventral pallidum, where neural activation may increase 'liking' expressions in response to sweetness. Similar pleasure coding and incentive salience networks have also been identified in humans. (C) The so-called "pleasure" electrodes in rodents and humans are unlikely to have elicited true pleasure but perhaps only incentive salience or 'wanting.' (D) The cortical localization of pleasure coding may reach an apex in various regions of the orbitofrontal cortex that differentiate subjective pleasantness from valence processing of aspects the same stimulus, such as a pleasant food.

234

receptors on neurons within a hotspot, and caused a doubling or tripling of the number of hedonic 'liking' reactions normally elicited by a pleasant sucrose taste (Figure 10.2A; Smith et al., 2010).

Hedonic hotspots are anatomically distributed but closely interact to form a functional integrated circuit. The circuit obeys control rules that are largely hierarchical and organized into brain levels. Top levels function together as a cooperative heterarchy, so that, for example, multiple unanimous favorable simultaneous "votes" from participating hotspots in the nucleus accumbens and ventral pallidum are required for opioid stimulation in either forebrain site to enhance 'liking' above normal (Smith & Berridge, 2007).

In contrast, regions decoding pleasure are found mostly in the cortex. Hedonic evaluation of pleasure valence is anatomically distinguishable from precursor operations such as sensory computations, suggesting existence of a hedonic cortex proper (Figure 10.2B; Kringelbach, 2004). Hedonic cortex involves regions such as the orbitofrontal, insula, medial prefrontal and cingulate cortices (Amodio & Frith, 2006; Beckmann, Johansen-Berg, & Rushworth, 2009; Craig, 2002; Kringelbach, 2005; see Barrett et al., Chapter 4, and Cunningham, Dunfield, & Stillman, Chapter 7, this volume), which a wealth of human neuroimaging studies have shown to code for hedonic evaluations (including anticipation, appraisal, experience, and memory of pleasurable stimuli), and which have close anatomical links to subcortical hedonic hotspots.

Pleasure encoding may reach an apex of cortical localization in a midanterior subregion within the orbitofrontal cortex, where neuroimaging activity correlates strongly to subjective pleasantness ratings of food varieties (Kringelbach et al., 2003) and to other pleasures such as sexual orgasm (Georgiadis et al., 2006), drugs (Völlm et al., 2004), chocolate (Small, Zatorre, Dagher, Evans, & Jones-Gotman, 2001), emotional experiences (Wilson-Mendenhall, Barrett, & Barsalou, 2013), object identification (Shenhav, Barrett, & Bar, 2013), and music (Blood & Zatorre, 2001; Salimpoor et al., 2013). Most importantly, midanterior orbitofrontal activity tracks changes in subjective pleasure, such as a decline in palatability when the reward value of one food was reduced by eating it to satiety (while remaining high in response to another food; Kringelbach, 2005; Kringelbach et al., 2003). The midanterior subregion of orbitofrontal cortex is thus a prime candidate for the coding of subjective experience of pleasure (Kringelbach, 2005; see Figure 10.2D).

Another coding site for positive hedonics in orbitofrontal cortex is along its medial edge that has activity related to the valence of positive and negative events (Kringelbach & Rolls, 2004), contrasted to lateral portions that have been suggested to code unpleasant events (O'Doherty, Kringelbach, Rolls, Hornak, & Andrews, 2001), although the activity in the lateral part is more likely to reflect a signal to escape the situation rather than displeasure per se (Hornak et al., 2004; Iversen & Mishkin, 1970; Kringel-bach & Rolls, 2003, 2004).

The medial–lateral hedonic gradient in the orbitofrontal cortex inter-acts with an abstraction–concreteness gradient in the posterior–anterior dimension, so that more complex or abstract reinforcers (e.g., monetary gain and loss; O'Doherty et al., 2001) are represented more anteriorly in the orbitofrontal cortex than less complex sensory rewards (e.g., taste; Small et al., 2001). The medial region does not, however, appear to change its activity with reinforcer devaluation, so it may not reflect the full dynam-ics of pleasure.

Some studies have also shown lateralization of affect or hemispheric differences in humans, with the left hemisphere of prefrontal cortex some-times being implicated more in positive affect than the right hemisphere (Davidson, 2004). For example, individuals who give higher ratings of sub-jective well-being may have higher activity in left prefrontal cortex, and left subcortical striatal activity also is more tightly linked to pleasantness ratings in some studies than right-side activity (Kuhn & Gallinat, 2012; Lawrence, Hinton, Parkinson, & Lawrence, 2012; Price & Harmon-Jones, 2011). However, many other studies have found more equal bilateral activ-ity patterns, so the precise role of lateralization in pleasure still remains somewhat unclear.

Wanting Mechanisms

In addition to 'liking' mechanisms, pleasure is translated into motivational processes in part by activating a second component of reward, which turns out to be psychologically distinct from pleasure, even if it is often also considered to occur together with pleasant events. This second compo-nent, termed 'wanting' or incentive salience, makes stimuli attractive when attributed to them by mesolimbic brain systems (Berridge & Robinson, 2003). Incentive salience depends in particular on mesolimbic dopamine neurotransmission between select regions of the pleasure network, although other neurotransmitters and structures also are involved.

Importantly, incentive salience does not involve hedonic impact or pleasure 'liking' (Berridge, 2007). This is why an individual can 'want' a reward without necessarily 'liking' that same reward. Irrational 'wanting' without liking can occur especially in addiction via incentive-sensitization of the mesolimbic dopamine system and connected structures (Robinson & Berridge, 2003). At the extreme, the addict may come to 'want' what is neither 'liked' nor expected to be liked, a dissociation that is possible because 'wanting' mechanisms are largely subcortical and separable from cortically mediated declarative expectation and conscious planning. This is one reason why addicts may compulsively 'want' to take drugs even if, at a more cognitive and conscious level, they do not want to do so.

Learning Mechanisms

In addition to the 'wanting' and 'liking' components mentioned earlier, learning is important for linking these components over time and usually, but not exclusively, follows consumption.

Powerful learning mechanisms are involved when the consumption of a highly liked food causes an adverse effect, such as an allergic reaction. People learn to avoid this liked substance in the future to avoid the negative outcome. Memories obtained through this Pavlovian learning remain stable over time until devaluation or until new information becomes available (Smith, Berridge, & Aldridge, 2011; Zhang, Berridge, Tindell, Smith, & Aldridge, 2009).

'Wanting' is known to exhibit dynamic fluctuation corresponding to hunger states, for example, but it can also shift from a reward food stimulus to a conditioned stimulus or cue. This cue itself can be highly wanted and become a motivational magnet. The immense attractive properties of such a motivational magnet can be seen when it is hard to ignore the cue (e.g., rats will try to consume an inedible cue that predicts the arrival of food instead of the food itself; Berridge, 2012).

'Wanting' and 'liking' are difficult to tease apart in human psychological studies, and there is an ongoing debate regarding how to best dissociate them (Finlayson & Dalton, 2012; Havermans, 2012). Some of the best successes have come from drug-related studies, in which wanting or liking ratings of cocaine, heroin, or other drugs can be dissociated from each other, especially by dopamine-related pharmacological manipulations (Evans et al., 2006; Leyton, 2010). Perhaps the most robust clinical phenomenon is incentive sensitization in addiction. Addicts may strongly 'want' to take a drug, even when they know they will not 'like' the drug very much, when they do not like it once they have taken it, when they know that taking it may have serious detrimental consequences on the quality of their life, and even when they are no longer experiencing any withdrawal symptoms (e.g., after quitting the drug and completing detox, they relapse once again; Robinson & Berridge, 2003). Additionally, neural signatures within the brain for 'wanting' and 'liking' can be successfully dissociated by various pharmacological manipulations (e.g., dopamine levels in select brain regions; Smith et al., 2011).

In humans, it is more difficult to dissociate wanting and liking (Finlayson & Dalton, 2012) but some progress has been made (Dai, Brendl, & Ariely, 2010). As an example, we introduced a behavioral paradigm in which human participants indicate their subjective liking of a stimulus, as well as their wanting, measured by the amount of effort they are willing to expend to prolong or shorten the exposure to the stimulus (Parsons, Young, Kumari, Stein, & Kringelbach, 2011). This paradigm demonstrates that even though men and women differ in their liking ratings of baby faces, they have similar viewing times (as a measure of wanting indicated by exerted effort to influence viewing times).

In humans, neuroimaging offers a route to investigate the partly separable liking, wanting, and learning components in the human brain with spatiotemporal monitoring of activity patterns in the different cortical regions regulating each of these components.

Learning is an important component in decision making relative to eating-related behavior, when the brain must compare and evaluate the predicted reward value of various behaviors. This processing can be complex, because the estimations vary in quality depending on the sampling rate of the behavior and the variance of reward distributions. It is difficult to provide a reliable estimate of the reward value of a food that appears to be highly desirable and highly nutrititious but that is only rarely available and varies significantly in quality.

This raises a classic problem in animal learning of how to optimize behavior such that the amount of exploration is balanced with the amount of exploitation, where exploration is the time spent sampling the outcome of different behaviors, and exploitation is the time spent using existing behaviors with known reward values.

Ultimately, pleasure can be thought of as an important tool to control this balancing act between exploitation and exploration. As mentioned earlier, evidence from neuroimaging studies has linked regions of the human brain—in particular the orbitofrontal cortex—to various aspects of eating and especially to the representation of the subjective pleasantness of foods (Kringelbach, 2004).

Brain Networks for Resource Allocation

Overall, as reviewed earlier, the data gathered from animal and human studies support the existence of reward networks with important subcomponents of wanting, liking, and learning. While it is tempting to work out the circuitry of brain regions in these networks in isolation, it is pertinent to take a more global brain perspective on how to interpret the changes found in brain activity (Lindquist & Barrett, 2012; Oosterwijk, Touroutoglou, & Lindquist, Chapter 5, this volume).

In particular it is important to integrate these reward networks with activity in widely distributed brain networks, often called *resting state networks*. We have previously speculated that activity in one of these brain resting state networks, the so-called *default mode network* (Gusnard & Raichle, 2001; Raichle et al., 2001) is closely linked to reward processing and may have an important role in shaping our overall well-being (Kringelbach & Berridge, 2009).

The last few years have seen a shift in the focus of modern neuroimaging from the study of extrinsic to intrinsic brain activity (Biswal et al., 2010). This change has been brought about by the realization that while the vast majority of neuroimaging studies have been devoted to studying task-related changes in brain activity, the additional energy associated with this activity is remarkable low, often less than 5% (Raichle & Mintun, 2006). Instead, the majority of brain energy consumption study is devoted to intrinsic brain activity.

Such intrinsic brain activity was mapped during the resting period in cognitive studies in which researchers found a network of brain regions with remarkably high rates of change in metabolic markers such as cerebral blood flow, oxygen extraction, and blood oxygen level dependent (BOLD) functional magnetic resonance imaging (fMRI) (Lou et al., 1999). In this network of brain regions termed the default mode network, the main regions showed the largest deactivations during extrinsic cognitive tasks (Gusnard & Raichle, 2001; Raichle et al., 2001).

Subsequent sophisticated independent component analyses of resting state patterns have identified at least seven networks that stay coherent over several minutes (Damoiseaux et al., 2006). Based on their brain components, these networks have been classified in (1) primary input–output networks (including sensorimotor, visual, and auditory regions), (2) higher integrative networks (including attention, language, default mode, and executive regions; Beckmann, DeLuca, Devlin, & Smith, 2005), and (3) cortical–subcortical networks (including structures such as the thalamus, basal ganglia, and cerebellum; Fox & Raichle, 2007). Interestingly, regions of the default mode network remain tightly coherent but tend to show negative correlations with task-positive regions in the other networks.

The intrinsic activity of the human brain must be closely related to the large-scale anatomical connectivity between brain regions (Barrett & Satpute, 2013). Techniques such diffusion spectrum imaging and graph theory have revealed that the human brain exhibits a special kind of topology known as *small-world architecture* (Watts & Strogatz, 1998), which is characterized by high levels of local clustering among neighboring nodes (Bullmore & Sporns, 2009; Hagmann et al., 2007). Some nodes have higher connectivity in comparison with other nodes and are called *hubs* (He et al., 2009). The default mode network mostly consists of hubs, and in particular, ventromedial prefrontal/medial orbitofrontal, precuneus, and posterior cingulate cortices have been proposed to form the structural core (Hagmann et al., 2008).

Knowledge about the workings of these resting state networks is necessary in order to understand the fundamentals of how our brains work and particularly the processing that uses memory-dependent self-reference, which is important for binding together these networks (e.g., Corbetta,

Patel, & Shulman, 2008; Seeley et al., 2007). We have proposed the existence of a common paralimbic network that serves to regulate and balance the dynamic resource allocation needed to ensure survival (Lou et al., 2011). This process is guided by processes linked to awareness, attention, and emotion in order to support memory-dependent self-reference, which in narrative self-consciousness is extended into adjacent neocortical regions. Recent evidence from human lesion studies has demonstrated that medial prefrontal cortex is necessary for self-reference (Philippi, Duff, Denburg, Tranel, & Rudrauf, 2012a), although self-awareness has also been found to persist even with extensive bilateral brain damage to insula, anterior cingulate, and medial prefrontal cortices (Philippi et al., 2012b).

Critically, sensory inputs such as vision, hearing, taste, smell, and touch (linked to survival-related rewards such as food and sex) and their subsequent hedonic evaluation have the potential to shift the focus of the brain networks temporarily to allow for efficient processing and control over behaviors (Berridge & Kringelbach, 2008). The paralimbic network helps to ensure that the processing remains balanced over longer time periods across many reward cycles.

Implications for Emotional Disorders

Emotional disorders are all too common and often are linked to problems with core affect that arise from the unbalancing of the neural processing that underlies the pleasure cycle. This is turn leads to unbalanced resource allocation for the resting state networks of the brain or other networks involved in emotion and self-concept, which is found in many brain and neuropsychiatric disorders. For example, resting state networks have been found to undergo changes in affective disorders such as depression (Broyd *et al.*, 2009; Greicius, 2008; van Eimeren, Monchi, Ballanger, & Strafella, 2009).

In terms of emotional disorders, anhedonia, the lack of pleasure, is one of the most important symptoms. We have previously proposed that anhedonia can be viewed as acute and sometimes chronic unbalancing of the brain networks supporting the pleasure cycle (Kringelbach & Berridge, 2009; Kringelbach, Green, & Aziz, 2011).

Although anhedonia is expressed differently across individual patients, and sometimes even across time within the same patient, such as in bipolar disorder (Nelson, Gebauer, LaBrie, & Shaffer, 2009), there are clear differences between the imbalances in, for example, affective and addictive disorders.

In the normal brain, wanting, liking, and learning processes are balanced over time. A breakdown of the balance between these processes can lead to various expressions of anhedonia. On the one hand, imbalance can lead to a reduced ability to pursue and experience pleasure, as seen, for example, in the affective disorders. On the other hand, this progressive decrease in wanting and liking is markedly different from the imbalance leading to addictive and impulse control disorders (e.g., in which 'wanting' to take drugs grows over time, independent of 'liking' for drugs, as suggested by the incentive sensitization model of addiction; Robinson & Berridge, 1993).

Conclusion

In this chapter we have put forward the hypothesis that pleasure helps to optimize the survival-related decision making involved in brain resource allocation. We have made important progress in understanding the underlying neural processing of reward. In particular, we have begun to investigate mechanisms underlying the full pleasure cycle, particularly the brain processing that initiates, sustains, and terminates the various phases of wanting, liking, and satiety.

Many brain disorders arise from the unbalancing of these reward mechanisms, which in turn has repercussions for the resource allocation of more general resting state networks. The growing understanding of partly dissociable mechanisms of 'wanting' and 'liking' have led to a better understanding of differences in anhedonia found in affective versus addictive disorders. In affective disorders such as monopolar depression, anhedonia is usually manifested in decreases in both wanting and liking, whereas addictive disorders often lead to an increase in wanting, with a simultaneous decrease in liking. This new understanding may in time lead to new and more targeted treatments. Similarly, a fuller understanding how wanting processes can act as motivational magnets for desired rewards may also benefit the treatment of patients with consummatory behavior problems.

More generally, however, this new understanding of pleasure may in the fullness of time help to achieve more balanced states of well-being. For example, one view is that hedonic happiness could be conceived of as 'liking' without 'wanting'; that is, a state of pleasure without disruptive desires, a state of contentment (Kringelbach & Berridge, 2009).

At the same time, balanced 'wanting' and 'liking' processing can facilitate engagement with the world. It is important to avoid too much 'wanting,' which can readily spiral into maladaptive consummatory patterns, such as those found in addiction, that may be a direct route to great unhappiness. Maximization of any of the underlying processes leads to unbalanced states that are unsustainable. Instead, a route to positive well-being seems to be the best way to balance the many demands on our brains, so that we can use our time to engage meaningfully with the fullness of what life has to offer.

ACKNOWLEDGMENTS

Our research has been supported by grants from the TrygFonden Charitable Foundation to Morten L. Kringelbach and from the National Institute of Mental Health and the National Institute on Drug Abuse to Kent C. Berridge. This chapter is derived and adapted from our recent articles.

REFERENCES

Amodio, D. M., & Frith, C. D. (2006). Meeting of minds: The medial frontal cortex and social cognition. *Nature Reviews Neuroscience, 7,* 268–277.

Aragona, B. J., Liu, Y., Yu, Y. J., Curtis, J. T., Detwiler, J. M., Insel, T. R., et al. (2006). Nucleus accumbens dopamine differentially mediates the formation and maintenance of monogamous pair bonds. *Nature Neuroscience, 9,* 133–139.

Atzil, S., Hendler, T., & Feldman, R. (2011). Specifying the neurobiological basis of human attachment: Brain, hormones, and behavior in synchronous and intrusive mothers. *Neuropsychopharmacology, 36,* 2603–2615.

Barrett, L. F., & Satpute, A. B. (2013). Large-scale brain networks in affective and social neuroscience: Towards an integrative functional architecture of the brain. *Current Opinion in Neurobiology, 23*(3), 361–372.

Beckmann, C. F., DeLuca, M., Devlin, J. T., & Smith, S. M. (2005). Investigations into resting-state connectivity using independent component analysis. *Philosophical Transactions of the Royal Society of London B: Biological Sciences, 360,* 1001–1013.

Beckmann, M., Johansen-Berg, H., & Rushworth, M. F. (2009). Connectivity-based parcellation of human cingulate cortex and its relation to functional specialization. *Journal of Neuroscience, 29,* 1175–1190.

Berridge, K. C. (1996). Food reward: Brain substrates of wanting and liking. *Neuroscience and Biobehavioral Reviews, 20,* 1–25.

Berridge, K. C. (2007). The debate over dopamine's role in reward: The case for incentive salience. *Psychopharmacology, 191,* 391–431.

Berridge, K. C. (2012). From prediction error to incentive salience: Mesolimbic computation of reward motivation. *European Journal of Neuroscience, 35*(7), 1124–1143.

Berridge, K. C., & Kringelbach, M. L. (2008). Affective neuroscience of pleasure: Reward in humans and animals. *Psychopharmacology, 199,* 457–480.

Berridge, K. C., & Robinson, T. E. (2003). Parsing reward. *Trends in Neurosciences, 26,* 507–513.

Biswal, B. B., Mennes, M., Zuo, X. N., Gohel, S., Kelly, C., Smith, S. M., et al. (2010). Toward discovery science of human brain function. *Proceedings of the National Academy of Sciences USA, 107,* 4734–4739.

Blood, A. J., & Zatorre, R. J. (2001). Intensely pleasurable responses to music correlate with activity in brain regions implicated in reward and emotion. *Proceedings of the National Academy of Sciences USA, 98,* 11818–11823.

Britton, J. C., Phan, K. L., Taylor, S. F., Welsh, R. C., Berridge, K. C., & Liberzon,

I. (2006). Neural correlates of social and nonsocial emotions: An fMRI study. *NeuroImage, 31,* 397–409.

Broyd, S. J., Demanuele, C., Debener, S., Helps, S. K., James, C. J., & Sonuga-Barke, E. J. (2009). Default-mode brain dysfunction in mental disorders: A systematic review. *Neuroscience and Biobehavioral Reviews, 33,* 279–296.

Bullmore, E., & Sporns, O. (2009). Complex brain networks: Graph theoretical analysis of structural and functional systems. *Nature Reviews Neuroscience, 10,* 186–198.

Cardinal, R. N., Parkinson, J. A., Hall, J., & Everitt, B. J. (2002). Emotion and motivation: The role of the amygdala, ventral striatum, and prefrontal cortex. *Neuroscience and Biobehavioral Reviews, 26,* 321–352.

Corbetta, M., Patel, G., & Shulman, G. L. (2008). The reorienting system of the human brain: From environment to theory of mind. *Neuron, 58,* 306–324.

Craig, A. D. (2002). Opinion: How do you feel? Interoception: The sense of the physiological condition of the body. *Nature Reviews Neuroscience, 3,* 655–666.

Dai, X., Brendl, C. M., & Ariely, D. (2010). Wanting, liking, and preference construction. *Emotion, 10,* 324–334.

Damoiseaux, J. S., Rombouts, S. A. R. B., Barkhof, F., Scheltens, P., Stam, C. J., Smith, S. M., et al. (2006). Consistent resting-state networks across healthy subjects. *Proceedings of the National Academy of Sciences USA, 103,* 13848–13853.

Darwin, C. (1872). *The expression of the emotions in man and animals.* Chicago: University of Chicago Press.

Davidson, R. J. (2004). Well-being and affective style: Neural substrates and biobehavioural correlates. *Philosophical Transactions of the Royal Society of London B: Biological Sciences, 359,* 1395–1411.

De Araujo, I. E. T., Kringelbach, M. L., Rolls, E. T., & Hobden, P. (2003a). The representation of umami taste in the human brain. *Journal of Neurophysiology, 90*(1), 313–319.

De Araujo, I. E. T., Kringelbach, M. L., Rolls, E. T., & McGlone, F. (2003b). Human cortical responses to water in the mouth, and the effects of thirst. *Journal of Neurophysiology, 90,* 1865–1876.

Evans, A. H., Pavese, N., Lawrence, A. D., Tai, Y. F., Appel, S., Doder, M., et al. (2006). Compulsive drug use linked to sensitized ventral striatal dopamine transmission. *Annals of Neurology, 59,* 852–858.

Everitt, B. J., Belin, D., Economidou, D., Pelloux, Y., Dalley, J. W., & Robbins, T. W. (2008). Neural mechanisms underlying the vulnerability to develop compulsive drug-seeking habits and addiction. *Philosophical Transactions of the Royal Society of London B: Biological Sciences, 363,* 3125–3135.

Everitt, B. J., & Robbins, T. W. (2005). Neural systems of reinforcement for drug addiction: From actions to habits to compulsion. *Nature Neuroscience, 8,* 1481–1489.

Finlayson, G., & Dalton, M. (2012). Current progress in the assessment of "liking" vs. "wanting" food in human appetite: Comment on "You say it's liking, I say it's wanting . . . ": On the difficulty of disentangling food reward in man. *Appetite, 58,* 373–378; discussion 252–375.

Fox, M. D., & Raichle, M. E. (2007). Spontaneous fluctuations in brain activity observed with functional magnetic resonance imaging. *Nature Reviews Neuroscience, 8,* 700–711.

Frijda, N. (2010). On the nature and function of pleasure. In M. L. Kringelbach & K. C. Berridge (Eds.), *Pleasures of the brain* (pp. 99–112). New York: Oxford University Press.

Friston, K., & Kiebel, S. (2009). Predictive coding under the free-energy principle. *Philosophical Transactions of the Royal Society of London B: Biological Sciences, 364,* 1211–1221.

Frith, U., & Frith, C. (2010). The social brain: Allowing humans to boldly go where no other species has been. *Philosophical Transactions of the Royal Society of London B: Biological Sciences, 365,* 165–176.

Georgiadis, J. R., Kortekaas, R., Kuipers, R., Nieuwenburg, A., Pruim, J., Reinders, A. A., et al. (2006). Regional cerebral blood flow changes associated with clitorally induced orgasm in healthy women. *European Journal of Neuroscience, 24,* 3305–3316.

Georgiadis, J. R., & Kringelbach, M. L. (2012). The human sexual response cycle: Brain imaging evidence linking sex to other pleasures. *Progress in Neurobiology, 98,* 49–81.

Green, A. L., Pereira, E. A., & Aziz, T. Z. (2010). Deep brain stimulation and pleasure. In M. L. Kringelbach & K. C. Berridge (Eds.), *Pleasures of the brain* (pp. 302–319). New York: Oxford University Press.

Greicius, M. (2008). Resting-state functional connectivity in neuropsychiatric disorders. *Current Opinion in Neurology, 21,* 424–430.

Gusnard, D. A., & Raichle, M. E. (2001). Searching for a baseline: Functional imaging and the resting human brain. *Nature Reviews Neuroscience, 2,* 685–694.

Hagmann, P., Cammoun, L., Gigandet, X., Meuli, R., Honey, C. J., Wedeen, V. J., et al. (2008). Mapping the structural core of human cerebral cortex. *PLoS Biology, 6,* e159.

Hagmann, P., Kurant, M., Gigandet, X., Thiran, P., Wedeen, V. J., Meuli, R., et al. (2007). Mapping human whole-brain structural networks with diffusion MRI. *PLoS ONE, 2,* e597.

Havermans, R. C. (2012). How to tell where "liking" ends and "wanting" begins. *Appetite, 58,* 252–255.

He, Y., Wang, J., Wang, L., Chen, Z. J., Yan, C., Yang, H., et al. (2009). Uncovering intrinsic modular organization of spontaneous brain activity in humans. *PLoS ONE, 4,* e5226.

Hornak, J., O'Doherty, J., Bramham, J., Rolls, E. T., Morris, R. G., Bullock, P. R., et al. (2004). Reward-related reversal learning after surgical excisions in orbitofrontal and dorsolateral prefrontal cortex in humans. *Journal of Cognitive Neuroscience, 16,* 463–478.

Iversen, S. D., & Mishkin, M. (1970). Perseverative interference in monkeys following selective lesions of the inferior prefrontal convexity. *Experimental Brain Research, 11,* 376–386.

Kelley, A. E., & Berridge, K. C. (2002). The neuroscience of natural rewards: Relevance to addictive drugs. *Journal of Neuroscience, 22,* 3306–3311.

King-Casas, B., Tomlin, D., Anen, C., Camerer, C. F., Quartz, S. R., & Montague,

P. R. (2005). Getting to know you: Reputation and trust in a two-person economic exchange. *Science, 308*, 78–83.

Koob, G. F., & Volkow, N. D. (2010). Neurocircuitry of addiction. *Neuropsychopharmacology, 35*, 217–238.

Kringelbach, M. L. (2004). Food for thought: Hedonic experience beyond homeostasis in the human brain. *Neuroscience, 126*, 807–819.

Kringelbach, M. L. (2005). The orbitofrontal cortex: Linking reward to hedonic experience. *Nature Reviews Neuroscience, 6*, 691–702.

Kringelbach, M. L. (2010). The hedonic brain: A functional neuroanatomy of human pleasure. In M. L. Kringelbach & K. C. Berridge (Eds.), *Pleasures of the brain* (pp. 202–221). New York: Oxford University Press.

Kringelbach, M. L., & Berridge, K. C. (2009). Towards a functional neuroanatomy of pleasure and happiness. *Trends in Cognitive Science, 13*, 479–487.

Kringelbach, M. L., & Berridge, K. C. (2010). *Pleasures of the brain*. New York: Oxford University Press.

Kringelbach, M. L., Green, A. L., & Aziz, T. Z. (2011). Balancing the brain: Resting state networks and deep brain stimulation. *Frontiers in Integrative Neuroscience, 5*, 8.

Kringelbach, M., Lehtonen, A., Squire, S., Harvey, A., Craske, M., Holliday, I., et al. (2008). A specific and rapid neural signature for parental instinct. *PLoS ONE, 3*, e1664.

Kringelbach, M. L., O'Doherty, J., Rolls, E. T., & Andrews, C. (2003). Activation of the human orbitofrontal cortex to a liquid food stimulus is correlated with its subjective pleasantness. *Cerebral Cortex, 13*, 1064–1071.

Kringelbach, M. L., & Rolls, E. T. (2003). Neural correlates of rapid context-dependent reversal learning in a simple model of human social interaction. *NeuroImage, 20*, 1371–1383.

Kringelbach, M. L., & Rolls, E. T. (2004). The functional neuroanatomy of the human orbitofrontal cortex: Evidence from neuroimaging and neuropsychology. *Progress in Neurobiology, 72*, 341–372.

Kringelbach, M. L., Stein, A., & van Hartevelt, T. J. (2012). The functional human neuroanatomy of food pleasure cycles. *Physiology and Behavior, 106*, 307–316.

Kuhn, S., & Gallinat, J. (2012). The neural correlates of subjective pleasantness. *NeuroImage, 61*, 289–294.

Lawrence, N. S., Hinton, E. C., Parkinson, J. A., & Lawrence, A. D. (2012). Nucleus accumbens response to food cues predicts subsequent snack consumption in women and increased body mass index in those with reduced self-control. *NeuroImage, 63*, 415–422.

Leknes, S., & Tracey, I. (2008). A common neurobiology for pain and pleasure. *Nature Reviews Neuroscience, 9*, 314–320.

Leknes, S., & Tracey, I. (2010). Pleasure and pain: Masters of mankind. In M. L. Kringelbach & K. C. Berridge (Eds.), *Pleasures of the brain* (pp. 320–335). New York: Oxford University Press.

Leyton, M. (2010) The neurobiology of desire: Dopamine and the regulation of mood and motivational states in humans. In M. L. Kringelbach & K. C. Berridge (Eds.), *Pleasures of the brain* (pp. 222–243). New York: Oxford University Press.

Lindquist, K. A., & Barrett, L. F. (2012). A functional architecture of the human brain: Emerging insights from the science of emotion. *Trends in Cognitive Sciences, 16,* 533–540.

Lindquist, K. A., Wager, T. D., Kober, H., Bliss-Moreau, E., & Barrett, L. F. (2012). The brain basis of emotion: A meta-analytic review. *Behavioral and Brain Sciences, 35,* 121–143.

Lorenz, K. (1943). Die angeborenen Formen Möglicher Erfahrung [Innate forms of potential experience]. *Zeitschrift für Tierpsychologie, 5,* 235–519.

Lou, H. C., Joensson, M., & Kringelbach, M. L. (2011). Yoga lessons for consciousness research: A paralimbic network balancing brain resource allocation. *Frontiers in Psychology, 2,* 366.

Lou, H. C., Kjaer, T. W., Friberg, L., Wildschiodtz, G., Holm, S., & Nowak, M. (1999). A [^{15}O]H$_2$O PET study of meditation and the resting state of normal consciousness. *Human Brain Mapping, 7,* 98–105.

Nelson, S. E., Gebauer, L., LaBrie, R. A., & Shaffer, H. J. (2009). Gambling problem symptom patterns and stability across individual and timeframe. *Psychology of Addictive Behaviors, 23,* 523–533.

O'Doherty, J., Kringelbach, M. L., Rolls, E. T., Hornak, J., & Andrews, C. (2001). Abstract reward and punishment representations in the human orbitofrontal cortex. *Nature Neuroscience, 4,* 95–102.

Panksepp, J. (1999) *Affective neuroscience.* Oxford, UK: Oxford University Press.

Parsons, C. E., Young, K. S., Kumari, N., Stein, A., & Kringelbach, M. L. (2011). The motivational salience of infant faces is similar for men and women. *PLoS ONE, 6,* e20632.

Parsons, C. E., Young, K. S., Murray, L., Stein, A., & Kringelbach, M. L. (2010). The functional neuroanatomy of the evolving parent–infant relationship. *Progress in Neurobiology, 91,* 220–241.

Peciña, S., Smith, K. S., & Berridge, K. C. (2006). Hedonic hot spots in the brain. *Neuroscientist, 12,* 500–511.

Philippi, C. L., Duff, M. C., Denburg, N. L., Tranel, D., & Rudrauf, D. (2012a). Medial PFC damage abolishes the self-reference effect. *Journal of Cognitive Neuroscience, 24,* 475–481.

Philippi, C. L., Feinstein, J. S., Khalsa, S. S., Damasio, A., Tranel, D., Landini, G., et al. (2012b). Preserved self-awareness following extensive bilateral brain damage to the insula, anterior cingulate, and medial prefrontal cortices. *PLoS ONE, 7,* e38413.

Posner, J., Russell, J. A., & Peterson, B. S. (2005). The circumplex model of affect: An integrative approach to affective neuroscience, cognitive development, and psychopathology. *Development and Psychopathology, 17,* 715–734.

Price, T. F., & Harmon-Jones, E. (2011). Approach motivational body postures lean toward left frontal brain activity. *Psychophysiology, 48,* 718–722.

Raichle, M. E., MacLeod, A. M., Snyder, A. Z., Powers, W. J., Gusnard, D. A., & Shulman, G. L. (2001). A default mode of brain function. *Proceedings of the National Academy of Sciences USA, 98,* 676–682.

Raichle, M. E., & Mintun, M. A. (2006). Brain work and brain imaging. *Annual Review of Neuroscience, 29,* 449–476.

Robinson, T. E., & Berridge, K. C. (1993). The neural basis of drug craving: An incentive-sensitization theory of addiction. *Brain Research Reviews, 18,* 247–291.

Robinson, T. E., & Berridge, K. C. (2003). Addiction. *Annual Review of Psychology, 54*, 25–53.

Russell, J. A., & Barrett, L. F. (1999). Core affect, prototypical emotional episodes, and other things called emotion: Dissecting the elephant. *Journal of Personality and Social Psychology, 76*, 805–819.

Ryle, G. (1954). Pleasure. *Proceedings of the Aristotelian Society, 28*, 135–146.

Salimpoor, V. N., Benovoy, M., Larcher, K., Dagher, A., & Zatorre, R. J. (2011). Anatomically distinct dopamine release during anticipation and experience of peak emotion to music. *Nature Neuroscence, 14*, 257–262.

Salimpoor, V. N., van den Bosch, I., Kovacevic, N., McIntosh, A. R., Dagher, A., & Zatorre, R. J. (2013). Interactions between the nucleus accumbens and auditory cortices predict music reward value. *Science, 340*, 216–219.

Seeley, W. W., Menon, V., Schatzberg, A. F., Keller, J., Glover, G. H., Kenna, H., et al. (2007). Dissociable intrinsic connectivity networks for salience processing and executive control. *Journal of Neuroscience, 27*, 2349–2356.

Shenhav, A., Barrett, L. F., & Bar, M. (2013). Affective value and associative processing share a cortical substrate. *Cognitive, Affective, and Behavioral Neuroscience, 13*, 46–59.

Skov, M. (2010). The pleasures of art. In M. L. Kringelbach & K. C. Berridge (Eds.), *Pleasures of the brain* (pp. 270–283). New York: Oxford University Press.

Small, D. M., Zatorre, R. J., Dagher, A., Evans, A. C., & Jones-Gotman, M. (2001). Changes in brain activity related to eating chocolate: From pleasure to aversion. *Brain, 124*, 1720–1733.

Smith, K. S., & Berridge, K. C. (2007). Opioid limbic circuit for reward: Interaction between hedonic hotspots of nucleus accumbens and ventral pallidum. *Journal of Neuroscience, 27*, 1594–1605.

Smith, K. S., Berridge, K. C., & Aldridge, J. W. (2011). Disentangling pleasure from incentive salience and learning signals in brain reward circuitry. *Proceedings of the National Academy of Sciences USA, 108*, E255–E264.

Smith, K. S., Mahler, S. V., Pecina, S., & Berridge, K. C. (2010). Hedonic hotspots: Generating sensory pleasure in the brain. In M. L. Kringelbach & K. C. Berridge (Eds.), *Pleasures of the brain* (pp. 27–49). New York: Oxford University Press.

Stein, A., Gath, D. H., Bucher, J., Bond, A., Day, A., & Cooper, P. J. (1991). The relationship between post-natal depression and mother–child interaction. *British Journal of Psychiatry, 158*, 46–52.

van Eimeren, T., Monchi, O., Ballanger, B., & Strafella, A. P. (2009). Dysfunction of the default mode network in Parkinson disease: A functional magnetic resonance imaging study. *Archives of Neurology, 66*, 877–883.

Völlm, B. A., de Araujo, I. E. T., Cowen, P. J., Rolls, E. T., Kringelbach, M. L., Smith, K. A., et al. (2004). Methamphetamine activates reward circuitry in drug naïve human subjects. *Neuropsychopharmacology, 29*, 1715–1722.

Vuust, P., & Kringelbach, M. L. (2010). The pleasure of music. In M. L. Kringelbach & K. C. Berridge (Eds.), *Pleasures of the brain* (pp. 255–269). New York: Oxford University Press.

Watson, K. K., Shepherd, S. V., & Platt, M. L. (2010). Neuroethology of pleasure. In M. L. Kringelbach & K. C. Berridge (Eds.), *Pleasures of the brain* (pp. 85–95). New York: Oxford University Press.

Watts, D., & Strogatz, S. (1998). Collective dynamics of "small-world" networks. *Nature, 393*, 440–442.

Wilson-Mendenhall, C. D., Barrett, L. F., & Barsalou, L. W. (2013). Neural evidence that human emotions share core affective properties. *Psychological Science, 24*(6), 947–956.

Zhang, J., Berridge, K. C., Tindell, A. J., Smith, K. S., & Aldridge, J. W. (2009). A neural computational model of incentive salience. *PLoS Computational Biology, 5*, e1000437.

CHAPTER 11

Mesolimbic Dopamine and Emotion

A Complex Contribution to a Complex Phenomenon

JOHN D. SALAMONE
MERCÈ CORREA
PATRICK A. RANDALL
ERIC J. NUNES

Background: The "Anhedonia" Hypothesis of Dopamine Function

For several years, one of the most popular ideas originating from the behavioral neuroscience literature has been that dopamine (DA), particularly in ventral striatum/nucleus accumbens, mediates the "rewarding" effects of positive reinforcers such as food, water, sex, and drugs of abuse. After originating in the animal literature, with a focus on the effects of DA antagonists on operant responding reinforced by food or intracranial self-stimulation (e.g., Wise, 1982), this hypothesis has been extended into virtually every realm of neuroscience (e.g., Peterson, 2005). Moreover, this idea has fully permeated the popular media, including film and the Internet. Years ago it was common to hear the term "pop psychology" used to refer to the popularization of psychological terms in the media. One could argue that the DA hypothesis of "reward" has become a modern-day example of "pop neuroscience," used to explain our reactions to all pleasurable stimuli, as well as our marketing choices and sexual or political preferences. For example, an Internet search of just one magazine (*The Atlantic*) reveals seven articles in 2012 alone that discuss how DA mediates pleasure or "reward."

Yet despite its popularity, there are numerous problems with the DA hypothesis of "reward" (sometimes this hypothesis is also referred to as the "anhedonia" hypothesis, because DA antagonists are said to blunt the hedonic impact of reinforcing stimuli; for an overview of the history of this hypothesis, see Wise, 2008). Some of these problems are terminological and conceptual, while others are empirical. Within the field of emotion research, it is probably true that no debate has garnered more interest than the issue of whether positive and negative affect are generated within biologically independent systems (for a review, see Barrett & Bliss-Moreau, 2009). At the center of the argument in favor of the independence view is the claim that dopamine mediates reward, or pleasure. In this chapter we review the theory and evidence challenging the utility of the concept that ventral striatal DA mediates "reward" or hedonia, and point to the rather complex role that mesolimbic DA plays in emotion and motivation.

What Is the Relation between "Reward" and "Hedonia"?

What is "reward"? At the outset, we should stated that there is no standard definition or usage of this term, despite the fact that it is so widely employed. Although *reward* can be used as a synonym for *positive reinforcer* when it refers to a stimulus, the term *reward* also has many additional connotations (Cannon & Bseikri, 2004; Salamone, Correa, Farrar, & Mingote, 2007; Salamone & Correa, 2012). Several investigators have noted that usage of this term seems to evoke ideas related to emotion and motivation (White, 1989; Stellar, 2001; Everitt & Robbins, 2005). Initial studies that laid the foundation of the DA hypothesis of "reward" emphasized these emotional processes in suggesting that interference with DA transmission produced "anhedonia" (Wise, 1982; Wise & Raptis, 1985; Wise, Spindler, de Wit, & Gerberg, 1978). The hypothesized "reward" functions of DA have been particularly popular in the drug abuse and self-administration literatures (e.g., Gardner, 1992). More recently, Everitt and Robbins (2005) observed that the use of the term *reward* emphasizes the "subjective, attributional aspects" of reinforcing stimuli. Thus, many researchers use the term *reward* as a thinly veiled synonym for *pleasure* or *hedonia*. Of course, this is not the only usage; *reward* also is used as a synonym for *reinforcement learning*, or as a general term referring to all aspects of appetitive learning, motivation, and emotion. There are three major problems with this: (1) It is virtually impossible to test the hypothesis that DA mediates *reward* when the term can mean so many different things; (2) when used in a very general way (i.e., to describe all processes related in some way to appetitive motivation), *reward* lumps together a number of processes that are easily distinct and dissociable from each other, some of which are mediated by DA, and others that are not; and (3) the idea that *reward* means "pleasure" is so omnipresent that use of the term *reward* tends to evoke the idea of pleasure or hedonia, even if this is not intended by the author (Salamone & Correa, 2012).

Does DA Mediate Pleasure or Hedonia?

Results from Animal Studies

Despite its popularity, the idea that interference with DA systems causes "anhedonia" is highly controversial, and there is considerable evidence against it. Although sucrose consumption or preference is sometimes used as a measure of food-related hedonia (e.g., Johnson & Kenney, 2010), there are several reasons why consumption or preference measures per se are not reliable indices of the emotional state. For example, if sucrose consumption is impaired by a particular treatment, it may reflect changes in a number of different processes other than emotion, including oral motor function, approach to the drinking tube, or sensorimotor responsiveness (Muscat & Willner, 1989; Berridge, 2000, 2007; Sederholm, Johnson, Brodin, & Södersten, 2002; Salamone & Correa, 2002). In order to address these concerns, one of the tests that has become widely accepted as a measure hedonic reactivity to sweet solutions is the taste reactivity paradigm. Over the last several years, a substantial body of research from Berridge and colleagues has demonstrated that systemic administration of DA antagonists, whole forebrain DA depletions, or local depletions of nucleus accumbens DA fail to blunt appetitive taste reactivity for food (Berridge & Robinson, 1998, 2003; Berridge, 2007). Furthermore, manipulations that elevate extracellular DA, including knockdown of the DA transporter (Peciña, Cagniard, Berridge, Aldridge, & Zhuang, 2003) and microinjections of the stimulant drug amphetamine directly into nucleus accumbens (Smith, Berridge, & Aldridge, 2011), failed to enhance appetitive taste reactivity for sucrose. Although nucleus accumbens shell DA D2 receptors appeared to regulate aversive taste reactivity, and stimulation of DA D2 receptors in the brainstem suppressed sucrose consumption, neither population of receptors mediated the hedonic display of taste (Sederholm et al., 2002). These findings and others have led Berridge and Robinson (1998, 2003) to conclude that brain DA does not mediate "liking" (i.e., the hedonic reaction to food). Nevertheless, these authors have suggested that DA systems are involved in "wanting" (i.e., incentive motivation) of natural and drug rewards (see Berridge, 2007).

A superficial review of some articles in the DA literature may leave one with the impression that ventral striatal/nucleus accumbens DA is selectively involved in hedonic processes, appetitive motivation, and reinforcement-related learning, but not in aspects of aversive emotion or motivation. For example, it has been stated that increases in DA release are only associated with appetitive stimuli, not aversive ones (e.g., Burgdorf & Panksepp, 2006). Nevertheless, such a suggestion is not supported by the literature. Neurochemical markers of accumbens DA transmission, such as extracellular levels of DA as measured by microdialysis, are elevated in response to a diverse variety of aversive conditions, including foot shock, tail shock, tail pinch, restraint stress, instrumental avoidance, conditioned aversive stimuli, anxiogenic drugs, and social defeat stress (Salamone, 1994, 1996; McCullough, Sokolowski, & Salamone, 1993; Tidey & Miczek, 1996; Datla, Ahier, Young, Gray, & Joseph, 2002; Young, 2004; Marinelli, Pascucci, Bernardi, Puglisi-Allegra, & Mercuri, 2005). Although the slow time resolution of microdiaysis methods makes it difficult to establish specific relations between neurochemical changes and transient behavioral or environmental events, several investigators have used electrophysiological and voltammetric methods (i.e., electrochemical methods that detect transient changes in extracellular DA) to obtain markers of fast phasic DA activity. For many years, it was thought that activity of putative ventral tegmental DA neurons was not increased by aversive stimuli. However, Guarraci and Kapp (1999) showed that putative ventral tegmental DA neurons responded to the conditioned stimulus during Pavlovian fear conditioning, and subsequently, Anstrom and Woodward (2005) reported that virtually all putative ventral tegmental DA neurons from which they recorded showed increased activity during restraint stress. More recent studies have confirmed that the electrophysiological activity of putative or identified DA neurons is increased by aversive or stressful conditions (Brischoux, Chakraborty, Brierley, & Ungless, 2009; Matsumoto & Hikosaka, 2009; Bromberg-Martin, Matsumoto, & Hikosaka, 2010; Schulz, 2010; Lammel, Ion, Roeper, & Malenka, 2011). Although Roitman, Wheeler, Wightman, and Carelli (2008) reported that an aversive taste stimulus (quinine) decreased DA transients in nucleus accumbens as measured by voltammetry, Anstrom, Miczek, and Budygin (2009) observed that social defeat stress was accompanied by increases in fast phasic DA activity, as measured by both electrophysiology and voltammetry.

Although it often is stated that interference with DA transmission impairs "reward"-related learning, a substantial literature also implicates DA systems in the behavioral response to aversive stimuli or stressful conditions, and in aversive learning. These studies go back several decades (Salamone, 1994) and have continued up to more recent reports (Faure, Reynolds, Richard, & Berridge, 2008; Zweifel et al., 2011). Considerable evidence indicates that interference with DA transmission can impair the acquisition or performance of aversively motivated behavior. In fact, for many years, DA antagonists underwent preclinical screening for assessment of potential antipsychotic activity based partly on their ability to blunt avoidance behavior (Salamone, 1994). Accumbens DA depletions impair shock avoidance lever pressing (i.e., Sidman avoidance; McCullough et al., 1993). Systemic or intra-accumbens injections of DA antagonists also disrupt the acquisition of place aversion and taste aversion (Acquas & Di Chiara, 1991; Fenu, Bassareo, & Di Chiara, 2001), as well as fear conditioning (Inoue, Izumi, Maki, Muraki, & Koyama, 2000; Pezze & Feldon, 2004). Zweifel et al. (2011) reported that knockout of N-methyl-D-aspartate (NMDA) receptors, which acts to reduce fast phasic DA release, impaired the acquisition of cue-dependent fear conditioning. Furthermore, an emerging body of work has demonstrated that rats showing greater response to conditioned cues (sign-trackers) display different patterns of dopaminergic adaptation to training than do animals that are more responsive to the primary reinforcer (goal trackers; Flagel, Watson, Robinson, & Akil, 2007). Interestingly, the rats that show greater Pavlovian conditioned approach to an appetitive stimulus, and show greater incentive conditioning to drug cues, also tend to show greater fear in response to cues predicting shock, and greater contextual fear conditioning (Morrow, Maren, & Robinson, 2011).

In summary, research from the animal literature does not indicate that mesolimbic DA shows increased activity solely in response to stimuli or conditions that are marked by positive hedonic valence. Furthermore, the involvement of DA in instrumental behavior, learning, or motivation is not unique to appetitively motivated tasks. Finally, there is considerable evidence that interference with DA transmission does not blunt hedonic reactivity to taste stimuli. Taken together, these findings sharply challenge the long-held belief that mesolimbic DA is a critical mediator of pleasure or hedonia.

Results from Human Studies

Several lines of evidence indicate that there are many problems with the idea that DA systems mediate pleasure (Barrett, 2006; Salamone et al., 2007). For example, patients with Parkinson's disease, who have a severe DA depletion, were reported not to have significant alterations in the perceived pleasantness of gustatory stimuli (Sienkiewicz-Jarosz et al., 2005). In an early article focusing on the role of DA in the hedonic reaction to drugs of abuse, Gunne, Anggard, and Jonsson (1972) reported that the euphoric effects of amphetamine could be blocked by DA antagonism. Nevertheless, considerable research over the last few years has challenged this notion. Gawin (1986) studied the effects of DA antagonism in cocaine users, and these patients actually reported continued euphoria from cocaine, as well as lengthened cocaine binges. Brauer and de Wit (1997) investigated the effects of the DA antagonist pimozide, and reported that this drug failed to blunt amphetamine-stimulated euphoria. Neither the typical antipsychotic (and DA D2 antagonist) haloperidol nor the atypical antipsychotic risperidone suppressed the positive self-reported effects of methamphetamine (Wachtel, Ortengren, & de Wit, 2002). Furthermore, the DA D1 antagonist ecopipam failed to attenuate the self-administration and subjective euphoria induced by cocaine (Haney, Ward, Foltin, & Fischman, 2001; Nann-Vernotica, Donny, Bigelow, & Walsh, 2001). Leyton, Casey, Delaney, Kolivakis, and Benkelfat (2005) demonstrated that catecholamine depletion induced by feeding people a phenylalanine/tyrosine-free diet did not reduce cocaine self-administration or cocaine-induced self-reported euphoria. A recent article from the same laboratory described the ability of catecholamine synthesis inhibition to differentiate between different aspects of motivation and emotion in humans (Venugopalan et al., 2011). In this article, the investigators manipulated DA transmission by transiently inhibiting catecholamine synthesis with phenylalanine/tyrosine depletion, and access to cigarette smoking was used as a reinforcer. Inhibition of catecholamine synthesis did not attenuate self-reported craving for cigarettes, nor did it blunt smoking-induced hedonic responses. Nevertheless, it did lower progressive ratio break points for cigarette reinforcement (i.e., the number of operant responses in which the people would engage to obtain the cigarettes), indicating that people with reduced DA synthesis showed a reduced willingness to work for cigarettes.

Imaging methods have allowed for *in vivo* assessment of the responsiveness to appetitive and aversive stimuli in DA terminal areas in humans. Several studies have focused on emotional stimuli, and, as in the early animal research, a common view is that accumbens/ventral striatal activity as measured in imaging studies is closely associated with pleasure (e.g., Peterson, 2005; Keedwell, Andrew, Williams, Brammer, & Phillips, 2005; Sarchiapone et al., 2006). In fact, it is not clear whether the imaging response is greater in response to the primary motivational stimulus, to cues that predict the occurrence of that stimulus, or to the instrumental action. For example, Knutson, Fong, Adams, Varner, and Hommer (2001; Knutson, Fong, Bennett, Adams, & Hommer, 2003) reported that accumbens functional magnetic resonance imaging (fMRI) activation was evident in people performing a gambling task, but that the increased activity was associated with reward prediction or anticipation rather than presentation of the monetary reward per se. O'Doherty, Deichmann, Critchley, and Dolan (2002) observed that anticipation of glucose delivery was associated with increased fMRI activation in midbrain and striatal DA areas, but that these areas did not respond to glucose delivery. In addition, a recent imaging article indicated that doses of the DA precursor L-dihydroxyphenylalanine (L-dopa) that enhanced the striatal representation of appetitively motivated actions did not affect the neural representation of reinforcement value (Guitart-Masip et al., 2012). Evidence from imaging studies also indicates that the response of ventral striatum to anticipation of motivationally or emotionally significant stimuli is not unique to appetitive conditions. Jensen et al. (2003) showed that anticipation of an aversive cutaneous stimulus was associated with fMRI activation of ventral striatum.

Activation of accumbens fMRI responses was related to emotional intensity for both positive and aversive conditions (Phan et al., 2004).

Vietnam War veterans with posttraumatic stress disorder demonstrated increased blood flow in nucleus accumbens in response to the presentation of aversive stimuli (i.e., combat sounds; Liberzon et al., 1999). Aharon, Becerra, Chabris, and Borsook (2006) observed that distinct subregions of the accumbens undergo temporally dependent activation or inhibition of fMRI signals in response to a painful thermal stimulus, which may be related to the perception or anticipation of the stressor. Human imaging studies indicate that ventral striatal blood-oxygen-level-dependent (BOLD) responses, as measured by fMRI, are increased in response to prediction errors regardless of whether the stimulus predicted rewarding or aversive events (Jensen et al., 2007), and that aversive prediction errors were blocked by the DA antagonist haloperidol (Menon et al., 2007). Baliki, Geha, Fields, and Apkarian (2010) reported that in normal subjects, phasic BOLD responses occurred at both the onset and offset of a painful thermal stimulus. Levita et al. (2009) used fMRI to delineate brain response to the onset and offset of unpleasant and pleasant auditory stimuli in the absence of any learning or motor responses; they observed that increased nucleus accumbens activity was present for the onset of both pleasant and unpleasant stimuli. Delgado, Jou, and Phelps (2011) demonstrated that ventral striatal BOLD responses were increased during aversive conditioning to a primary aversive stimulus (shock) as well as monetary loss. Although most imaging studies do not deal directly with DA per se, Preussner, Champagne, Meaney, and Dagher (2004) used positron emission tomography (PET) measurements of *in vivo* raclopride displacement to assess DA release in humans, and observed that exposure to psychosocial stress increased markers of extracellular DA in the ventral striatum in a manner that was correlated with increased cortisol release.

To summarize, research with human subjects, like that with animals, also has failed to support the idea that DA systems, or the ventral striatum/nucleus accumbens, respond uniquely or selectively to pleasurable stimuli or conditions that are marked by positive hedonic valence. Furthermore, the preponderance of evidence indicates that interference with DA transmission in humans does not selectively affect self-reported pleasure or euphoria in response to primary motivational stimuli or drugs of abuse. Together with the animal studies, these findings provide a strong challenge to the hypothesis that mesolimbic DA or the ventral striatal region is a critical mediator of pleasure or hedonia.

DA Transmission as a Vital Contributor to Motivational Processes and an Ingredient in Emotional Processes

As reviewed earlier, DA transmission in the nucleus accumbens does not appear to be a specific marker of hedonic reactivity. Furthermore, evidence indicates that accumbens DA activity does not mediate primary motivation or appetite for natural stimuli such as food. Although it is generally agreed that whole-forebrain DA depletions impair food intake, this effect is closely linked to depletions or antagonism of DA in the sensorimotor or motor-related areas of lateral or ventrolateral neostriatum, but not the nucleus accumbens (Koob, Riley, Smith, & Robbins, 1978; Salamone, Mahan, & Rogers, 1993). Baldo, Sadeghian, Basso, and Kelley (2002) reported that D1 and D2 antagonists injected into either core or shell subregions of nucleus accumbens at doses that suppressed locomotor activity failed to affect food intake. Moreover, the effects of DA antagonists or accumbens DA depletions on food-reinforced instrumental behavior differ substantially from the effects of appetite suppressant drugs (Salamone & Correa, 2002; Sink, Vemuri, Olszewska, Makriyannis, & Salamone, 2008), and from reinforcer devaluations such as prefeeding (Salamone et al., 1991; Aberman & Salamone 1999; Pardo et al., 2012). Furthermore, the DA antagonist flupenthixol did not affect the palatability of food reward or the increase in palatability induced by the upshift in motivational state produced by increased food deprivation (Wassum, Ostlund, Balleine, & Maidment, 2011). Moreover, the long-held view about DA as a critical neural mechanism underlying addiction is being revised, and DA is now seen as being more related to its involvement in the initial reinforcing characteristics of drugs. It has become more common to view addiction in terms of neostriatal habit-formation mechanisms built on extensive drug taking, which can be relatively independent of instrumental reinforcement contingencies or the initial motivational characteristics of drug reinforcers (Belin, Jonkman, Dickinson, Robbins, & Everitt, 2009). These emerging views about the neural basis of drug addiction, and its potential treatment, have moved well beyond the original concepts offered by the DA hypothesis of "reward."

So, if nucleus accumbens DA does not mediate hedonic responses to stimuli such as food or drugs of abuse, and does not mediate primary motivation or appetite for food, then what functions does it perform? A thorough discussion of this topic is beyond the scope of this chapter (see Salamone & Correa, 2012), but we provide a brief summary. A significant body of evidence indicates that accumbens DA depletions or antagonism leave core aspects of food-induced hedonia, appetite, or primary food motivation intact but do affect critical features of the instrumental (i.e., food-seeking) behavior. Nucleus accumbens DA is particularly important for mediating activational aspects of motivation (i.e., behavioral activation; Koob et al., 1978; Robbins & Koob, 1980; Salamone, 1988, 1991; Salamone, Correa, Mingote, & Weber, 2005; Salamone et al., 2007; Calaminus & Hauber, 2007; Lex & Hauber, 2010), exertion of effort during instrumental behavior (Salamone, Cousins, & Bucher, 1994; Salamone, Correa, Nunes, Randall, & Pardo, 2012; Salamone et al., 2007; Treadway et al., 2012), Pavlovian responsiveness to instrumental transfer and to conditioned stimuli (Wyvell & Berridge, 2000; Everitt & Robbins, 2005; Lex

& Hauber, 2008), incentive salience (Berridge, 2007); flexible approach behavior (Nicola, 2010), energy expenditure and regulation (Salamone, 1987; Beeler, Frazier, & Zhuang, 2012), and exploitation of reward learning (Beeler, Daw, Frazier, & Zhuang, 2010). Putting all these related ideas together, it has been suggested that nucleus accumbens DA helps organisms overcome the "psychological distance" that separates them from significant stimuli (Salamone & Correa, 2012). In other words, accumbens DA transmission facilitates the process of enabling organisms to surmount various obstacles (e.g., physical distance, time, probability, instrumental requirements) that separate them from these motivations or events. These functions obviously represent critical aspects of motivation, but they are quite different from maintaining that DA is some kind of "pleasure chemical" or that DA systems mediate "reward" or hedonia.

In view of the clear evidence linking DA transmission to aspects of motivation, what does this say about dopaminergic involvement in emotion? Is DA irrelevant as an ingredient in emotional states? Not necessarily. Burgdorf and Panksepp (2006) suggested that ventral striatal mechanisms are not related to "pleasure" or "consummatory reward" in the traditional sense, but instead are involved in anticipatory or appetitive energizing effects of stimuli. More recently, Panksepp (2011) has described how emotional networks in the brain are interwoven with motivational systems involved in patterns of behavior such as seeking, rage, or panic. Thus, it is possible that mesolimbic DA, while acting as a vital mediator of several important aspects of motivation, also contributes to the emotions experienced during seeking or avoidance behavior. In addition, it is possible that DA participates in the intensity or arousal dimension of emotions, as opposed to the valence dimension (Russell & Barrett, 1999; Phan et al., 2004). Finally, DA transmission in the nucleus accumbens may generate internal stimuli consistent with feelings of self-reported energy or efficacy (i.e., "I can obtain this" or "I can avoid this"; Salamone, 1991; Nesse & Berridge, 1997). Examples of this include the omnipotence and power that cocaine addicts report as the main feelings the drug produces (Sherer, Kumor, & Jaffe, 1989), and the concept of self-perceived fitness (Newlin, 2002). These speculations all points to a potential role for nucleus accumbens DA as an ingredient in the emotional stew, albeit one that may affect taste quite differently depending on the rest of the ingredients.

A rejection of the idea that mesolimbic DA mediates hedonia or euphoria also can help to reshape concepts about the involvement of this system in psychopathology, and shed light on the nature of emotional disruptions seen across various disorders. For example, it no longer seems tenable to maintain that reduced DA transmission is the fundamental cause of anhedonia (in terms of an inability to experience pleasure) in depression. Indeed, there are several problems with this. As reviewed by Treadway and Zald (2011), multiple studies have shown that the hedonic responses of depressed patients to the direct experience of pleasurable stimuli appear to be relatively intact. Instead, many depressed people have more clear difficulties with pursuit of motivational stimuli, exertion of effort, and motivational anticipation. In fact, it can be argued that in many instances depressed patients are mislabeled as anhedonic, when their more fundamental pathologies may be related to psychomotor retardation, anergia or motivational apathy. Considerable evidence indicates that DA systems are involved in these motivational symptoms of depression (Salamone, Correa, Mingote, Weber, & Farrar, 2006; Salamone et al., 2007; Treadway & Zald, 2011). Thus, mesolimbic DA and related brain circuits could be contributing substantially to the symptomatology of depression, but in a manner quite different from that outlined by the DA hypothesis of "reward."

REFERENCES

Aberman, J. E., & Salamone, J. D. (1999). Nucleus accumbens dopamine depletions make rats more sensitive to high ratio requirements but do not impair primary food reinforcement. *Neuroscience, 92,* 545–552.

Acquas, E., & Di Chiara, G. (1991). D1 receptor blockade stereospecifically impairs the acquisition of drug-conditioned place preference and place aversion. *Behavioural Pharmacology, 5,* 555–569.

Aharon, I., Becerra, L., Chabris, C. F., & Borsook, D. (2006). Noxious heat induces fMRI activation in two anatomically distinct clusters within the nucleus accumbens. *Neuroscience Letters, 392,* 159–164.

Anstrom, K. K., Miczek, K. A., & Budygin, E. A. (2009). Increased phasic dopamine signaling in the mesolimbic bathway during social defeat in rats. *Neuroscience, 161,* 3–12.

Anstrom, K. K., & Woodward, D. J. (2005). Restraint increases dopaminergic burst firing in awake rats. *Neuropsychopharmacology, 30,* 1832–1840.

Baldo, B. A., Sadeghian, K., Basso, A. M., & Kelley, A. E. (2002). Effects of selective dopamine D1 or D2 receptor blockade within nucleus accumbens subregions on ingestive behavior and associated motor activity. *Behavioural Brain Research, 137,* 165–177.

Baliki, M. N., Geha, P. Y., Fields, H. L., & Apkarian, A. V. (2010). Predicting value of pain and analgesia: Nucleus accumbens response to noxious stimuli changes in the presence of chronic pain. *Neuron, 66,* 149–160.

Barrett, L. F. (2006). Are emotions natural kinds? *Perspectives on Psychological Science, 1,* 28–58.

Barrett, L. F., & Bliss-Moreau, E. (2009). Affect as a psychological primitive. *Advances in Experimental Social Psychology, 41,* 167–218.

Beeler, J. A., Daw, N., Frazier, C. R., & Zhuang, X. (2010). Tonic dopamine modulates exploitation of reward learning. *Frontiers in Behavioral Neuroscience, 4,* 170.

Beeler, J., Frazier, C. R. M., & Zhuang, X. (2012). Putting desire on a budget: Dopamine and energy expenditure, reconciling reward and resources. *Frontiers in Integrative Neuroscience, 6,* 49.

Belin, D., Jonkman, S., Dickinson, A., Robbins, T. W., & Everitt, B. J. (2009). Parallel and interactive learning processes within the basal ganglia: Relevance for the understanding of addiction. *Behavioural Brain Research, 199,* 89–102.

Berridge, K. C. (2000). Measuring hedonic impact in animals and infants: Microstructure of affective taste reactivity patterns. *Neuroscience and Biobehavioral Reviews, 24,* 173–198.

Berridge, K. C. (2007). The debate over dopamine's role in reward: The case for incentive salience. *Psychopharmacology, 191,* 391–431.

Berridge, K. C., & Robinson, T. E. (1998). What is the role of dopamine in reward: Hedonic impact, reward learning, or incentive salience? *Brain Research Reviews, 28,* 309–369.

Berridge, K. C., & Robinson, T. E. (2003). Parsing reward. *Trends in Neurosciences, 26,* 507–513.

Brauer, L. H., & de Wit, H. (1997). High dose pimozide does not block amphetamine-induced euphoria in normal volunteers. *Pharmacology Biochemistry and Behavior, 56,* 265–272.

Brischoux, F., Chakraborty, S., Brierley, D. I., & Ungless, M. A. (2009). Phasic excitation of dopamine neurons in ventral VTA by noxious stimuli. *Proceedings of the National Academy of Sciences USA, 106,* 4894–4899.

Bromberg-Martin, E. S., Matsumoto, M., & Hikosaka, O. (2010). Dopamine in motivational control: Rewarding, aversive, and alerting. *Neuron, 68,* 815–834.

Burgdorf, J., & Panksepp, J. (2006). The neurobiology of positive emotions. *Neuroscience and Biobehavioral Reviews, 30,* 173–187.

Calaminus, C., & Hauber, W. (2007). Intact discrimination reversal learning but slowed responding to reward-predictive cues after dopamine D1 and D2 receptor blockade in the nucleus accumbens of rats. *Psychopharmacology, 191,* 551–566.

Cannon, C. M., & Bseikri, M. R. (2004). Is dopamine required for natural reward? *Physiology and Behavior, 81,* 741–748.

Datla, K. P., Ahier, R. G., Young, A. M., Gray, J. A., & Joseph, M. H. (2002). Conditioned appetitive stimulus increases extracellular dopamine in the nucleus accumbens of the rat. *European Journal of Neuroscience, 16,* 1987–1993.

Delgado, M. R., Jou, R. L., & Phelps, E. A. (2011). Neural systems underlying aversive conditioning in humans with primary and secondary reinforcers. *Frontiers in Neuroscience, 5,* 71.

Everitt, B. J., & Robbins, T. W. (2005). Neural systems of reinforcement for drug addiction: From actions to habits to compulsion. *Nature Neuroscience, 8,* 1481–1489.

Faure, A., Reynolds, S. M., Richard, J. M., & Berridge, K. C. (2008). Mesolimbic dopamine in desire and dread: Enabling motivation to be generated by localized glutamate disruptions in nucleus accumbens. *Journal of Neuroscience, 28,* 7184–7192.

Fenu, S., Bassareo, V., & Di Chiara, G. (2001). A role for dopamine D1 receptors of the nucleus accumbens shell in conditioned taste aversion learning. *Journal of Neuroscience, 21,* 6897–6904.

Flagel, S. B., Watson, S. J., Robinson, T. E., & Akil, H. (2007). Individual differences in the propensity to approach signals vs goals promote different adaptations in the dopamine system of rats. *Psychopharmacology, 191*, 599–607.

Gardner, E. L. (1992). Brain reward mechanisms. In J. H. Lowinson, P. Ruiz, & R. B. Millman (Eds.), *Substance abuse* (pp. 70–99). New York: Williams & Wilkins.

Gawin, F. H. (1986). Neuroleptic reduction of cocaine-induced paranoia but not euphoria? *Psychopharmacology, 90*, 142–143.

Guarraci, F. A., & Kapp, B. S. (1999). An electrophysiological characterization of ventral tegmental area dopaminergic neurons during differential Pavlovian fear conditioning in the awake rabbit. *Behavioural Brain Research, 99*, 169–179.

Guitart-Masip, M., Chowdhury, R., Sharot, T., Dayan, P., Duzel, E., & Dolan, R. J. (2012). Action controls dopaminergic enhancement of reward representations. *Proceedings of the National Academy of Sciences, 109*, 7511–7516.

Gunne, L. M., Anggard, E., & Jonsson, L. E. (1972). Clinical trials with amphetamine-blocking drugs. *Schweizer Archiv für Neurologie, Neurochirurgie und Psychiatrie, 75*, 225–226.

Haney, M., Ward, A. S., Foltin, R. W., & Fischman, M. W. (2001). Effects of ecopipam, a selective dopamine D1 antagonist, on smoked cocaine self-administration by humans. *Psychopharmacology, 155*, 330–337.

Inoue, T., Izumi, T., Maki, Y., Muraki, I., & Koyama, T. (2000). Effect of dopamine D1/5 antagonist SCH 23390 on the acquisition of conditioned fear. *Pharmacology Biochemistry and Behavior, 66*, 573–578.

Jensen, J., McIntosh, A. R., Crawley, A. P., Mikulis, D. J., Remington, G., & Kapur, S. (2003). Direct activation of the ventral striatum in anticipation of aversive stimuli. *Neuron, 40*, 1251–1257.

Jensen, J., Smith, A. J., Willeit, M., Crawley, A. P., Mikulis, D. J., Vitcu, I., et al. (2007). Separate brain regions code for salience vs. valence during reward prediction in humans. *Human Brain Mapping, 28*, 294–302.

Johnson, P. M., & Kenney, P. J. (2010). Dopamine D2 receptors in addiction-like reward dysfunction and compulsive eating in obese rats. *Nature Neuroscience, 13*, 635–641.

Keedwell, P. A., Andrew, C., Williams, S. C., Brammer, M. J., & Phillips, M. L. (2005). The neural correlates of anhedonia in major depressive disorder. *Biological Psychiatry, 58*, 843–853.

Knutson, B., Fong, G. W., Adams, C. M., Varner, J. L., & Hommer, D. (2001). Dissociation of reward anticipation and outcome with event-related fMRI. *NeuroReport,12*, 3683–3687.

Knutson, B., Fong, G. W., Bennett, S. M., Adams, C. M., & Hommer, D. (2003). A region of mesial prefrontal cortex tracks monetarily rewarding outcomes: Characterization with rapid event-related fMRI. *NeuroImage, 18*, 263–272.

Koob, G. F., Riley, S. J., Smith, S. C., & Robbins, T. W. (1978). Effects of 6-hydroxydopamine lesions of the nucleus accumbens septi and olfactory tubercle on feeding, locomotor activity, and amphetamine anorexia in the rat. *Journal of Comparative Physiological Psychology, 92*, 917–927.

Lammel, S., Ion, D. I., Roeper, J., & Malenka, R. C. (2011). Projection-specific modulation of dopamine neuron synapses by aversive and rewarding stimuli. *Neuron, 70*, 855–862.

Levita, L., Hare, T. A., Voss, H. U., Glover, G., Ballon, D. J., & Casey, B. J. (2009). The bivalent side of the nucleus accumbens. *NeuroImage, 44*, 1178–1187.

Lex, A., & Hauber, W. (2008). Dopamine D1 and D2 receptors in the nucleus accumbens core and shell mediate Pavlovian-instrumental transfer. *Learning and Memory, 15*, 483–491.

Lex, B., & Hauber, W. (2010). The role of nucleus accumbens dopamine in outcome encoding in instrumental and Pavlovian conditioning. *Neurobiology of Learning and Memory, 93*, 283–290.

Leyton, M., Casey, K. F., Delaney, J. S., Kolivakis, T., & Benkelfat, C. (2005). Cocaine craving, euphoria, and self-administration: A preliminary study of the effect of catecholamine precursor depletion. *Behavioral Neuroscience, 119*, 1619–1627.

Liberzon, I., Taylor, S. F., Amdur, R., Jung, T. D., Chamberlain, K. R., Minoshima, S., et al. (1999). Brain activation in PTSD in response to trauma-related stimuli. *Biological Psychiatry, 45*, 817–826.

Marinelli, S., Pascucci, T., Bernardi, G., Puglisi-Allegra, S., & Mercuri, N. B. (2005). Activation of TRPV1 in the VTA excites dopaminergic neurons and increases chemical- and noxious-induced dopamine release in the nucleus accumbens. *Neuropsychopharmacology, 30*, 864–870.

Matsumoto, M., & Hikosaka, O. (2009). Two types of dopamine neuron distinctly convey positive and negative motivational signals. *Nature, 459*, 837–841.

McCullough, L. D., Sokolowski, J. D., & Salamone, J. D. (1993). A neurochemical and behavioral investigation of the involvement of nucleus accumbens dopamine in instrumental avoidance. *Neuroscience, 52*, 919–925.

Menon, M., Jensen, J., Vitcu, I., Graff-Guerrero, A., Crawley, A., Smith, M. A., et al. (2007). Temporal difference modeling of the blood-oxygen level dependent response during aversive conditioning in humans: Effects of dopaminergic modulation. *Biological Psychiatry, 62*, 765–772.

Morrow, J. D., Maren, S., & Robinson, T. E. (2011). Individual variation in the propensity to attribute incentive salience to an appetitive cue predicts the propensity to attribute motivational salience to an aversive cue. *Behavioural Brain Research, 220*, 238–243.

Muscat, R., & Willner, P. (1989). Effects of dopamine receptor antagonists on sucrose consumption and preference. *Psychopharmacology (Berlin), 99*, 98–102.

Nann-Vernotica, E., Donny, E. C., Bigelow, G. E., & Walsh, S. L. (2001). Repeated administration of the D1/5 antagonist ecopipam fails to attenuate the subjective effects of cocaine. *Psychopharmacology, 155*, 338–347.

Nesse, R. M., & Berridge, K. C. (1997). Psychoactive drug use in evolutionary perspective. *Science, 278*, 63–66.

Newlin, D. B. (2002). The self-perceived survival ability and reproductive fitness (SPFit) theory of substance use disorders. *Addiction, 97*, 427–445.

Nicola, S. M. (2010). The flexible approach hypothesis: Unification of effort and cue-responding hypotheses for the role of nucleus accumbens dopamine in the activation of reward-seeking behavior. *Journal of Neuroscience, 30*, 16585–16600.

O'Doherty, J. P., Deichmann, R., Critchley, H. D., & Dolan, R. J. (2002). Neural responses during anticipation of a primary taste reward. *Neuron, 33*, 815–826.

Panksepp, J. (2011). Cross-species affective neuroscience decoding of the primal affective experiences of humans and related animals. *PLoS ONE, 6,* e21236.

Pardo, M., Lopez-Cruz, L., Valverde, O., Ledent, C., Baqi, Y., Müller, C. E., et al. (2012). Adenosine A_{2A} receptor antagonism and genetic deletion attenuate the effects of dopamine D2 antagonism on effort-based decision making in mice. *Neuropharmacology, 62,* 2068–2077.

Peciña, S., Cagniard, B., Berridge, K. C., Aldridge, J. W., & Zhuang, X. (2003). Hyperdopaminergic mutant mice have higher "wanting" but not "liking" for sweet rewards. *Journal of Neuroscience, 23,* 9395–9402.

Peterson, R. L. (2005). The neuroscience of investing: fMRI of the reward system. *Brain Research Bulletin, 67,* 391–397.

Pezze, M. A., & Feldon, J. (2004). Mesolimbic dopaminergic pathways in fear conditioning. *Progress in Neurobiology, 74,* 301–320.

Phan, K. L., Taylor, S. F., Welsh, R. C., Ho, S. H., Britton, J. C., & Liberzon, I. (2004). Neural correlates of individual ratings of emotional salience: A trial-related fMRI study. *NeuroImage, 21,* 768–780.

Pruessner, J. C., Champagne, F., Meaney, M. J., & Dagher, A. (2004). Dopamine release in response to a psychological stress in humans and its relationship to early life maternal care: A positron emission tomography study using [^{11}C] raclopride. *Journal of Neuroscience, 24,* 2825–2831.

Robbins, T. W., & Koob, G. F. (1980). Selective disruption of displacement behaviour by lesions of the mesolimbic dopamine system. *Nature, 285,* 409–412.

Roitman, M. F., Wheeler, R. A., Wightman, R. M., & Carelli, R. M. (2008). Real-time chemical responses in the nucleus accumbens differentiate rewarding and aversive stimuli. *Nature Neuroscience, 11,* 1376–1377.

Russell, J. A., & Barrett, L. F. (1999). Core affect, prototypical emotional episodes, and other things called emotion: Dissecting the elephant. *Journal of Personality and Social Psychology, 76,* 805–819.

Salamone, J. D. (1987). The actions of neuroleptic drugs on appetitive instrumental behaviors. In L. L. Iversen, S. D. Iversen, & S. H. Snyder (Eds.), *Handbook of psychopharmacology* (pp. 575–608). New York: Plenum Press.

Salamone, J. D. (1988). Dopaminergic involvement in activational aspects of motivation: Effects of haloperidol on schedule induced activity, feeding and foraging in rats. *Psychobiology, 16,* 196–206.

Salamone, J. D. (1991). Behavioral pharmacology of dopamine systems: A new synthesis. In P. Willner & J. Scheel-Kruger (Eds.), *The mesolimbic dopamine system: From motivation to action* (pp. 599–613). Cambridge, UK: Cambridge University Press.

Salamone, J. D. (1994). The involvement of nucleus accumbens dopamine in appetitive and aversive motivation. *Behavioural Brain Research, 61,* 117–133.

Salamone, J. D. (1996). The behavioral neurochemistry of motivation: Methodological and conceptual issues in studies of the dynamic activity of nucleus accumbens dopamine. *Journal of Neuroscience Methods, 64,* 137–149.

Salamone, J. D., & Correa, M. (2002). Motivational views of reinforcement: Implications for understanding the behavioral functions of nucleus accumbens dopamine. *Behavioural Brain Research, 137,* 3–25.

Salamone, J. D., & Correa, M. (2012). The mysterious motivational functions of mesolimbic dopamine. *Neuron, 276*(3), 470–485.

Salamone, J. D., Correa, M., Farrar, A. M., & Mingote, S. M. (2007). Effort-related functions of nucleus accumbens dopamine and associated forebrain circuits. *Psychopharmacology, 191*, 461–482.

Salamone, J. D., Correa, M., Mingote, S. M., & Weber, S. M. (2005). Beyond the reward hypothesis: Alternative functions of nucleus accumbens dopamine. *Current Opinion in Pharmacology, 5*, 34–41.

Salamone, J. D., Correa, M., Mingote, S. M., Weber, S. M., & Farrar, A. M. (2006). Nucleus accumbens dopamine and the forebrain circuitry involved in behavioral activation and effort-related decision making: Implications of understanding anergia and psychomotor slowing and depression. *Current Psychiatry Reviews, 2*, 267–280.

Salamone, J. D., Correa, M., Nunes, E. J., Randall, P. A., & Pardo, M. (2012). The behavioral pharmacology of effort-related choice behavior: Dopamine, adenosine and beyond. *Journal of the Experimental Analysis of Behavior, 97*, 125–146.

Salamone, J. D., Cousins, M. S., & Bucher, S. (1994). Anhedonia or anergia?: Effects of haloperidol and nucleus accumbens dopamine depletion on instrumental response selection in a T-maze cost/benefit procedure. *Behavioural Brain Research, 65*, 221–229.

Salamone, J. D., Mahan, K., & Rogers, S. (1993). Ventrolateral striatal dopamine depletions impair feeding and food handling in rats. *Pharmacology Biochemistry and Behavior, 44*, 605–610.

Salamone, J. D., Steinpreis, R. E., McCullough, L. D., Smith, P., Grebel, D., & Mahan, K. (1991). Haloperidol and nucleus accumbens dopamine depletion suppress lever pressing for food but increase free food consumption in a novel food choice procedure. *Psychopharmacology, 104*, 515–521.

Sarchiapone, M., Carli, V., Camardese, G., Cuomo, C., Di Guida, D., Calgagni, M. L., et al. (2006). Dopamine transporter binding in depressed patients with anhedonia. *Psychiatry Research: Neuroimaging, 147*, 243–248.

Schultz, W. (2010). Dopamine signals for reward value and risk: Basic and recent data. *Behavioral and Brain Functions, 6*, 24.

Sederholm, F., Johnson, A. E., Brodin, U., & Södersten, P. (2002). Dopamine D(2) receptors and ingestive behavior: Brainstem mediates inhibition of intraoral intake and accumbens mediates aversive taste behavior in male rats. *Psychopharmacology, 160*, 161–169.

Sherer, M. A., Kumor, K. M., & Jaffe, J. H. (1989). Effects of intravenous cocaine are partially attenuated by haloperidol. *Psychiatry Research, 27*, 117–125.

Sienkiewicz-Jarosz, H., Scinska, A., Kuran, W., Ryglewicz, D., Rogowski, A., Wrobel, E., et al. (2005). Taste responses in patients with Parkinson's disease. *Journal of Neurology, Neurosurgery, and Psychiatry, 76*, 40–46.

Sink, K. S., Vemuri, V. K., Olszewska, T., Makriyannis, A., & Salamone, J. D. (2008). Cannabinoid CB1 antagonists and dopamine antagonists produce different effects on a task involving response allocation and effort-related choice in food-seeking behavior. *Psychopharmacology, 196*, 565–574.

Smith, K. S., Berridge, K. C., & Aldridge, J. W. (2011). Disentangling pleasure from incentive salience and learning signals in brain reward circuitry. *Proceedings of the National Academy of Sciences USA, 108*, E255–E264.

Stellar, J. R. (2001). Reward. In P. Winn (Ed.), *Dictionary of biological psychology* (p. 679). London: Routledge.

Tidey, J. W., & Miczek, K. A. (1996). Social defeat stress selectively alters mesocorticolimbic dopamine release: An *in vivo* microdialysis study. *Brain Research, 721,* 140–149.

Treadway, M. T., Buckholtz, J. W., Cowan, R. L., Woodward, N. D., Li, R., Ansari, M. S., et al. (2012). Dopaminergic mechanisms of individual differences in human effort-based decision-making. *Journal of Neuroscience, 32,* 6170–6176.

Treadway, M. T., & Zald, D. H. (2011). Reconsidering anhedonia in depression: Lessons from translational neuroscience. *Neuroscience and Biobehavioral Reviews, 35,* 537–555.

Venugopalan, V. V., Casey, K. F., O'Hara, C., O'Loughlin, J., Benkelfat, C., Fellows, L. K., et al. (2011). Acute phenylalanine/tyrosine depletion reduces motivation to smoke cigarettes across stages of addiction. *Neuropsychopharmacology, 36,* 2469–2476.

Wachtel, S. R., Ortengren, A., & de Wit, H. (2002). The effects of acute haloperidol or risperidone on subjective responses to methamphetamine in healthy volunteers. *Drug and Alcohol Dependence, 68,* 23–33.

Wassum, K. M., Ostlund, S. B., Balleine, B. W., & Maidment, N. T. (2011). Differential dependence of Pavlovian incentive motivation and instrumental incentive learning processes on dopamine signaling. *Learning and Memory, 18,* 475–483.

White, N. M. (1989). Reward or reinforcement: What's the difference? *Neuroscience and Biobehavioral Reviews, 13,* 181–186.

Wise, R. A. (1982). Neuroleptics and operant behavior: The anhedonia hypothesis. *Behavioral and Brain Sciences, 5,* 39–87.

Wise, R. A. (2008). Dopamine and reward: The anhedonia hypothesis—30 years on. *Neurotoxicity Research, 14,* 169–183.

Wise, R. A., & Raptis, L. (1985). Effects of pre-feeding on food-approach latency and food consumption speed in food deprived rats. *Physiology and Behavior, 35,* 961–963.

Wise, R. A., Spindler, J., deWit, H., & Gerberg, G. J. (1978). Neuroleptic-induced "anhedonia" in rats: Pimozide blocks reward quality of food. *Science, 201,* 262–264.

Wyvell, C. L., & Berridge, K. C. (2001). Incentive sensitization by previous amphetamine exposure: Increased cue-triggered "wanting" for sucrose reward. *Journal of Neuroscience, 21,* 7831–7840.

Young, A. M. (2004). Increased extracellular dopamine in nucleus accumbens in response to unconditioned and conditioned aversive stimuli: Studies using 1 min microdialysis in rats. *Journal of Neuroscience Methods, 138,* 57–63.

Zweifel, L. S., Fadok, J. P., Argilli, E., Garelick, M. G., Jones, G. L., Dickerson, T. M., et al. (2011). Activation of dopamine neurons is critical for aversive conditioning and prevention of generalized anxiety. *Nature Neuroscience, 14,* 620–626.

CHAPTER 12

An Approach to Mapping the Neurophysiological State of the Body to Affective Experience

IAN R. KLECKNER
KAREN S. QUIGLEY

Your heart races, your mouth is dry, your palms are sweaty, and you are breathing quickly. When a bodily state like this is functional and adaptive, it provides the physiological support required for goal-directed action (e.g., physical activity or enhanced attention to optimize cognitive performance). Alternatively, we can interpret these physiological changes in ourselves in other ways, such as feelings of excitement (e.g., if we are riding a roller coaster) or as physical symptoms of an illness (e.g., if we just ate some questionable food). Thus, ostensibly similar bodily sensations can be experienced differently depending on context and expectations. But within a given context, how consistently and specifically do particular bodily states map to particular affective experiences? And what biological substrates and mechanisms support the process by which bodily change informs experience? To begin to answer these questions, we present an approach to mapping the neurophysiological state of the body to affective experience. To inform these issues we consider functional principles related to peripheral physiology and to the central nervous system (CNS) that affect the mapping process, thereby extending prior discussions of the psychological and neural features of affect (Barrett & Bliss-Moreau, 2009).

1. *If emotions are psychological events constructed from more basic ingredients, then what are the key ingredients from which emotions are constructed? Are they specific to emotion or are they general ingredients of the mind? Which, if any, are specific to humans?*

We think ingredients involved in construction of emotion are general ingredients of the mind, because the neurobiological processes (e.g., lateral inhibition) and organizational features of the CNS (e.g., heterarchical structure) do not appear to be specialized for any particular mental state. We think it is not clear whether any ingredients are specific for humans. However, we see at least two important ways in which the quality and/or implementation of psychological ingredients might be significantly different in humans compared to other animals. First, regarding core affect, Craig (2002, 2011) hypothesized that primates (including humans) may have an important stream of information from the body not found in nonprimate mammalian species (i.e., primates have a well-developed insula and a sympathetic afferent system in addition to the parasympathetic afferent system). If future evidence further supports this claim, then primates could have a more nuanced representation of their neurophysiological state, providing a richer sensory stream for making inferences about the world (perhaps analogous to the "superior" olfactory system of dogs relative to humans). Second, the use of language appears to be qualitatively different in humans compared to animals (e.g., chimpanzees or dolphins; See Fitch, 2005). First, in a social setting, human language allows a mental state to be communicated without the aid of other sensory information (e.g., a text message). When the individual(s) receiving that information share a language and meaning structures (i.e., conceptualizations) of the communicated mental state, then a closely related mental state can be generated in the person receiving the communication. Second, the use of language may increase the granularity of mental states, thereby increasing the number of distinct mental states that can be experienced.

2. *What brings these ingredients together in the construction of an emotion? Which combinations are emotions and which are not (and how do we know)?*

Functional networks that span a wide spatial area in the brain provide neurophysiological processes that can support the combination of ingredients (e.g., a neuronal workspace or functional connections with small- and large-world properties; Baars, 2005). Within these large-scale networks, synchronous neural activity that oscillates at 10-120 Hz across wide swaths of brain may be a mechanism by which information is integrated across dispersed regions (Senkowski, Schneider, Foxe, & Engel, 2008). A particular mental state may result from the coactivation of multiple functional modules (i.e., circuits of neurons that temporarily function together). Importantly, brain regions can be part of multiple modules. In this way, a circuit is "modular in the moment," not

(continued)

in a hardwired, permanent sense. By extension, we contend that these functionally modular networks can serve as the neural bases of psychological ingredients, as proposed by our colleagues in their discussion of the neural basis of a construction framework for emotion (e.g., Barrett & Satpute, 2013; Lindquist, Wager, Kober, Bliss-Moreau, & Barrett, 2012). To create a mental state or experience, these functionally defined networks become temporarily linked, perhaps through the processes described briefly here and in our chapter.

We define emotion here as a reportable mental experience that has a consciously accessible affective quality and is categorized as a feeling state. Individuals in each culture have different terms to describe these categorically defined feeling states; thus, the category boundaries will be fluid across individuals, and even more fluid across cultures (see Barrett, 2006, for a discussion). The ingredients minimally required for an emotional mental state are (1) the state of core affect (i.e., a feeling described by valence and arousal related to the neurophysiological state of the body), (2) an attentional process by which the core affect state is foregrounded (attention may or may not be related to a change in core affect), and (3) a conceptual process that categorizes the core affective state (or a change in core affective state).

3. *How important is variability (across instances within an emotion category, and in the categories that exist across cultures)? Is this variance epiphenomenal or a thing to be explained? To the extent that it makes sense, it would be desirable to address issues such as universality and evolution.*

We think variability is critically important to a constructionist view of emotion. Naturally occurring variation in core affect, for example, will influence the kinds of affective statistical regularities that co-occur with a person's feeling states and become linked to that individual's learned emotion concepts. Those concepts will have some similarity across individuals within a cultural context because of shared cultural norms, including explicit and directed learning about emotion concepts (e.g., a child is taught that when another person smiles, it means that person feels happy). But individuals will also vary in their emotional concepts because of specific personal histories (e.g., a child who grows up with a depressed parent may have different emotional concepts than a child who does not).

This variability is a thing to be explained. It will be useful to identify how psychological ingredients vary across individuals within a culture, and across cultures, because such variation may help us to further define the nature of each of the ingredients.

Emotions can be considered in the context of two types of evolution: genetic evolution (i.e., natural selection) and cultural evolution (i.e., propagation of "memes" or information copied across individuals generally via the process of imitation; Dawkins, 1989). Via genetic evolution, mental states (including emotions) will be selected for or against by virtue of how they allow an organism to produce reproductively viable offspring (e.g., by increasing the

(continued)

chances of its own or its offspring's survival, or by attracting a mate). Via cultural evolution, features of emotional states can be transmitted even if those ideas do not influence natural selection of genes (although they can). Hence, due to different selective pressures in different environments, a pattern of emotional reactivity that enhances survival and reproductive outcomes (i.e., genetically) or that is intrinsically salient (i.e., culturally) can differ across cultures. In this sense, we would not expect emotions to be universal across cultures.

4. *What constitutes strong evidence to support a psychological construction to emotion? Point to or summarize empirical evidence that supports your model or outline what a key experiment would look like. What would falsify your model?*

In our view, psychological theory should be constrained by the operating principles that govern the PNS and CNS (e.g., a systems biological approach). By extension, emotion theories must be able to address how emotions are generated using neurobiologically plausible mechanisms. Furthermore, comparison of constructionist and nonconstructionist perspectives requires using paradigms to compare emotion inductions both *with* and *without* explicitly labeling emotional experience. This is difficult because researchers often include manipulation checks on emotion inductions in which the participant conceptualizes discrete emotions (e.g., "How much did the stimulus make you feel anxious, afraid, sad, happy, etc.?"). From a psychological constructionist perspective, it is critical to consider both the nature of any manipulation checks (i.e., only affective or including discrete emotion terms) and their timing (e.g., if the participant is asked only after an initial emotion induction).

Using an appropriate design for comparing different emotion theories, we think quantitative model selection methods would help formalize the comparison process (e.g., Pitt, Myung, & Zhang, 2002). In this approach, experimentally observed data are estimated by each quantitative model of emotion, each of which has a set of explicit neuropsychological mechanisms. For example, a given model may estimate a participant's self-reported mental state by considering his or her physiological activity, neural activity, self-reported affect, conceptual knowledge, and so forth, using a mapping procedure like that in Figure 12.1. Each model is then assessed for its accuracy in estimating observations and its complexity (simpler is better) and models that are both less accurate and more complex will be disfavored (as opposed to being falsified outright). Thus far, quantitative models of emotion have been implemented with pattern classification (which lacks an explicit neurobiological mechanism; e.g., Kragel & LaBar, 2013) and appraisal approaches (e.g., Marsella, Gratch, & Petta, 2010), but not constructionist approaches. We think this field would benefit from comparing quantitative emotion models inspired by neurobiological mechanisms.

Before describing our approach to mapping the neurophysiological state of the body to affective experience, we briefly provide an overview of an existing psychological constructionist theoretical framework for understanding emotional and affective experience. Psychological constructionist theories posit that all mental states (e.g., feelings, thoughts, perceptions) are constructed from the same set of basic psychological ingredients. Many constructionist models posit that one basic ingredient is *core affect*, which is the consciously accessible representation of one's overall bodily state. Core affect is based on both internal and external sensations, and has features of both valence (pleasure vs. displeasure) and arousal (activated vs. deactivated); core affect therefore relies on the current and ever-changing neurophysiological state of the body and the brain, which we discuss in more detail below (Barrett, 2006; Barrett & Bliss-Moreau, 2009; Russell, 2003; Russell, Chapter 8, this volume; Russell & Barrett, 1999). Another psychological ingredient of interest for constructing emotional experiences is *conceptualization* (or more specifically *categorization*), which influences how core affect and other sensory input are categorized and experienced (e.g., as an emotion, a thought, a perception). In a psychological constructionist view, a mental state is changed when the features of one or more psychological ingredients are changed and/or when the psychological ingredients are combined in a different way. Various constructionist models differ on the identity of the psychological ingredients and how they combine to form a mental state and, to date, the mechanisms supporting the construction process are unknown (Barrett, 2011; Cacioppo, Berntson, & Klein, 1992; James, 1890; Mandler, 1984; Russell, 2003; Schachter & Singer, 1962; for a review, see Gendron & Barrett, 2009). We focus in this chapter on core affect, which we consider a psychological ingredient in accord with prior theory (e.g., Barrett & Bliss-Moreau, 2009; Barrett & Satpute, 2013; Lindquist & Barrett, 2012), and we discuss how to map physical measures of the neurophysiological state to psychological-level phenomena such as psychological ingredients.

In this chapter we first present our general approach for mapping central and peripheral neurophysiological measures to core affect and affective experience. Next, we discuss several broad principles of peripheral physiological function, what we have learned from prior efforts to map peripheral neurophysiological measures to affective experience, and how these principles and the reviewed evidence inform the mapping process. We then discuss several broad principles of central neurophysiological function, what prior efforts at mapping reveal, and how these inform our proposed mapping process. We conclude by considering how psychological construction frames hypotheses and studies aimed at understanding the mechanisms of emotional content, both at the level of the ingredient of interest here, core affect, and at the level of emotional experience.

An Approach to Mapping Neurophysiological States to Psychological Ingredients and Affective Experience

The history of psychology is replete with attempts to map physical states to psychological ones as a way to estimate features of a conscious mental state that cannot be observed directly. The "reverse inference" problem has been discussed relative to inferring psychological states from measures of the brain (e.g., Barrett & Satpute, 2013; Lindquist & Barrett, 2012; Poldrack, 2006, 2008, 2011; Sarter, Berntson, & Cacioppo, 1996), and from measures of the body (e.g., Cacioppo & Tassinary, 1990; Kreibig, 2010). As we discuss below, we cannot use physical measures to make strong psychophysiological inferences until we understand the likely limited conditions (e.g., specific contexts) under which these maps can be relatively specific and reliable (Cacioppo & Tassinary, 1990).

Figure 12.1 illustrates our approach for mapping neurophysiological states[1] of the periphery and the central nervous system (CNS) to psychological ingredients; this approach is motivated by prior discussions of inferring psychological states from peripheral physiological measures (Cacioppo & Tassinary, 1990) and from CNS states (Barrett, 2011). The first step in this general approach is to specify the peripheral, central, and psychological states of interest (circles in Figure 12.1, top row; e.g., sympathetic activity, respiration rate, synchronous neural activity, affect). Together, the peripheral and central states constitute the overall neurophysiological state (represented in Figure 12.1 by enclosing the separate peripheral and central states within a single rounded rectangle). Next, peripheral and/or central neurophysiological measures (decagons in Figure 12.1, bottom row) must be examined across multiple studies to determine which sets of neurophysiological measures are most consistently and specifically related to the psychological ingredient of interest (in Figure 12.1, dashed lines map measures in the bottom row to states in the top row). Consistent with prior discussions (Cacioppo & Tassinary, 1990), we propose that core affect maps most reliably to a multivariate pattern of neurophysiological components. A mental state arises when a person makes meaning of his or her internal context (or neurophysiological state) situated within a particular setting and given his or her personal learning history (Barrett, Wilson-Mendenhall, & Barsalou, Chapter 4, this volume). As such, we predict that many related but nonidentical neurophysiological states can map to the same affective mental state, and that a given neurophysiological state can map to several different affective states (i.e., a many-to-many mapping between neurophysiological state and affective state). However, this does not mean that there is an unpredictable or limitless set of many-to-many mappings. Instead, we propose that some mappings are more likely than others (e.g., greater electrodermal activity is more likely to be associated with a high arousal core affective state than with a low arousal one).

There are some caveats to the mapping process. First, each measured variable or set of variables provides an estimate of only some features of the neurophysiological state (i.e., not the entire neurophysiological state). The validity and reliability of the physiological measures as estimates of the true physiological state vary due to measurement issues such as limited spatial resolution, limited temporal resolution, and limited precision, and because the process of measurement can change the system under study. For example, any given measurement of sympathetic activity (e.g., a change in skin conductance or a change in pre-ejection period) can only provide an approximation of sympathetic activity, which is often inaccurately assumed to be uniform across the body despite considerable evidence for specific regional control (for reviews see Jänig & Häbler, 2003; Morrison, 2001). The second caveat is that the set of measurements available for mapping are typically incomplete because it is not feasible to measure every potentially relevant feature of the neurophysiological state, the psychological ingredients, and the mental state (i.e., the mapping of the bottom row in Figure 12.1 to the top row). However, newer technology has made it easier than ever to measure peripheral and central neurophysiology simultaneously, which permits better estimates of the overall neurophysiological state (e.g., Harrison, Gray, Gianaros, & Critchley, 2010; Henderson et al., 2012).

How Do Organizational Features of the Peripheral Nervous System Affect the Mapping of Neurophysiological Measures to Affective Experience?

Several principles governing the peripheral nervous system (PNS) and other peripheral tissues provide important constraints on mapping the neurophysiological state to affective experience. We provide here just a few illustrative examples (for more examples, see Berntson, Cacioppo, & Quigley, 1991, 1993; Jennings & Gianaros, 2007; Quigley, Lindquist, & Barrett, 2013). First, peripheral neurophysiological changes are controlled by the CNS but also impact the CNS via afferent, feedback mechanisms. Efferent physiological control of peripheral bodily functions occurs predominantly by way of the autonomic nervous system (ANS); the enteric nervous system (Mayer, 2011); and the endocrine, the immune, and skeletomotor systems. The afferent sensory mechanisms include not only the afferents of the ANS (see CNS section) and circulating endocrine and immune mediators (Cameron, 2009; Lane et al., 2009), but also afferents of the proprioceptive and kinesthetic systems (Johnson, Babis, Soultanis, & Soucacos, 2008), and the nociceptive (pain) system (Craig, 2003). For example, descending pain control systems modulate or "gate" ascending signals, demonstrating that a normally functioning pain system has both afferent and efferent signals that are critical to normal pain perception (Brooks, Zambreanu, Godinez,

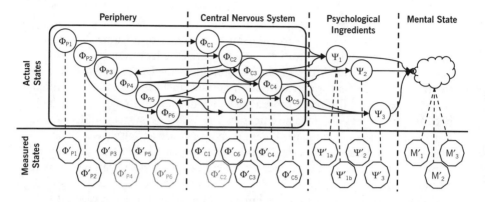

FIGURE 12.1. An example model that illustrates how specific neurophysiological components within the periphery and the CNS map to psychological ingredients, which are involved in the construction of mental states. The top row in the first column illustrates that in the periphery, each peripheral neurophysiological component is designated $\Phi_{P1}, \Phi_{P2}, \Phi_{P3}, \ldots, \Phi_{Pn}$ and corresponds to one or more specific features of particular biological components in the periphery (e.g., the sympathetic activation to muscles in the right hand). The top row in the second column illustrates that in the CNS, each central neurophysiological component is designated $\Phi_{C1}, \Phi_{C2}, \Phi_{C3}, \ldots, \Phi_{Cn}$ and corresponds to specific features of particular biological components in the CNS (e.g., the neural activity of the anterior insula). The rounded rectangle that encloses the states in the periphery and the CNS signifies that these components are part of the overall neurophysiological state. The top row in the third column illustrates psychological ingredients ($\Psi_1, \Psi_2, \Psi_3, \ldots, \Psi_n$; e.g., core affect) to which peripheral and CNS components map. There is potential for each neurophysiological component to map to a given psychological ingredient, but it is possible that some of them do not. It is also possible that some neurophysiological components map to multiple psychological ingredients. The top row in the fourth column illustrates that all of the psychological ingredients combine to construct a mental state. Different properties of those psychological ingredients and/ or different contribution strengths of each ingredient may be associated with different mental states. The bottom row illustrates that experimental measurements estimate certain aspects of certain actual components. Measured components are illustrated as decagons and are denoted with a prime (e.g., Φ'_{P1} is the measurement of Φ_{P1}). In the periphery and the CNS, each component is associated with one potential measurement (Φ_{P4}, Φ_{P6}, and Φ_{C2} are gray because they are not measured). But certain psychological ingredients can be characterized by measuring different features (e.g., core affect is described by valence *and* arousal). Similarly, mental states can be measured using self-reports. The mechanistic relationships among the actual components should propagate to the relationships among the measured components, but for simplicity these lines are not shown. Finally, although this figure shows only one set of components and relationships, a variety of models can be proposed under this framework by considering the following possibilities. Each component in the periphery (1) may or may not directly influence other peripheral components, (2) may or may not directly influence CNS components, (3) may or

Craig, & Tracey, 2005; Melzack & Wall, 1965). These afferent and efferent signals synchronize bodily states with goal-directed behavior and are often accompanied by affective feelings.

Second, because both afferent and efferent neural signaling occurs in close temporal succession during emotional experience, ANS measures alone cannot distinguish between a psychological construction perspective (which emphasizes that afferent information is critical to constructing an emotional episode) and a discrete emotion perspective (which emphasizes that efferent effects on the viscera are triggered by an emotional episode). Cannon's critique of the James–Lange view of emotion centered on the idea that afferent ANS input to the CNS was thought to be too slow and insensitive to be perceived as a feeling state (Cannon, 1927, p. 112). But the delays in bodily feedback are less than what Cannon assumed, because the CNS not only changes its activation with incoming afferent information about a new stimulus, but it also processes ongoing changes in the context to generate predictions about what new stimulus or event could appear (Barrett & Bar, 2009). When accuracy of the prediction is better, the organism can respond more quickly to other incoming sensory changes (see discussion below for more on the predictive nature of the brain).

A third organizational principle that is critical to mapping physical measures to psychological states is that the PNS supports physical action as well as cognitive demands, and both can sometimes influence affective experience. For example, changes in metabolic need in exercising muscles (or in muscles being prepared for action) strongly drive changes in blood flow and associated changes in heart rate. Over and above these physically mediated changes in heart rate, there is the so-called "additional heart rate," which is attributable to psychological effects (e.g., Turner & Carroll, 1985). For example, using ambulatory measures of heart rate, we can assess these much smaller psychological effects only after accounting for the larger metabolic effects on heart rate that occur during active daily life (e.g., Wilhelm, Pfaltz, Grossman, & Roth, 2006; Wilhelm & Roth, 1998). Thus, we might expect that changes in core affect will mostly reflect these changes in metabolic need, but this is not the case. Rather, our conceptual system can adjust for these relationships, such that when exercising, we are

---

may not directly influence psychological ingredients, and (4) may or may not be measured. Each state in the CNS (1) may or may not directly influence peripheral components, (2) may or may not directly influence other CNS components, (3) may or may not directly influence psychological ingredients, and (4) may or may not be measured. Each psychological ingredient (1) is involved in the construction of a mental state, and (2) may or may not be measured. Moreover, the strength of each connection (i.e., the weight of each line) must either be defined a priori or be determined by fitting observed data.

more likely to conceptualize physiological changes as being due to exercise rather than to feelings of anxiety. When we are less aware of metabolically related bodily changes, however, affective changes due to metabolic activity can be misattributed to a spurious source or conceptualized as an emotional state (e.g., after crossing a precarious footbridge, participants perceived a potential romantic partner as more attractive; Dutton & Aron, 1974).

Fourth, the basal physiological state of systems in the body can influence how the viscera respond to psychological manipulations, and they in turn influence the extent to which an affective manipulation can alter affective experience. For example, the myoelectrical activity of the stomach can be changed by a stressor task (Stern, Vasey, Hu, & Koch, 1991) or by stimuli that cause nausea (e.g., Harrison et al., 2010; Stern, Ray, & Quigley, 2001; Uijtdehaage, Stern, & Koch, 1992). However, the effects of these manipulations differ depending on the kind and amount of food or liquid in the stomach when the affective induction occurs (Levanon, Zhang, Orr, & Chen, 1998; Uijtdehaage et al., 1992). Similarly, posture can influence the functional dynamic range across which visceral changes (e.g., a change in heart rate) can occur; when a participant is lying down, sitting, or standing, his or her basal sympathetic activity is relatively low, intermediate, or high, respectively. Thus, sympathetic activity can increase the most from a lying down position (with an appropriate stimulus), and can decrease the most from a standing position (Berntson, Cacioppo, Binkley, et al., 1994; Berntson, Cacioppo, & Quigley, 1994; Cacioppo et al., 1994). Taken together, these organizational principles of the PNS provide important limitations to consistent mapping of the peripheral neurophysiological state to core affect and to affective experience.

How Can Peripheral Physiological States Be Measured?

Because there is an extensive literature on psychophysiological methodologies and because of space constraints, we provide here only a brief overview of these measures (for more information, see Cacioppo, Tassinary, & Berntson, 2007; Cohen, Kessler, & Gordon, 1997; Stern et al., 2001). In the psychology laboratory we can noninvasively assess cardiac and vascular function (e.g., using the electrocardiogram, impedance cardiogram, and measures of blood pressure and flow), gastrointestinal function (using the electrogastrogram), eccrine sweat gland function (i.e., electrodermal activity), pupillary diameter, and sexual function. Furthermore, neurophysiological features that can be measured in the blood, lymph, or other biological fluids may contribute to core affect (for a review, see Lee, Hwang, Cheon, & Jung, 2012). Some measures of possible interest include humoral factors such as oxytocin, testosterone, and cortisol (Shirtcliff et al., 2000), immune cells and molecules (McDade et al., 2000), neuromodulators such as nitric oxide and its metabolites (Tsikas, 2005), telomeres (Lin & Yan, 2007), and messenger ribonucleic acid (mRNA).

There are also a few extant methods for assessing both objective and subjective facets of afferent somatovisceral function (i.e., interoception or internal perception) in some peripheral organ systems (e.g., cardiovascular, gastrointestinal, and respiratory; Table 12.1). These measures are of two distinct types and frequently reveal divergent outcomes (e.g., Critchley, 2004). One type is *interoceptive sensitivity*, which is the psychophysically defined ability to detect a viscerosensory signal from the body. The other type is *bodily* (or *interoceptive*) *awareness*, which is subjective awareness of the body, which is additionally influenced by concepts about one's body, such as illness representations (e.g., Cameron, Leventhal, & Leventhal, 1993), state and trait tendencies to experience negative affect (e.g., Howren & Suls, 2011), and self-focused attention (e.g., Gendolla, Abele, Andrei, Spurk, & Richter, 2005). Although these are distinct concepts measured using different methods (Table 12.1), they are often mistakenly described as reflecting the identical concept (for a discussion of this problem, see Ceunen, van Diest, & Vyaelen, 2013). Also, although it is frequently assumed that interoceptive abilities are similar across visceral systems within an individual, we are aware of only three studies that have rigorously tested this assumption: Two groups found concordance across physiological systems (Whitehead & Drescher, 1980, using detection of heartbeats and gastrointestinal motility, and Herbert, Muth, Pollatos, & Herbert, 2012, using heartbeat tracking and a water load test for gastrointestinal sensitivity), whereas the another (Harver, Katkin, & Bloch, 1993, using heartbeats and respiratory resistance) did not. Especially because afferent information is key to a constructionist account of emotion, further studies are needed to determine whether interoceptive abilities generalize across organ systems, and new methods will be required to permit online assessments of how both interoceptive input and viscerosensory abilities change across time, rather than the current methodologies that provide only a minimal snapshot of trait-like information about viscerosensory abilities.

How Have Prior Studies Mapped the Peripheral Neurophysiological State to Core Affect?

Prior studies have frequently attempted to map neurophysiological changes to either discrete emotion states or to affective features such as arousal, valence, or approach–avoidance motivational state. For example, changes in the arousal feature of core affect often covary with sympathetically mediated peripheral physiological measures, but only when potential confounds

TABLE 12.1. Selected Methods for Assessing Interoceptive Sensitivity and Bodily Awareness

Construct	Method	Description	Recommended references
Interoceptive sensitivity	Cardiac detection tasks	*Modified Whitehead procedure:* A series of heartbeats is measured and tones are presented to either coincide or not coincide with the perception of those heartbeats in the periphery. In each trial, the participant indicates whether a series of beats and tones (usually 10) were coincident or not. Signal detection parameters of sensitivity and bias can be quantified over multiple trials (usually 30–100).	*Modified Whitehead method:* e.g., Barrett, Quigley, Bliss-Moreau, & Aronson (2004); Critchley, Wiens, Rotshtein, Ohman, & Dolan (2004)
			Method of constant stimuli: e.g., Brener, Liu, & Ring (1993); Wiens & Palmer (2001)
		Method of constant stimuli: A series of time intervals between the measured heartbeat and an auditory stimulus are presented (like the modified Whitehead procedure, but using a large number of heartbeat-tone intervals). The temporal interval in which a participant has maximum detectability is assessed, and from that value, good versus poor detection ability or sensitivity is determined. In both methods, participants are asked to not touch their bodies or use other direct ways to feel their heartbeats.	*Reviews of methods:* Jones (1994); Vaitl (1996)
	Gastrointestinal detection tasks	Most current studies utilize a balloon inflated to a specific pressure in the esophagus, stomach, or colon to determine sensory thresholds (e.g., first detection or onset of pain). In a less commonly used task, gastric contractions are measured using a swallowed pressure sensor introduced into the lumen of a part of the gastrointestinal tract (typically, the fundus of the stomach). In each trial, the participant determines whether or not auditory tones coincide with a gastric contraction.	*Distension methods:* Truong, Naliboff, & Chang (2008)
			Methods for detecting motility: Griggs & Stunkard (1964); Stunkard & Koch (1964)
	Respiratory tasks	*Respiratory resistance:* Individuals breathe normal room air through a tube containing filters that produce amounts of respiratory resistance during normal breathing. Multiple	*Methods for detecting respiratory resistance:* e.g., Dahme (1996); Harver et al. (1993)

	different resistances are used to determine the threshold for reporting resistance to airflow. *Carbon dioxide (CO_2) detection:* Participants breathe through a closed system in which various concentrations of CO_2 are introduced into the breathed airstream. Higher concentrations of CO_2 lead to a greater sensation of dyspnea (the subjective sense of trouble breathing). Sensitivity to changes in CO_2 concentration is measured.	*Methods for assessing sensitivity to increases in CO_2;* e.g., Bogaerts et al. (2005, 2008); Stegen et al. (1998)
Bodily (or interoceptive) awareness		
Heartbeat tracking method	Using three or four different time periods (e.g., 25, 35, 45, and 55 seconds), individuals are asked to report the total number of heartbeats felt between tones sounded at the beginning and end of each of these epochs. Individuals are asked not to touch their body or use other direct ways to feel their heartbeats. Accuracy is measured by comparing the number of actual and reported heartbeats.	e.g., Herbert, Pollatos, Flor, Enck, & Schandry (2010); Pollatos, Herbert, Kaufmann, Auer, & Schandry (2007); Pollatos, Kirsch, & Schandry (2005)
Self-report of autonomic or bodily awareness	Many self-report measures exist to provide a subjective measure of the ability to sense some aspect of one's bodily state. Some of these measures attempt to assess specific autonomically mediated bodily awareness, while others assess bodily awareness more broadly.	*Autonomic awareness:* e.g., Mandler, Mandler, & Uviller (1958); *http://terpconnect.umd.edul~sporges/body/body.txt* (retrieved January 8, 2013) *Overall bodily awareness:* Private Body Consciousness subscale of the Body Consciousness Questionnaire (Miller, Murphy, & Buss, 1981); Body Awareness Questionnaire (Shields, Mallory, & Simon, 1989); and Body Vigilance Scale (Schmidt, Lerew, & Trakowski, 1997) *Reviews of measures and methodological issues:* Jones (1994); Mehling et al. (2009); Pennebaker & Hoover (1984)

are held constant, including physical (e.g., posture), cognitive (e.g., mental effort), and environmental (e.g., room temperature) factors. For example, fear and sadness were distinguished by both nonspecific skin conductance responses and tonic skin conductance level in the meta-analysis of emotion studies by Cacioppo, Berntson, Larsen, Poehlmann, and Ito (2000); however, these findings could have been due to differences in arousal, appetitive versus defensive strategy (i.e., valence; Lang, Bradley, & Cuthbert, 1990), or discrete emotion states. The meta-analysis did not reveal evidence of specific ANS responses for discrete emotions, at least as assessed using single ANS measures, and concluded that differentiation might occur for inductions that varied in valence (e.g., negative emotional states producing greater ANS activation than positive ones). This meta-analysis did not, however, code for possible differences in the intensity of arousal across the emotion inductions in the reviewed studies, making it difficult to determine when emotional valence could have been confounded by differences in arousal. In another example, programmatic work by Lang, Bradley, and colleagues (e.g., Bradley & Lang, 2007; Lang et al., 1990) on the affective modulation of the startle reflex demonstrated the importance of both arousal and valence of images used as an affective foreground, with negatively valent images enhancing the startle reflex amplitude (when arousal is held constant) and greater arousal enhancing the startle reflex (when valence is held constant). Also, several recent literature reviews or meta-analyses also have explored whether discrete emotions have consistent and specific physiological response profiles (Kreibig, 2010; Lench, Flores, & Bench, 2011; Mauss & Robinson, 2009; Stemmler, 2004). In those reviews that looked for consistency and specificity of discrete emotions across studies, the results tended to reveal relatively few consistent and unique patterns across studies and across discrete emotions, particularly when using the tools of meta-analysis (see also Barrett, Wilson-Mendenhall, & Barsalou, Chapter 4, this volume; Cacioppo et al., 2000; Lindquist, Siegel, Quigley, & Barrett, 2013; Mauss & Robinson, 2009; for discussion, see Quigley & Barrett, 2014).

Using a multivariate pattern classification or cluster analysis, investigators have distinguished at better than chance levels among some discrete emotional states using peripheral autonomic measures, at least within contextually constrained datasets in which potential confounding factors are held constant (e.g., Christie & Friedman, 2004; Kolodyazhniy, Kreibig, Gross, Roth, & Wilhelm, 2011; Kragel & Labar, 2013; Kreibig, Wilhelm, Roth, & Gross, 2007; Stephens, Christie, & Friedman, 2010; for a review of these methods, see Novak, Mihelj, & Munih, 2012). These investigators do not, however, typically reveal the set of physiological responses that are purported to distinguish each discrete emotion that would provide a set of explicit hypotheses for testing in future studies. Furthermore, these studies use paradigms in which there is explicit conceptualization of the discrete emotions assessed (e.g., frequent manipulation checks that include discrete emotion terms); therefore, these paradigms cannot distinguish between models predicting that reliable ANS patterns are triggered by a discrete emotion episode and models predicting that emotional episodes arise from the conceptualization of changed bodily state and other contextual information (i.e., constructionist view).

We suggest that more theoretical traction will be gained by comparing results from paradigms that can distinguish between a discrete emotions view and a psychological constructionist view. For example, one could compare results across paradigms in which discrete emotion states are conceptualized and those in which they are not. The prediction from a psychological constructionist view is that without conceptualization, ANS patterns will not consistently differentiate all discrete emotion states, but that patterns of ANS-mediated physiological responses may differentiate features of core affective states (e.g., a high-arousal negative state vs. a low-arousal negative state). To develop an inclusive and more general mapping from the neurophysiological state to the core affective state, we need to conduct studies that have variable contextual features (posture, affect induction method, etc.; Quigley et al., 2013), because context has a significant effect on the reliability of the mapping (e.g., Stemmler, 1989; Stemmler, Heldmann, Pauls, & Scherer, 2001).

How Do Organizational Features of the CNS Impact the Mapping of Central Neurophysiological Measures to Affective Experience?

In this section, we review CNS principles that apply to core affect and how these relate to the process of mapping the neurophysiological state to affective experience. Here we highlight three key principles of the CNS: its heterarchical structure, how it stores information, and its predictive functions. As illustrated in Figure 12.1, both the periphery and the CNS have important physical features that can be mapped to the psychological ingredient of core affect. In contrast to peripheral physiology though, the CNS is unique because patterns of neural activation across brain areas can be compared using a common metric (via the firing of neurons, which can be measured using neuroimaging, electrophysiology, etc.).

First, neural networks are arranged in a heterarchical structure, wherein lower-level circuits and higher-level circuits not only interact via intermediate-level circuits, but also interact directly, even across considerable distances in the brain (Figure 12.2; Berntson & Cacioppo, 2008). The heterarchical arrangement has three practical implications:

1. Functional redundancy—neural activation along many separate neural pathways can produce the same output.
2. Functional robustness—inhibition or loss of some neural elements (e.g., neurons or small circuits) can be compensated via changes in other neural elements. For example, some individuals can have a seemingly normal mental life despite loss of peripheral afferent neurons (Heims, Critchley, Dolan, Mathias, & Cipolotti, 2004; Wiens, 2005).
3. Functional conflicts—which can arise between different levels, for example, psychological states such as the desire to be healthy motivate an individual to keep exercising despite the presence of pain due to fatigue in the muscles (Ekkekakis, Parfitt, & Petruzzello, 2011).

Second, the way we understand how the CNS represents information such as the body's peripheral state, core affect, and so on, depends on the level of analysis: molecular (not discussed here), individual neuron, small

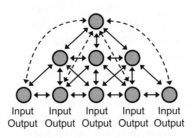

Input   Input   Input   Input   Input
Output Output Output Output Output

FIGURE 12.2. Neural networks are heterarchical, which means that interactions can bridge neural elements at adjacent levels (solid lines) and interactions can bridge neural elements more than one level apart (dashed lines). In this neural system, more caudal circuits operate with unimodal sensory input and motor output (e.g., a neural circuit at the spinal level implements the reflex to withdraw from a painful stimulus), and more rostral circuits operate with multimodal representations of sensory input (e.g., a neural circuit within the cortex utilizes the insula as a hub for associating information from the body with other multimodal sensory information). For simplicity, this schematic only shows three levels, but these neural circuits in humans are better described using many more levels (e.g., if each neuron links adjacent levels, then the CNS–peripheral system requires at least five levels: the peripheral tissue, the spinal cord, the thalamus, the insula, and the frontal cortex; some paths between the periphery and the cortex require more than four synapses and therefore more than five levels). Here, we use "levels" to describe the anatomical arrangement of different brain areas (rostral is higher, caudal is lower), but see Swanson (2012) for an alternative to describing the brain using "levels." Adapted from Berntson and Cacioppo (2008). Copyright 2008 by The Guilford Press. Adapted by permission.

population of neurons, or large distributed neural network. In individual neurons, almost all of the information is encoded by the neuronal firing rate within a relatively short time window (about 20 milliseconds; for a review, see Rolls & Treves, 2011). In a small population of neurons (e.g., 15 neurons, and perhaps more), the firing rate of some individual neurons encodes the features described by a set of many other neurons (designated "hierarchical convergence"; for a review, see Meredith, 2002; Rolls & Treves, 2011). In relatively large distributed neural networks of the brain, information is encoded by the synchronous neural activity that occurs in a given time window (usually tens of milliseconds).[2] More generally, synchronous oscillations of both neural activity and local electric fields play a critical role in many descriptions of multimodal associations (e.g., Senkowski, Schneider, Foxe, & Engel, 2008) and large-scale neural computations (e.g., Buzsáki, 2010; Fries, 2009; Guidolin, Albertin, Guescini, Fuxe, & Agnati, 2011). However, the precise causes and functional implications of synchronous oscillations are still being explored (Rolls & Treves, 2011). Also, information can be altered at any of these levels if excitatory or inhibitory synapses are added or removed (i.e., via synaptic plasticity), or if chemical effectors modulate neural activity (Cameron, 2009; Lane et al., 2009). Finally, although single-neuron recordings have been related to core affect (e.g., Rolls, Grabenhorst, & Franco, 2009), it is likely that large distributed networks will better capture the relevant features and complexities of psychological ingredients and mental states (Barrett & Satpute, 2013; Oosterwijk, Touroutoglou, & Lindquist, Chapter 5, this volume).

Third, the CNS uses relatively sparse sensory inputs and prior knowledge to form a more complete, albeit approximated, representation of the sensory world (for a review, see Clark, 2013). This is analogous to imagining the appearance of a dark and unfamiliar room by touching the walls and the furniture inside it. The brain predicts not only across space but also over time, such that representations of current and prior sensory inputs are extrapolated to predict future sensory input. Importantly, the CNS hypothetically stores the differences between its current and expected sensory states to make more accurate predictions in the future. This principle has been quantitatively applied to psychological phenomena using an approach called *predictive coding* (Bastos et al., 2012; Bubic, von Cramon, & Schubotz, 2010; Friston, 2010; for a model of visceral perception inspired by predictive coding, see Seth, Suzuki, & Critchley, 2011). These ideas also appear in a model that describes how predictions about the visual world are informed by changes in core affect (Barrett & Bar, 2009). Ideas consistent with predictive coding also explain how anxiety and depression hypothetically result from prolonged uncertainty about the future, which can occur when inputs from the periphery of the body to the CNS are too "noisy," thus yielding a predicted bodily state that is not informative (Paulus & Stein, 2010). More generally, some constructionist theories consider the brain as a predictive organ because this view can mechanistically explain conceptual knowledge as a collection of possible sensory and motor patterns (i.e., predictions) inspired by current sensory input.

What Features of the Body's Peripheral State Are Conveyed to the CNS?

The following is a brief overview of peripheral physiological features that are conveyed to the CNS; this evidence has been reviewed in greater detail elsewhere (Adam, 1998; Cameron, 2001, 2009; Craig, 2002; Vaitl, 1996). Information about the peripheral physiological states of organs, muscles, and joints is carried by afferent sensory neurons that are sensitive to one or more properties (or changes in properties) such as temperature, physical deformation, and concentrations of chemical effectors (e.g., acids, oxygen, adenosine triphosphate [ATP], hormones, and immunological molecules; Cameron, 2009; Lane et al., 2009). Electrical stimulation studies suggest these afferent neurons carry information that can be experienced as coolness, warmth, pain, itch, visceral sensations, sensual touch, hunger, thirst, air hunger, and so forth (Craig, 2002, 2003). Independent of the features that are conveyed to the CNS, the CNS representation of the peripheral state of the body is also influenced by the distribution of afferent fibers in the periphery and by circulating chemicals detected in the CNS. As a corollary, some physical changes in the body may not be conveyed to the CNS, and when this occurs, these changes cannot impact core affect (e.g., Φ_{P3} in Figure 12.1. For example, age-related impairments in interoceptive sensitivity (Khalsa, Rudrauf, & Tranel, 2009) and changes in emotional experience (for a review, see Mendes, 2010) may reflect age-related limitations of the afferent systems in conveying peripheral changes to the CNS. Taken together from a constructionist view, mental states are influenced by how extensively peripheral features such as temperature, chemical concentrations, and so forth can be represented in the CNS, which depends on many factors such as the distribution and functionality of neurons that can detect those features.

Where in the CNS Is the Body's Peripheral State Represented?

Although many CNS functions are carried out via distributed networks that span widespread brain regions, several CNS structures play prominent roles in representing the body's peripheral state at various levels in the neural heterarchy (Figures 12.3 and 12.4). Functional neuroanatomical evidence for the connections forming the heterarchy have been gleaned from spatially and temporally detailed invasive studies of nonhuman animals, less-detailed noninvasive studies of humans (e.g., using neuroimaging), and a relatively small number of invasive studies of humans. More extensive

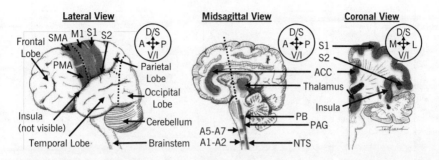

FIGURE 12.3. Many basic neuroanatomical structures are important for how the CNS represents the body's peripheral state. In the lateral view, the dotted lines separate the lobes of the brain. In the midsagittal view, the vertical dotted line indicates the anterior–posterior position of the coronal view, which only shows the right hemisphere. This figure is a schematic as the gyri and sulci patterns are only guidelines. Although there are many other important brain structures related to how the CNS represents the body's peripheral state, only some structures are shown and discussed in this chapter. Each set of crosshairs designates anatomical directions: dorsal/superior (D/S), ventral/inferior (V/I), anterior (A), posterior (P), medial (M), and lateral (L). Anatomical abbreviations are provided in the caption for Figure 12.4.

reviews of this evidence can be found elsewhere (Adam, 1998; Cameron, 2002; Cervero & Foreman, 1990; Craig, 2002, 2003; Lane et al., 2009; Nieuwenhuys, Voogd, & van Huijzen, 2008).

It is helpful to consider the neuroanatomy of the brainstem, limbic system, cortex, and other regions that subserves the processing of afferent signals from the body.[3] Within peripheral tissues such as organs, muscles, and joints, afferent neuronal axonal fibers project to the CNS via either sympathetic or parasympathetic afferent pathways. Most of the parasympathetic afferents run through the vagus nerve, which conveys general visceral and gustatory information from organs in the thorax to the brainstem at the nucleus tractus solitarius (NTS; Loewy, 1990; Nieuwenhuys et al., 2008, Chapter 16). Other parasympathetic afferents and the sympathetic afferents project via two separate fiber tracts in the spinal cord: the lamina I and lamina V spinothalamic tracts. The anatomical distinction between lamina I and lamina V afferents is important because they each convey different, although partially overlapping, information; lamina I fibers carry modality-specific information about sharp pain, temperature, and metabolic state (Craig, 2002) and lamina V fibers carry multimodal information about touch, proprioception, and slow, dull, burning pain (Craig, 2003). At the level of the brainstem, neurons originating in lamina I of the cord and vagal afferents that synapse in the NTS play a role in not only sensing

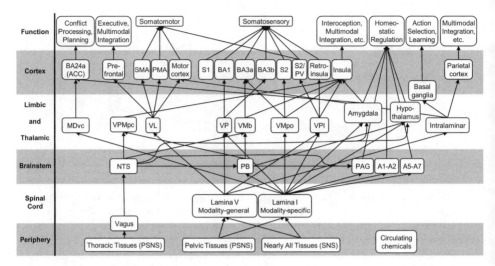

FIGURE 12.4. Neural pathways from the body's peripheral tissues to the CNS traverse several key levels: the periphery, the spinal cord, the brainstem, the limbic and thalamic structures, and the cortex. At each level, the body's peripheral state is represented via a network of neurons. Key structures at each level serve as relay hubs that link adjacent networks. For simplicity, only some structures and projections are shown, although many other structures and ascending and descending projections are important for representing and regulating the body's peripheral state. Also for simplicity, many nuclei have sectors that are not shown (e.g,. both VPMpc and PB contain medial and lateral sectors). Hence, different projections that are drawn to the same nucleus are not necessarily integrated (e.g., projections from NTS and PB remain segregated within the VPMpc as they project to the medial and lateral sectors, respectively, and these distinct sectors of the VPMpc project to distinct subregions of the insula; see Figure 12.5). This figure summarizes neuroanatomical connections described in three reviews (Craig, 2002, 2003; Nieuwenhuys et al., 2008, Chapter 15). A1, A2, A5, and A7 refer to the particular groups of catecholamine cells. ACC, anterior cingulate cortex; BA, Brodmann area; MDvc, ventral caudal part of the mediodorsal nucleus; NTS, nucleus tractus solitarius; PAG, periaqueductal gray; PB, parabrachial nucleus; PMA, premotor area; PSNS, parasympathetic nervous system; PV, parietal ventral; S1, primary somatosensory cortex; S2, secondary somatosensory cortex; SMA, supplementary motor area; SNS, sympathetic nervous system; VL, ventral lateral nucleus; Vmb, ventromedial basal nucleus; VMpo, ventromedial posterior nucleus; VP, ventral posterior complex; VPI, ventral posterior inferior nucleus; VPMpc, parvocellular part of the ventral posteromedial nucleus.

but also regulating the body's peripheral state via projections to homeo-static regions including catecholamine cell groups A1–A2 and A5–A7, the parabrachial nucleus (PB), and the periaqueductal gray (PAG; Craig, 2002; Nieuwenhuys et al., 2008, Chapter 16).

At the heterarchical level above the cord, the next important set of neural structures, collectively designated the limbic system, link the brain-stem and cortex and support functions critical to the survival of the organ-ism (i.e., forming memories, processing visceral information, support-ing social behavior; Mesulam, 2000; Nieuwenhuys et al., 2008, Chapter 23). Researchers do not entirely agree upon the structures making up the limbic system, but typically they include the hypothalamus, the corticoid structures (septal region, substantia innominata, amygdala, and perhaps olfactory nucleus), the allocortical structures (hippocampus and piriform cortex), the paralimbic structures (insula, orbitofrontal cortex [OFC], tem-poral pole, cingulate, rhinal cortices, and parahippocampal structures), the ventral striatum, the ventral pallidum, the ventral tegmental area of Tsai, the habenula, and some nuclei of the thalamus (Mesulam, 2000). An important characteristic of limbic structures such as the amygdala and the hippocampus is that they appear to encode the significance or novelty of a stimulus as opposed to its sensory properties per se. Thus, the limbic system filters information arriving from the periphery of the body and the external world preferentially processing information that appears salient to the organism; this selectivity reduces metabolically expensive cortical processing of irrelevant information. As per the heterarchical structure of the CNS, limbic tissue receives information about the body's peripheral state from many levels: circulating chemicals in the blood, brainstem struc-tures (e.g., the NTS and the PAG), and cortical structures (e.g., the insula). The subcortical limbic structures project to multiple regions of the cortex, where information about the body's peripheral state and its salience is com-bined with other sensory information and conceptual knowledge.

At the cortical level, three key structures support the representation of the body's peripheral state via inputs from thalamic nuclei: insula, somato-sensory cortex, and anterior cingulate cortex (ACC). The insula is con-sidered the brain's primary interoceptive cortex due to the multitude of projections it receives from the lamina I spinothalamic tract by way of the posterior part of the ventromedial thalamic nucleus (VMpo; Craig, 2002). More generally, the insula supports many diverse functions, in that it con-tains the primary sensory cortices for gustation, general viscerosensation, somatosensation (pain and temperature), and the vestibular sense, and because it has widespread bidirectional connections within itself and with many other brain structures (Figure 12.5; Nieuwenhuys, 2012). Another cortical structure related to representing the body's peripheral state is the somatosensory cortex, which receives input from several thalamic nuclei and supports perception of touch, proprioception, and pain (Craig, 2003),

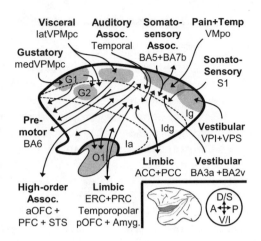

FIGURE 12.5. Tract tracing studies of the monkey insula reveal an extensive set of neural connections that project into, out of, and within the insula to support primary sensory functions, multimodal association functions, and more generally to serve as a hub in distributed networks that span the brain. Based on cytoarchitecture, the insula is divided into three regions: the agranular region (Ia), the dysgranular region (Idg), and the granular region (Ig; separated by dashed lines), which correspond to the absence, scarcity, and presence, respectively, of an internal granular layer (layer IV). The insula contains four primary sensory cortices (shown in gray) with each receiving input from a thalamic nucleus: gustatory (G1; input from medial VPMpc), visceral (input from lateral VPMpc), somatosensory (pain and temperature; input from VMpo), and vestibular (input from VPI and the ventral posterior superior nucleus [VPS]). The insula is also multisensory, because it receives input from several adjacent primary sensory cortices: olfactory (O1), somatosensory (S1), and vestibular (BA3a and BA2v). The insula also contains secondary gustatory cortex (G2). Moreover, the insula receives input from other multimodal association regions: auditory association (temporal cortex), somatosensory association (BA5 and BA7b), and higher-order association (anterior orbitofrontal cortex [aOFC], prefrontal cortex [PFC], and the superior temporal sulcus [STS]). Finally, the insula can encode features of salience and motivation via projections from (and in some cases to) limbic regions such as the entorhinal cortex (ERC), perirhinal cortex (PRC), temporopolar cortex, amygdala (Amyg.), anterior cingulate cortex (ACC), and posterior cingulate cortex (PCC). As mentioned in the text, the regions and projections shown here for the monkey insula may not map directly to the human insula, which is less well understood. For simplicity, the afferent and efferent projections are merely drawn to the correct cytoarchitecturally defined region (Ia, Idg, and/or Ig) and not to the exact site within each region. Also for simplicity, the dense short-range intrainsular projections are not shown (intrainsular projections are ~1 mm long, whereas the monkey insula is ~50 mm long; Augustine, 1996). Finally for clarity, only the left insula is shown. The inset shows a lateral view of an inflated monkey brain with the visible part of the insula shaded darker. The crosshairs designate anatomical directions: dorsal/superior (D/S), ventral/inferior (V/I), anterior (A), and posterior (P). Anatomical abbreviations are provided in the caption for Figure 12.4. Adapted from Nieuwenhuys (2012). Copyright 2012 by Elsevier. Adapted by permission.

and contains a detailed somatotopic map of the body (Nieuwenhuys et al., 2008 , Chapter 16). The role of the somatosensory cortex in interoception was highlighted in a study that compared heart rate detection performance in healthy participants and a patient with insula and ACC damage, and suggested that the perception of cardiac sensations is mediated by two independent pathways: one to the insula and ACC, and another to the somatosensory cortex (Khalsa, Rudrauf, Feinstein, & Tranel, 2009). A final cortical structure related to representing the body's peripheral state is the ACC, which receives primary sensory input encoding the body's peripheral state via the ventral caudal part of the medial dorsal thalamic nucleus (MDvc). The ACC supports many other functions and is typically associated with conflict processing, planning, motivation, and autonomic control (Weston, 2012). Together, the insula, somatosensory cortex, and ACC play key roles in representing the body's peripheral state and are therefore candidate hubs in neural networks related to core affect.

Practically, the characteristics of the neural structures or circuits that represent the body's peripheral state may help to provide constraints on the process of mapping the body's peripheral state to core affect or other psychological phenomena, such as affective experience. For example, both the thalamic nucleus VMpo, which receives interoceptive input from the lamina I spinothalamic tract and projects to the insula, and the anterior portion of the insula are larger in humans than in other primates and subprimates (Blomqvist, Zhang, & Craig, 2000; Craig, 2002, 2011; but for a counterpoint to purported unique portions of the human insula, see Nieuwenhuys, 2012, and for the human brain, more generally, see Finlay & Workman, 2013). Hypothetically, a phylogenetically newer and more differentiated VMpo and anterior insula combined with a more complex set of cortical structures may allow humans unique access to the body's peripheral state such that self-awareness is possible (for a review, see Craig, 2002, 2011). Also, from a constructionist perspective, more complex and differentiated interoceptive neural architecture may permit a richer emotional life by representing a greater number of distinct body states (in contrast, relatively poor discrimination between body states would make more body states experienced as identical to one another, thus limiting how changes in the body could influence affective experience).

How Have Prior Studies Mapped the Central Neurophysiological State to Core Affect?

The representation of core affect in the CNS hypothetically requires integrating the representations of interoceptive information about the body and exteroceptive information about the world (i.e., context) to make meaning of these sensory inputs. Our discussion of this integration extends prior theory describing how the CNS supports core affect (Barrett & Bliss-Moreau, 2009) by considering two neurobiological mechanisms by which the CNS stores information. First, across a smaller spatial scale, information encoded by a set of neurons can instead be encoded by a single association neuron (designated hierarchical convergence; for a review, see Meredith, 2002; Rolls & Treves, 2011). Second, across a larger spatial scale, integration could occur via synchronous neural activity across multiple brain regions, including (1) nuclei of the thalamus that relay sensory inputs, (2) limbic circuitry for interoceptive and exteroceptive information (e.g., hypothalamus, amygdala, hippocampus, ventral striatum, and paralimbic structures such as OFC, insula, and cingulate cortex), (3) primary sensory regions for interoception (insula, somatosensory cortex, ACC, and limbic circuitry), (4) primary sensory regions for exteroception (visual cortex, auditory cortex, gustatory cortex, olfactory cortex), and (5) multimodal association regions (for a review of large-scale integration, see Senkowski et al., 2008). Thus, core affect could be represented in the CNS when neurons in these distant brain regions fire synchronously (at a frequency on the order of 10-120 Hz).

Two recent meta-analytic reviews have assessed the neuroimaging literature to examine the potential neuroanatomical and functional bases of core affect. These reviews used different methodological and theoretical approaches to assess the potential neural correlates of discrete emotions (Lindquist, Wager, Kober, Bliss-Moreau, & Barrett, 2012; Vytal & Hamann, 2010) and for a broader review, see (Hamann, 2012; Oosterwijk et al., Chapter 5, this volume). Vytal and Hamann (2010) took a basic emotion perspective and suggested that there were differences in the neural activation maps when they contrasted multiple pairs of basic emotions (e.g., anger minus fear). Lindquist et al. (2012) took a constructionist perspective that yielded two key outcomes: First, they suggested that a basic emotion view is not supported because although some regions showed consistent activation with a particular emotion (e.g., amygdala with fear), the activation was not specific to that emotion (amygdala activation was also associated with disgust, happiness, anger, sadness, etc.). Second, they identified seven functional networks that may provide the neural substrates for psychological ingredients that together construct all types of mental states (not just discrete emotion states; see Table 5.1 (pp. 118–119) in Oosterwijk et al., Chapter 5, this volume).

Other neuroimaging studies specifically motivated by a psychological constructionist approach have provided useful evidence for mapping the features of core affect, namely valence and arousal, to particular regions of the brain (e.g., Wilson-Mendenhall, Barrett, & Barsalou, 2013). In this study, the researchers induced emotional states using imagery, such that the valence and arousal of the induced state varied within an emotion category (e.g., pleasant fear and unpleasant fear). Both within and across inductions of fear, sadness, and happiness, neural activity in the medial OFC correlated with experienced valence, and neural activity in the left amygdala correlated with experienced arousal. These results are consistent with prior studies that implicate the medial OFC and amygdala as encoding valence and arousal of simple sensory stimuli (Rolls, 2010). But, importantly, these results also support the idea that certain neural substrates support core affect regardless of the category of emotion experienced. For additional examples detailing the neural circuitry that supports affective states, see Kringelbach & Berridge (Chapter 10, this volume) for neural mechanisms of liking and wanting, and Salamone, Correa, Randall, and Nunes (Chapter 11, this volume) for how dopamine signaling contributes to emotion.

Finally, to learn more about mapping the neurophysiological state to core affect, we need a better understanding of how information is stored and manipulated in the CNS (i.e., the neural syntax; Buzsáki, 2010; Rolls & Treves, 2011). At this point, large-world neural properties and synchronized oscillations are current candidates for describing how information can be integrated across different brain networks (Baars, 2005) or different sensory modalities (Klemen & Chambers, 2012), and are therefore candidates for how psychological ingredients may combine to produce a mental state.

How Can a Psychological Construction View and the Ingredient of Core Affect Help Us to Better Understand Emotional Experience?

Considering the principles of peripheral and central neurophysiological organization outlined earlier, we see several reasons why a psychological constructionist approach is advantageous for a science of *how* mental states such as emotions arise. First, psychological construction emphasizes the importance of the peripheral state of the body in *all* mental states. For example, as described earlier, mounting evidence indicates that the brain is a predictive organ (Barrett & Bar, 2009; Clark, 2013; Seth et al., 2011) with feedback from the body serving as a major mechanism by which we detect and predict impending changes in the world.

Second, it is becoming clear that brain processes do not parse along the fault lines of faculty psychological concepts such as memory or perception or emotion, but rather along the lines of more general processes such as core affect, conceptualization, executive function, and so forth. Importantly, principles of the CNS, such as its heterarchical organization, large-scale integration via large-world properties of networks or synchronous oscillations, and the brain's predictive nature, provide potential mechanisms to support the existence of, and interaction between, different psychological ingredients (Barrett & Satpute, 2013; Lindquist & Barrett, 2012).

Third, a constructionist view is consistent with the experimental observation from measures of the ANS that we would *not* expect to observe a single multivariate pattern of ANS responses that is invariant across two similar emotion instances (e.g., real-life anger induced by harassment from an experimenter vs. reimagining these feelings; Stemmler et al., 2001). In this example, the real-life anger task engendered a cardiovascular pattern that supported action (i.e., increased cardiac contractility and blood flow to the periphery),[4] whereas reimagination of the same content resulted in a cardiovascular pattern that did not support action (e.g., a small increase in cardiac contractility and peripheral vasoconstriction). Rather than seeing these as flaws to be explained away, a psychological constructionist approach considers these physiological differences to be important constraints, because other ingredients (e.g., conceptualization) produce "meaning" from the felt physiological changes, and context supplies part of how we determine that meaning.

Fourth, a psychological constructionist approach emphasizes not only that the mind is situated in a body, but also that conceptualization of core affect is situated within a social, cultural, historical, and current perceptual context (i.e., "situated conceptualizations"; Wilson-Mendenhall, Barrett, Simmons, & Barsalou, 2011). Therefore, the conceptual features of an emotion will have considerable similarities across individuals within a specific cultural context due to shared cultural influences (Barrett, 2012; see also Boiger & Mesquita, Chapter 15, this volume). On the other hand, individuals with different personal histories (e.g., those from stable vs. unstable households of origin) could have different habitually elicited patterns of core affect, or different tendencies to attend to and conceptualize particular patterns of core affective change. Again, contextual details are important in the experience of an emotion; they are not experimental noise.

By extension, these routinely observed contextual effects in emotional experience lead us to ask different research questions not contemplated by certain nonconstructionist perspectives. For example, recent studies demonstrate different brain patterns associated with different kinds of fear (e.g., fear in a dark alley vs. fear on a roller coaster; Wilson-Mendenhall et al., 2011, 2013). These studies suggest that although activation in specific brain regions may not be associated with particular discrete emotions, patterns of regional activation instead may have important and lawful relationships to affective features such as valence and arousal. Similarly, Lindquist and Barrett (2012) used modest changes in contextual cues to evoke an emotional experience of fear in one case but anger in another. They used a paradigm in which there was an experimental manipulation of the conceptualization process. Future studies could instead manipulate the neurophysiological state independent of conceptualization using pharmacology (e.g., Schachter & Singer, 1962), exercise (e.g., Ekkekakis et al., 2011), bodily manipulations (Niedenthal, 2007), biofeedback (e.g., Critchley, Melmed, Featherstone, Mathias, & Dolan, 2002), transcranial magnetic stimulation (Sack, 2006; Thut, Miniussi, & Gross, 2012), peripheral neural stimulation (e.g., Lange et al., 2011), or real-time neurofeedback (Weiskopf, 2012). Such studies could allow us to determine, for example, how much core affect has to change before a different concept is activated, and whether that results in a different emotional experience.

A final advantage of a psychological constructionist approach is that we can make predictions about where we would expect to find maximum distinctiveness between affective experiences. The first prediction is that an individual will have optimal ability to label a feeling state reliably when (1) the change in core affect is large, (2) the contextual cues in the environment are unambiguous, and (3) the conceptual system is unhindered (i.e., not under load). When these circumstances occur, the conceptualization of one emotion state versus another is predicted to be most reliable within an individual (in a given cultural context). Second, we expect that some, but not all, emotions will be associated (but not exclusively) with a related set of core affective patterns that are especially likely to be conceptualized as a particular emotion in specific contexts. Third, we expect that some emotion states with very similar core affective features (e.g., fear and anger) would be especially difficult to distinguish using neurophysiological measures, and are therefore frequently differentiated in the real world by contextual factors that assist the conceptualization process. Finally, we predict that certain notable changes in core affect will be very likely to be conceptualized as one emotion (e.g., high arousal, positive core affect conceptualized as joy), and very unlikely to be conceptualized as some other emotion (e.g., sadness, a low-arousal negative state). We will further refine these predictions as a better understanding of the neurophysiological state and conceptual processes producing affective experience emerges.

Conclusion

A key goal from a psychological constructionist perspective is to map features of biological substrates to the psychological ingredients that are combined to construct mental life. Here, we have proposed an approach by which psychological ingredients, especially core affect, can be mapped using measures of peripheral and central neurophysiological state (Figure 12.1). We also discussed how this mapping is constrained by neurophysiological principles operating within the periphery and the CNS. These principles are consistent with the constructionist emphasis on key roles for (1) afferent feedback from the periphery to the CNS, (2) contextual factors as relayed to the CNS by exteroceptive and interoceptive systems, (3) expectations based on prior knowledge (i.e., the predictive nature of the brain), and (4) CNS mechanisms that support the combination of psychological ingredients (i.e., synchronous oscillations and other large-scale properties that can link neural activity across distant networks). Even if the constructionist view is ultimately modified or replaced, new paradigms and evidence generated from this view will reveal critical gaps in our understanding of mental life. A multidisciplinary effort that addresses these gaps in knowledge will result in more complete, quantitative, and mechanistic models of affective experience.

ACKNOWLEDGMENTS

This work was supported by a National Institutes of Health Director's Pioneer Award (No. DP1OD003312) to Lisa Feldman Barrett and a National Institutes of Mental Health F32 NRSA postdoctoral award (No. F32MH096533-01A1) to Ian R. Kleckner. Thanks to Kevin Bickart, Ajay Satpute, Amber Simmons, Christy Wilson-Mendenhall, and the editors of this volume for helpful comments on this chapter.

NOTES

1. We define the neurophysiological state that contributes to core affect as all features of the current and ongoing biological processes within the body. We consider the body to include all biological components within the skin and the body cavities (e.g., the nasal cavity, the gastrointestinal tract, and the microbes therein). For historical reasons and for clarity of exposition, we distinguish between the CNS and the periphery of the body, and we acknowledge that this distinction is arbitrary and physiologically indefensible. But for didactic purposes, we consider the CNS to encompass all biological components within the brain and the spinal cord (e.g., neurons, glial cells, and neurochemicals in the cerebrospinal fluid). We then consider the periphery to be all those biological components within the skin, but outside the CNS, including the autonomic nervous system (ANS), enteric nervous system, endocrine system, immune system, muscles, joints, organs, gut, and gut microbiota.

2. Oscillatory activity at 10-120 Hz is typically measured using single neuron recordings, magnetoencephalography (MEG), or electroencephalography (EEG; Palva & Palva, 2012b), whereas functional magnetic resonance imaging (fMRI) is used to assess slower phenomena related to changes in relative oxygenation and blood flow (Logothetis, 2008; but see Palva & Palva, 2012a).

3. Although we focus on afferent projections from the body to the CNS, these networks also contain efferent projections that control the body's peripheral state at many levels, including the spinal cord, the brainstem, the limbic system, and the cortex.

4. This "action support" pattern is also reminiscent of a purportedly adaptive cardiovascular pattern observed during motivated performance tasks when the person finds the task stressful or challenging, but feels he or she has the resources to cope with it (a "challenge" response; for a review see Seery, 2011). Conversely, those who feel that they cannot cope with a significant stressor (a so-called "threat" response) show peripheral vasoconstriction that would be less compatible with subsequent whole-body motor activity.

REFERENCES

Adam, G. (1998). *Visceral perception*. New York: Springer-Verlag.

Augustine, J. R. (1996). Circuitry and functional aspects of the insular lobe in primates including humans. *Brain Research Reviews, 22*, 229–244.

Baars, B. J. (2005). Global workspace theory of consciousness: Toward a cognitive neuroscience of human experience. *Boundaries of Consciousness: Neurobiology and Neuropathology, 150*, 45–53.

Barrett, L. F. (2006). Solving the emotion paradox: Categorization and the experience of emotion. *Personality and Social Psychology Review, 10*, 20–46.

Barrett, L. F. (2009). The future of psychology: Connecting mind to brain. *Perspectives on Psychological Science, 4*(4), 326–339.

Barrett, L. F. (2011). Bridging token identity theory and supervenience theory through psychological construction. *Psychological Inquiry, 22*(2), 115–27.

Barrett, L. F. (2012). Emotions are real. *Emotion, 12*, 413–429.

Barrett, L. F., & Bar, M. (2009). See it with feeling: Affective predictions during object perception. *Philosophical Transactions of the Royal Society B: Biological Sciences, 364*, 1325–1334.

Barrett, L. F., & Bliss-Moreau, E. (2009). Affect as a psychological ingredient. *Advances in Experimental Social Psychology, 41*, 167–218.

Barrett, L. F., Quigley, K. S., Bliss-Moreau, E., & Aronson, K. R. (2004). Interoceptive sensitivity and self-reports of emotional experience. *Journal of Personality and Social Psychology, 87*, 684–697.

Barrett, L. F., & Satpute, A. (2013). Large-scale brain networks in affective and social neroscience: Towards an integrative functional architecture of the brain. *Current Opinion in Neurobiology, 23*, 361–372.

Bastos, A. M., Usrey, W. M., Adams, R. A., Mangun, G. R., Fries, P., & Friston, K. J. (2012). Canonical microcircuits for predictive coding. *Neuron, 76*(4), 695–711.

Berntson, G. G., & Cacioppo, J. T. (2008). The neuroevolution of motivation. In J. Y. Shah & W. L. Gardner (Eds.), *Handbook of motivation science* (pp. 188–200). New York: Guilford Press.

Berntson, G. G., Cacioppo, J. T., Binkley, P. F., Uchino, B. N., Quigley, K. S., & Fieldstone, A. (1994). Autonomic cardiac control: III. Psychological stress and cardiac response in autonomic space as revealed by pharmacological blockades. *Psychophysiology, 31*(6), 599–608.

Berntson, G. G., Cacioppo, J. T., & Quigley, K. S. (1991). Autonomic determinism: The modes of autonomic control, the doctrine of autonomic space, and the laws of autonomic constraint. *Psychological Review, 98*(4), 459–487.

Berntson, G. G., Cacioppo, J. T., & Quigley, K. S. (1993). Cardiac psychophysiology and autonomic space in humans: Empirical perspectives and conceptual implications. *Psychological Bulletin, 114*(2), 296–322.

Berntson, G. G., Cacioppo, J. T., & Quigley, K. S. (1994). Autonomic cardiac control: I. Estimation and validation from pharmacological blockades. *Psychophysiology, 31*(6), 572–585.

Blomqvist, A., Zhang, E. T., & Craig, A. D. (2000). Cytoarchitectonic and immunohistochemical characterization of a specific pain and temperature relay, the posterior portion of the ventral medial nucleus, in the human thalamus. *Brain, 123*(3), 601–619.

Bogaerts, K., Millen, A., Li, W., De Peuter, S., van Diest, I., Vlemincx, E., et al. (2008). High symptom reporters are less interoceptively accurate in a symptom-related context. *Journal of Psychosomatic Research, 65*, 417–424.

Bogaerts, K., Notebaert, K., van Diest, I., Devriese, S., De Peuter, S., & van den Bergh, O. (2005). Accuracy of respiratory symptom perception in different affective contexts. *Journal of Psychosomatic Research, 58*, 537–543.

Bradley, M. M., & Lang, P. J. (2007). Emotion and motivation. In J. T. Cacioppo, L. G. Tassinary, & G. Berntson (Eds.), *Handbook of psychophysiology* (pp. 581–607). New York: Cambridge University Press.

Brener, J., Liu, X., & Ring, C. (1993). A method of constant stimuli for examining heartbeat detection: Comparison with the Brener–Kluvitse and Whitehead methods. *Psychophysiology, 30*, 657–665.

Brooks, J. C. W., Zambreanu, L., Godinez, A., Craig, A. D. B., & Tracey, I. (2005). Somatotopic organisation of the human insula to painful heat studied with high resolution functional imaging. *NeuroImage, 27*, 201–209.

Bubic, A., von Cramon, D. Y., & Schubotz, R. I. (2010). Prediction, cognition and the brain. *Frontiers in Human Neuroscience, 4*, 25.

Buzsáki, G. (2010). Neural syntax: Cell assemblies, synapsembles, and readers. *Neuron, 68(3)*, 362–385.

Cacioppo, J. T., Berntson, G. G., Binkley, P. F., Quigley, K. S., Uchino, B. N., & Fieldstone, A. (1994). Autonomic cardiac control: II. Noninvasive indices and basal response as revealed by autonomic blockades. *Psychophysiology, 31(6)*, 586–598.

Cacioppo, J. T., Berntson, G. G., & Klein, D. J. (1992). What is an emotion?: The role of somatovisceral afference, with special emphasis on somatovisceral "illusions." *Review of Personality and Social Psychology, 14*, 63–98.

Cacioppo, J. T., Berntson, G. G., Larsen, J. T., Poehlmann, K. M., & Ito, T. A. (2000). The psychophysiology of emotion. In M. Lewis, J. M. Haviland-Jones, & L. F. Barrett (Eds.), *Handbook of emotion* (2nd ed., pp. 173–191). New York: Guilford Press.

Cacioppo, J. T., & Tassinary, L. G. (1990). Inferring psychological significance from physiological signals. *American Psychologist, 45(1)*, 16–28.

Cacioppo, J. T., Tassinary, L. G., & Berntson, G. G. (2007). *The handbook of psychophysiology* (3rd ed.). New York: Cambridge University Press.

Cameron, L., Leventhal, E. A., & Leventhal, H. (1993). Symptom representations and affect as determinants of care seeking in a community-dwelling, adult sample population. *Health Psychology, 12(3)*, 171–179.

Cameron, O. G. (2001). Interoception: The inside story—a model for psychosomatic processes. *Psychosomatic Medicine, 63(5)*, 697–710.

Cameron, O. G. (2002). *Visceral sensory neuroscience: Interoception.* New York: Oxford University Press.

Cameron, O. G. (2009). Visceral brain–body information transfer. *NeuroImage, 47(3)*, 787–794.

Cannon, W. B. (1927). The James–Lange theory of emotions: A critical examination and an alternative theory. *American Journal of Psychology, 39(1/4)*, 106–124.

Cervero, F., & Foreman, R. (1990). *Central regulation of autonomic functions.* New York: Oxford University Press.

Ceunen, E., van Diest, I., & Vyaelen, J. W. S. (2013). Accuracy and awareness of perception: Related, yet distinct (commentary on Herbert et al., 2012). *Biological Psychology, 92*(2), 426–427.

Christie, I. C., & Friedman, B. H. (2004). Autonomic specificity of discrete emotion and dimensions of affective space: A multivariate approach. *International Journal of Psychophysiology, 51*(2), 143–153.

Clark, A. (2013). Whatever next?: Predictive brains, situated agents, and the future of cognitive science. *Behavioral and Brain Sciences, 36*(3), 181–204.

Cohen, S., Kessler, R. C., & Gordon, L. U. (1997). *Measuring stress: A guide for health and social scientists.* New York: Oxford University Press.

Craig, A. D. (2002). How do you feel?: Interoception: The sense of the physiological condition of the body. *Nature Reviews Neuroscience, 3*(8), 655–666.

Craig, A. D. (2003). Pain mechanisms: Labeled lines versus convergence in central processing. *Annual Review of Neuroscience, 26*, 1–30.

Craig, A. D. (2009). How do you feel—now?: The anterior insula and human awareness. *Nature Reviews Neuroscience, 10*(1), 59–70.

Craig, A. D. (2011). Significance of the insula for the evolution of human awareness of feelings from the body. *New Perspectives on Neurobehavioral Evolution, 1225*, 72–82.

Critchley, H. D. (2004). The human cortex responds to an interoceptive challenge. *Proceedings of the National Academy of Sciences USA, 101*(17), 6333–6334.

Critchley, H. D., Melmed, R. N., Featherstone, E., Mathias, C. J., & Dolan, R. J. (2002). Volitional control of autonomic arousal: A functional magnetic resonance study. *NeuroImage, 16*(4), 909–919.

Critchley, H. D., Wiens, S., Rotshtein, P., Ohman, A., & Dolan, R. J. (2004). Neural systems supporting interoceptive awareness. *Nature Neuroscience, 7*, 189–195.

Dahme, B. (1996). Interoception of airway resistance in healthy and asthmatic subjects. *Biological Psychology, 43*(3), 247–248.

Dawkins, R. (1989). *The selfish gene.* Oxford, UK: Oxford University Press.

Dutton, D. G., & Aron, A. P. (1974). Some evidence for heightened sexual attraction under conditions of high anxiety. *Journal of Personality and Social Psychology, 30*(4), 510–517.

Ekkekakis, P., Parfitt, G., & Petruzzello, S. J. (2011). The pelasure and displeasure people feel when they exercise at different intensities: Decennial update and progress towards a tripartite rationale for exercise intensity prescription. *Sports Medicine, 41*(8), 641–671.

Finlay, B. L., & Workman, A. D. (2013). Human exceptionalism. *Trends in Cognitive Sciences, 17*(5), 199–201.

Fitch, W. T. (2005). The evolution of language: A comparative review. *Biology and Philosophy, 20*(2–3), 193–203.

Fries, P. (2009). Neuronal gamma-band synchronization as a fundamental process in cortical computation. *Annual Review of Neuroscience, 32*, 209–224.

Friston, K. (2010). The free-energy principle: A unified brain theory? *Nature Reviews Neuroscience, 11*, 127–138.

Gallos, L. K., Makse, H. A., & Sigman, M. (2012). A small world of weak ties provides optimal global integration of self-similar modules in functional brain networks. *Proceedings of the National Academy of Sciences, 109*(8), 2825–2830.

Gendolla, G. H. E., Abele, A. E., Andrei, A., Spurk, D., & Richter, M. (2005). Negative mood, self-focused attention, and the experience of physical symptoms: The joint impact hypothesis. *Emotion, 5*(2), 131–144.

Gendron, M., & Barrett, L. F. (2009). Reconstructing the past: A century of ideas about emotion in psychology. *Emotion Review, 1*(4), 316–339.

Griggs, R. C., & Stunkard, A. (1964). The interpretation of gastric motility: II. Sensitivity and bias in the perception of gastric motility. *Archives of General Psychiatry, 11*(1), 82–89.

Guidolin, D., Albertin, G., Guescini, M., Fuxe, K., & Agnati, L. F. (2011). Central nervous system and computation. *Quarterly Review of Biology, 86*(4), 265–285.

Hamann, S. (2012). Mapping discrete and dimensional emotions onto the brain: Controversies and consensus. *Trends in Cognitive Sciences, 16*(9), 458–466.

Harrison, N. A., Gray, M. A., Gianaros, P. J., & Critchley, H. D. (2010). The embodiment of emotional feelings in the brain. *Journal of Neuroscience, 30*, 12878–12884.

Harver, A., Katkin, E. S., & Bloch, E. (1993). Signal-detection outcomes on heartbeat and respiratory resistance detection tasks in male and female subjects. *Psychophysiology, 30*(3), 223–230.

Heims, H. C., Critchley, H. D., Dolan, R., Mathias, C. J., & Cipolotti, L. (2004). Social and motivational functioning is not critically dependent on feedback of autonomic responses: Neuropsychological evidence from patients with pure autonomic failure. *Neuropsychologia, 42*(14), 1979–1988.

Henderson, L. A., Stathis, A., James, C., Brown, R., McDonald, S., & Macefield, V. G. (2012). Real-time imaging of cortical areas involved in the generation of increases in skin sympathetic nerve activity when viewing emotionally charged images. *NeuroImage, 62*(1), 30–40.

Herbert, B. M., Muth, E. R., Pollatos, O., & Herbert, C. (2012). Interoception across modalities: On the relationship between cardiac awareness and the sensitivity for gastric functions. *PLoS ONE, 7*(5), e36646.

Herbert, B. M., Pollatos, O., Flor, H., Enck, P., & Schandry, R. (2010). Cardiac awareness and autonomic cardiac reactivity during emotional picture viewing and mental stress. *Psychophysiology, 47*, 342–354.

Howren, M. B., & Suls, J. (2011). The symptom perception hypothesis revised: Depression and anxiety play different roles in concurrent and retrospective physical symptom reporting. *Journal of Personality and Social Psychology, 100*, 182–195.

James, W. (1890). *The principles of psychology* (Vol. 2). New York: Holt.

Jänig, W., & Häbler, H. J. (2003). Neurophysiological analysis of target-related sympathetic pathways—from animal to human: Similarities and differences. *Acta Physiologica Scandinavica, 177*(3), 255–274.

Jennings, J. R., & Gianaros, P. J. (2007). Methodology. In J. T. Cacioppo, L. G. Tassinary, & G. G. Berntson (Eds.), *Handbook of psychophysiology* (3rd ed., pp. 812–833). New York: Cambridge University Press.

Johnson, E. O., Babis, G. C., Soultanis, K. C., & Soucacos, P. N. (2008). Functional neuroanatomy of proprioception. *Journal of Surgical Orthopaedic Advances, 17*(3), 159–164.

Jones, G. (1994). Perception of visceral sensations: A review of recent findings, methodologies, and future directions. *Advances in Psychophysiology, 5,* 55–191.

Khalsa, S. S., Rudrauf, D., Feinstein, J. S., & Tranel, D. (2009). The pathways of interoceptive awareness. *Nature Neuroscience, 12*(12), 1494–1496.

Khalsa, S. S., Rudrauf, D., & Tranel, D. (2009). Interoceptive awareness declines with age. *Psychophysiology, 46*(6), 1130–1136.

Klemen, J., & Chambers, C. D. (2012). Current perspectives and methods in studying neural mechanisms of multisensory interactions. *Neuroscience and Biobehavioral Reviews, 36*(1), 111–133.

Kolodyazhniy, V., Kreibig, S. D., Gross, J. J., Roth, W. T., & Wilhelm, F. H. (2011). An affective computing approach to physiological emotion specificity: Toward subject-independent and stimulus-independent classification of film-induced emotions. *Psychophysiology, 48*(7), 908–922.

Kragel, P. A., & LaBar, K. S. (2013). Multivariate pattern classification reveals autonomic and experiential representations of discrete emotions. *Emotion, 13*(4), 681–690.

Kreibig, S. D. (2010). Autonomic nervous system activity in emotion: A review. *Biological Psychology, 84*(3), 394–421.

Kreibig, S. D., Wilhelm, F. H., Roth, W. T., & Gross, J. J. (2007). Cardiovascular, electrodermal, and respiratory response patterns to fear- and sadness-inducing films. *Psychophysiology, 44*(5), 787–806.

Lane, R. D., Waldstein, S. R., Chesney, M. A., Jennings, J. R., Lovallo, W. R., Kozel, P. J., et al. (2009). The rebirth of neuroscience in psychosomatic medicine, part I: Historical context, methods, and relevant basic science. *Psychosomatic Medicine, 71,* 117–134.

Lang, P. J., Bradley, M. M., & Cuthbert, B. N. (1990). Emotion, attention, and the startle reflex. *Psychological Review, 97*(3), 377–395.

Lange, G., Janal, M. N., Maniker, A., FitzGibbons, J., Fobler, M., Cook, D., et al. (2011). Safety and efficacy of vagus nerve stimulation in fibromyalgia: A phase I/II proof of concept trial. *Pain Medicine, 12*(9), 1406–1413.

Lee, J.-H., Hwang, Y., Cheon, K.-A., & Jung, H.-I. (2012). Emotion-on-a-chip (EOC): Evolution of biochip technology to measure human emotion using body fluids. *Medical Hypotheses, 79*(6), 827–832.

Lench, H. C., Flores, S. A., & Bench, S. W. (2011). Discrete emotions predict changes in cognition, judgment, experience, behavior, and physiology: A meta-analysis of experimental emotion elicitations. *Psychological Bulletin, 137*(5), 834–855.

Levanon, D., Zhang, M., Orr, W. C., & Chen, J. D. Z. (1998). Effects of meal volume and composition on gastric myoelectrical activity. *American Journal of Physiology: Gastrointestinal and Liver Physiology, 274*(2), G430–G434.

Lin, K. W., & Yan, J. (2007). The telomere length dynamic and methods of its assessment. *Journal of Cellular and Molecular Medicine, 9*(4), 977–989.

Lindquist, K. A., & Barrett, L. F. (2012). A functional architecture of the human brain: Emerging insights from the science of emotion. *Trends in Cognitive Sciences, 16*(11), 533–540.

Lindquist, K. A., Siegel, E. H., Quigley, K. S., & Barrett, L. F. (2013). The hundred-year emotion war: Are emotions natural kinds or psychological constructions?: Comment on Lench, Flores, and Bench (2011). *Psychological Bulletin, 139*(1), 255–263.

Lindquist, K. A., Wager, T. D., Kober, H., Bliss-Moreau, E., & Barrett, L. F. (2012). The brain basis of emotion: A meta-analytic review. *Behavioral Brain Sciences, 35*(3), 121–143.

Loewy, A. D. (1990). Central autonomic pathways. In A. D. Loewy & K. M. Spyer (Eds.), *Central regulation of autonomic functions* (pp. 88–103). New York: Oxford University Press.

Logothetis, N. K. (2008). What we can do and what we cannot do with fMRI. *Nature, 453*(7197), 869–878.

Mandler, G. (1984). *Mind and body: Psychology of emotion and stress.* New York: Norton.

Mandler, G., Mandler, J. M., & Uviller, E. T. (1958). Autonomic feedback: The perception of autonomic activity. *Journal of Abnormal and Social Psychology, 56*(3), 367–373.

Marsella, S., Gratch, J., & Petta, P. (2010). Computational models of emotion. In K. R. Scherer, T. Banziger, & E. Roesch (Eds.), *A blueprint for affective computing: A sourcebook and manual* (pp. 21–46). New York: Oxford University Press.

Mauss, I. B., & Robinson, M. D. (2009). Measures of emotion: A review. *Cognition and Emotion, 23*(2), 209–237.

Mayer, E. a. (2011). Gut feelings: The emerging biology of gut-brain communication. *Nature Reviews Neuroscience, 12*, 453–466.

McDade, T. W., Stallings, J. F., Angold, A., Costello, E. J., Burleson, M., Cacioppo, J. T., et al. (2000). Epstein–Barr virus antibodies in whole blood spots: A minimally invasive method for assessing an aspect of cell-mediated immunity. *Psychosomatic Medicine, 62*(4), 560–568.

Mehling, W. E., Gopisetty, V., Daubenmier, J., Price, C. J., Hecht, F. M., & Stewart, A. (2009). Body awareness: Construct and self-report measures. *PLoS ONE, 4*, e5614.

Melzack, R., & Wall, P. D. (1965). Pain mechanisms: A new theory. *Science, 150*, 971–979.

Mendes, W. B. (2010). Weakened links between mind and body in older age: The case for maturational dualism in the experience of emotion. *Emotion Review, 2*, 240–244.

Meredith, M. A. (2002). On the neuronal basis for multisensory convergence: A brief overview. *Cognitive Brain Research, 14*(1), 31–40.

Mesulam, M. (2000). *Principles of behavioral and cognitive neurology.* New York: Oxford University Press.

Miller, L. C., Murphy, R., & Buss, A. H. (1981). Consciousness of body: Private and public. *Journal of Personality and Social Psychology, 41*(2), 397–406.

Morrison, S. F. (2001). Differential control of sympathetic outflow. *American Journal of Physiology: Regulatory, Integrative and Comparative Physiology, 281*, R683–R698.

Niedenthal, P. M. (2007). Embodying emotion. *Science, 316*(5827), 1002–1005.

Nieuwenhuys, R. (2012). The insular cortex: A review. *Progress in Brain Research, 195*, 123–163.

Nieuwenhuys, R., Voogd, J., & van Huijzen, C. (2008). *The human central nervous system.* Berlin: Springer-Verlag.

Novak, D., Mihelj, M., & Munih, M. (2012). A survey of methods for data fusion and system adaptation using autonomic nervous system responses in physiological computing. *Interacting with Computers, 24*(3), 154–172.

Palva, J. M., & Palva, S. (2012a). Infra-slow fluctuations in electrophysiological recordings, blood-oxygenation-level-dependent signals, and psychophysical time series. *NeuroImage, 62*(4), 2201–2211.

Palva, S., & Palva, J. M. (2012b). Discovering oscillatory interaction networks with M/EEG: Challenges and breakthroughs. *Trends in Cognitive Sciences, 16*(4), 219–230.

Paulus, M. P., & Stein, M. B. (2010). Interoception in anxiety and depression. *Brain Structure Function, 214*(5–6), 451–463.

Pennebaker, J. W., & Hoover, C. W. (1984). Visceral perception versus visceral detection: Disentangling methods and assumptions. *Biofeedback and Self-Regulation, 9*, 339–352.

Pitt, M. A., Myung, I. J., & Zhang, S. (2002). Toward a method of selecting among computational models of cognition. *Psychological Review, 109*(3), 472–491.

Poldrack, R. A. (2006). Can cognitive processes be inferred from neuroimaging data? *Trends in Cognitive Sciences, 10*(2), 59–63.

Poldrack, R. A. (2008). The role of fMRI in cognitive neuroscience: Where do we stand? *Current Opinion in Neurobiology, 18*(2), 223–227.

Poldrack, R. A. (2011). Inferring mental states from neuroimaging data: From reverse inference to large-scale decoding. *Neuron, 72*(5), 692–697.

Pollatos, O., Herbert, B. M., Kaufmann, C., Auer, D. P., & Schandry, R. (2007). Interoceptive awareness, anxiety and cardiovascular reactivity to isometric exercise. *International Journal of Psychophysiology, 65*, 167–173.

Pollatos, O., Kirsch, W., & Schandry, R. (2005). On the relationship between interoceptive awareness, emotional experience, and brain processes. *Cognitive Brain Research, 25*, 948–962.

Quigley, K. S., & Barrett, L. F. (2014). Is there consistency and specificity of autonomic changes during emotional episodes?: Guidance from the Conceptual Act Theory and psychophysiology. *Biological Psychology, 98*, 82–94.

Quigley, K. S., Lindquist, K. A., & Barrett, L. F. (2013). Inducing and measuring emotion and affect: Tips, tricks, and secrets. In H. T. Reis & C. M. Judd (Eds.), *Handbook of research methods in social and personality psychology* (pp. 220–250). New York: Cambridge University Press.

Rolls, E. T. (2010). The affective and cognitive processing of touch, oral texture, and temperature in the brain. *Neuroscience and Biobehavioral Reviews, 34*(2), 237–245.

Rolls, E. T., Grabenhorst, F., & Franco, L. (2009). Prediction of subjective affective state from brain activations. *Journal of Neurophysiology, 101*(3), 1294–1308.

Rolls, E. T., & Treves, A. (2011). The neuronal encoding of information in the brain. *Progress in Neurobiology, 95*(3), 448–490.

Russell, J. A. (2003). Core affect and the psychological construction of emotion. *Psychological Review, 110*, 145–172.

Russell, J. A., & Barrett, L. F. (1999). Core affect, prototypical emotional episodes, and other things called emotion: Dissecting the elephant. *Journal of Personality and Social Psychology, 76*(5), 805–819.

Sack, A. T. (2006). Transcranial magnetic stimulation, causal structure-function mapping and networks of functional relevance. *Current Opinion in Neurobiology, 16*(5), 593–599.

Sarter, M., Berntson, G. G., & Cacioppo, J. T. (1996). Brain imaging and cognitive neuroscience: Toward strong inference in attributing function to structure. *American Psychologist, 51*, 13–21.

Schachter, S., & Singer, J. E. (1962). Cognitive, social, and physiological determinants of emotional state. *Psychological Review, 69*, 379–399.

Schmidt, N. B., Lerew, D. R., & Trakowski, J. H. (1997). Body vigilance in panic disorder: Evaluating attention to bodily perturbations. *Journal of Consulting and Clinical Psychology, 65*(2), 214–220.

Seery, M. D. (2011). Challenge or threat?: Cardiovascular indexes of resilience and vulnerability to potential stress in humans. *Neuroscience and Biobehavioral Reviews, 35*(7), 1603–1610.

Senkowski, D., Schneider, T. R., Foxe, J. J., & Engel, A. K. (2008). Crossmodal binding through neural coherence: Implications for multisensory processing. *Trends in Neurosciences, 31*(8), 401–409.

Seth, A. K., Suzuki, K., & Critchley, H. D. (2011). An interoceptive predictive coding model of conscious presence. *Frontiers in Psychology, 2*, 395.

Shields, S. A., Mallory, M. E., & Simon, A. (1989). The Body Awareness Questionnaire: Reliability and validity. *Journal of Personality Assessment, 53*(4), 802–815.

Shirtcliff, E. A., Granger, D. A., Schwartz, E. B., Curran, M. J., Booth, A., & Overman, W. H. (2000). Assessing estradiol in biobehavioral studies using saliva and blood spots: Simple radioimmunoassay protocols, reliability, and comparative validity. *Hormones and Behavior, 38*(2), 137–147.

Stegen, K., Neujens, A., Crombez, G., Hermans, D., van de Woestijne, K. P., & van den Bergh, O. (1998). Negative affect, respiratory reactivity, and somatic complaints in a CO_2 enriched air inhalation paradigm. *Biological Psychology, 49*(1–2), 109–122.

Stemmler, G. (1989). The autonomic differentiation of emotions revisited: Convergent and discriminant validation. *Psychophysiology, 26*(6), 617–632.

Stemmler, G. (2004). Physiological processes during emotion. In P. Philippot & R. S. Feldman (Eds.), *The regulation of emotion* (pp. 33–70). Mahwah, NJ: Erlbaum.

Stemmler, G., Heldmann, M., Pauls, C. A., & Scherer, T. (2001). Constraints for emotion specificity in fear and anger: The context counts. *Psychophysiology, 38*(2), 275–291.

Stephens, C. L., Christie, I. C., & Friedman, B. H. (2010). Autonomic specificity of basic emotions: Evidence from pattern classification and cluster analysis. *Biological Psychology, 84*(3), 463–473.

Stern, R. M., Ray, W. J., & Quigley, K. S. (2001). *Psychophysiological recording* (2nd ed.). New York: Oxford University Press.

Stern, R. M., Vasey, M. W., Hu, S., & Koch, K. L. (1991). Effects of cold stress on gastric myoelectric activity. *Neurogastroenterology and Motility, 3*(4), 225–228.

Stunkard, A., & Koch, C. (1964). The interpretation of gastric motility: I. Apparent bias in the reports of hunger by obese persons. *Archives of General Psychiatry, 11*(1), 74–82.

Swanson, L. W. (2012). *Brain architecture: Understanding the basic plan* (2nd ed.). New York: Oxford University Press.

Thut, G., Miniussi, C., & Gross, J. (2012). The functional importance of rhythmic activity in the brain. *Current Biology, 22*(16), R658–R663.

Truong, T. T., Naliboff, B. D., & Chang, L. (2008). Novel techniques to study visceral hypersensitivity in irritable bowel syndrome. *Current Gastroenterology Reports, 10*(4), 369–378.

Tsikas, D. (2005). Review: Methods of quantitative analysis of the nitric oxide metabolites nitrite and nitrate in human biological fluids. *Free Radical Research, 39*(8), 797–815.

Turner, J. R., & Carroll, D. (1985). Heart rate and oxygen consumption during mental arithmetic, a video game, and graded exercise: Further evidence of metabolically-exaggerated cardiac adjustments? *Psychophysiology, 22*(3), 261–267.

Uijtdehaage, S. H. J., Stern, R. M., & Koch, K. L. (1992). Effects of eating on vection-induced motion sickness, cardiac vagal tone, and gastric myoelectric activity. *Psychophysiology, 29*(2), 193–201.

Vaitl, D. (1996). Interoception. *Biological Psychology, 42*, 1–27.

Vytal, K., & Hamann, S. (2010). Neuroimaging support for discrete neural correlates of basic emotions: A voxel-based meta-analysis. *Journal of Cognitive Neuroscience, 22*(12), 2864–2885.

Weiskopf, N. (2012). Real-time fMRI and its application to neurofeedback. *NeuroImage, 62*(2), 682–692.

Weston, C. S. (2012). Another major function of the anterior cingulate cortex: The representation of requirements. *Neuroscience and Biobehavioral Reviews, 36*(1), 90–110.

Whitehead, W. E., & Drescher, V. M. (1980). Perception of gastric contractions and self-control of gastric motility. *Psychophysiology, 17*(6), 552–558.

Wiens, S. (2005). Interoception in emotional experience. *Current Opinion in Neurology, 18*, 442–447.

Wiens, S., & Palmer, S. N. (2001). Quadratic trend analysis and heartbeat detection. *Biological Psychology, 58*, 159–175.

Wilhelm, F. H., Pfaltz, M. C., Grossman, P., & Roth, W. T. (2006). Distinguishing emotional from physical activation in ambulatory psychophysiological monitoring. *Biomedical Sciences Instrumentation, 42*, 458–463.

Wilhelm, F. H., & Roth, W. T. (1998). Using minute ventilation for ambulatory estimation of additional heart rate. *Biological Psychology, 49*(1), 137–150.

Wilson-Mendenhall, C. D., Barrett, L. F., & Barsalou, L. W. (2013). Neural evidence that human emotions share core affective properties. *Psychological Science, 24*(6), 947–956.

Wilson-Mendenhall, C. D., Barrett, L. F., Simmons, W. K., & Barsalou, L. W. (2011). Grounding emotion in situated conceptualization. *Neuropsychologia, 49*(5), 1105–1127.

PART IV

COMMENTARY AND CONSILIENCE

CHAPTER 13

Can an Appraisal Model Be Compatible with Psychological Constructionism?

ANDREW ORTONY
GERALD CLORE

In this chapter we argue that the account of emotion we proposed in *The Cognitive Structure of Emotions* (Ortony, Clore, & Collins, 1988) is quite compatible with the psychological constructionist approach to emotion that is the focus of this volume. And we believe this to be true even though our model (now widely referred to as the OCC model) is usually thought of as an appraisal theory. We begin with a brief overview of our model, and then present four sections whose contents relate to the four questions around which the chapters of this book are organized.

The OCC Model

At the most general level, we consider emotions to be affective reactions to significant psychological situations, and we consider affective reactions to be evaluations of any kind, including those that are implicit, automatic, and subcortical, as well as those that are explicit, conscious, and deliberative. For us, evaluation is the sine qua non of emotion. Whereas cognition concerns things such as the presence or absence of attributes, the truth or falsity of propositions, and categorization, emotion concerns the perception of the goodness or badness of things—evaluation. Thus we take it as axiomatic that where there is no (positive or negative) evaluation, there is no emotion.

1. *If emotions are psychological events constructed from more basic ingredients, then what are the key ingredients from which emotions are constructed? Are they specific to emotion or are they general ingredients of the mind? Which, if any, are specific to humans?*

Emotional reactions differ in both quality and quantity. We have distinguished emotions from non-emotions qualitatively by noting that they are internal (as opposed to external) mental (as opposed to physical) states (as opposed to nonstates, such as actions or dispositions) that primarily focus on affect (as opposed to cognition or behavior). These elements discriminate between good and less good candidates for emotion. Crossed with the degree of affect is another factor, namely, the *kind* of affective condition. We can distinguish four major kinds: emotions and moods (both of which are temporally constrained, the former with an object, the latter without), and attitudes and temperament (both of which are temporally unconstrained, with the former focused on objects, and the latter not). (See Figure 13.2 on p. 317.)

Although our own approach to emotion is an example of an appraisal theory, we see it as compatible also with a constructionist view. It characterizes specific emotions as undifferentiated affect that is constrained by the interpretation of the situation to which it is a response. Moreover, we see emotions as emergent conditions arising from somatic, cognitive, motivational–behavioral, and phenomenal reactions.

2. *What brings these ingredients together in the construction of an emotion? Which combinations are emotions and which are not (and how do we know)?*

Affective reactions are evaluations that can be multiply represented, for example, as embodied, enacted, expressed, and/or experienced evaluations. Emotions are affective reactions to psychologically important situations. A specific emotion reflects the specific nature of the situation it represents. Emotions are therefore psychological events with multiple facets, and like the proverbial blind men trying to describe an elephant, different investigators have tended to focus on different facets—some on physiological events, others on motivational or behavioral events, and still others on cognitive antecedents. These constituents of emotions are not themselves emotions, but jointly they do constitute an emotion. An emotion is a condition that emerges from the co-occurrence of these affective components. Appraisal theories are attempts to specify the kinds of characteristics that make these patterns one emotion rather than another. Identifying the processes responsible for seeing situations as having particular characteristics and for evaluating them as good or bad is not, one might argue, a special problem for emotion theory. Rather, it is a psychological question whose answer should draw on general principles of perception, cognition, categorization, and evaluation.

(continued)

3. *How important is variability (across instances within an emotion category, and in the categories that exist across cultures)? Is this variance epiphenomenal or a thing to be explained? To the extent that it makes sense, it would be desirable to address issues such as universality and evolution.*

The similarity or variability across peoples (or organisms) lies in the kinds of situations that different species and individuals (ages, cultures, etc.) within species find (or are capable of finding) psychologically significant. There are, of course, some universals among the kinds of situations with which living creatures must cope, including threat, competition, access to resources, access to mates, group inclusion, nurturance of young, and so on. Whereas the elicitation of some kind of response to threat is presumably universal, group inclusion is more characteristic of some social animals than others. The hypersocial nature of humans, along with our symbolic abilities means that we experience many more (and much more differentiated) emotions than do other animals. Hence, in contrast to traditional views, humans may be more rather than less emotional than other animals. In addition, we argue that emotions are situated, varying in innumerable ways to mark the particulars of the situation represented by the emotion. At the same time, however, there should be no variation in the deep structure of these representations that make a given type of emotion distinctive, and that allow it to organize experience, motivation, memory, and action.

4. *What constitutes strong evidence to support a psychological construction view of emotion? Point to or summarize empirical evidence that supports your model or outline what a key experiment would look like. What would falsify your model?*

Theories are generally assessed by inspecting the results of empirical tests of their predictions. In the case of constructionist theories of the appraisal variety, however, it is reasonable to ask whether they are testable in this way. The OCC account defines the emotion-eliciting situations for types of emotion, then tries to assimilate emotion tokens (words) to the specification of those psychologically important situations. The relative usefulness of such theories therefore depends on their coherence, comprehensiveness, and ease of application rather than their truth. Moreover, when appraisal theories have been tested, studies most commonly depend on responses to vignettes, which may tell us more about people's theories of emotion than about emotion itself. A problem faced in these tests also is that participants must agree on what constitutes a particular emotion. In addition to such qualitative criteria, however, the OCC model proposes sets of cognitive factors that are expected to govern the intensity of each emotion type. The virtue of such proposals is that they allow the model to be tested quantitatively, because they predict when a given emotion will be intense or mild. To date, only a limited number of empirical studies are available.

(continued)

> The main source of "evidence" for the model comes from computer simulations, which serve primarily to indicate the coherence of the theory, its ease of application, and the general plausibility of its predictions and proposals. The model has been widely used as the emotion module in a great variety of games, tutoring programs, and other software involving "believable agents." The realization that artificially intelligent agents must know about and be able to act on emotion knowledge has given rise to a subarea of cognitive science known as "affective computing," within which the OCC model is prominent. None of the "evidence" unique to the theory, however, speaks to whether emotions are emergent or not.

Affective reactions can occur at various levels and in multiple modes ranging from low-level approach–avoidance impulses to complex evaluative judgments, experiences, expressions, and actions. As a result of iterative reprocessing (Cunningham, Dunfield, & Stillman, Chapter 7, this volume; Cunningham & Zelazo, 2007), the situational context and its interpretation give shape and definition to what would otherwise be amorphous, undifferentiated affective responses. Specific emotions differ from each other in terms of the psychological situations to which they are related and the extent to which and the way they are cognitively elaborated. The constellation of key elements in such a situation serves as the object of the emotion, directing and constraining emotional thought and action (Clore & Ortony, 2008).

The OCC model is an attempt to specify these key situational elements precisely, but with sufficient generality to encompass all instances of a given emotion type. That is, it seeks to characterize the structure of the situational construals—the appraisals—that are associated with one kind of emotion rather than another. The structure of the model, therefore, mirrors the structure of the construed situations associated with the different emotion types.[1] Figure 13.1 shows the important features of the model, which organizes and gives the specifications of 22 emotion types (e.g., resentment emotions, pride emotions) in six categories (e.g., fortunes-of-others emotions, attribution emotions). Associated with each of the 22 emotion types are words (tokens) whose corresponding emotions share the same eliciting conditions. Thus, emotion types such as distress and anger (along with a set of associated tokens; e.g., depressed and sad, and irritation and fury), are evaluative states whose eliciting conditions are focused on the elements of the psychological situations they represent. Examples of such elements are whether the construed situation is about event outcomes or actions and whether such actions are perceived as being one's own or another's.

The OCC model posits three different sources of value on which appraisals are based, and it views the structure of emotional space in terms

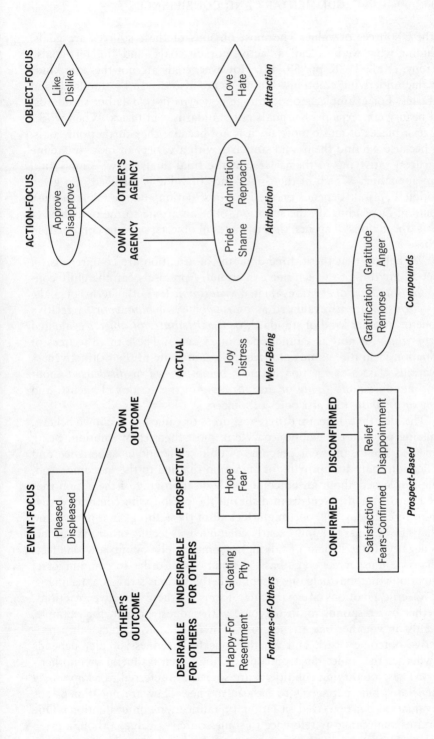

FIGURE 13.1. The OCC model specifies three kinds of affective reactions (in rectangular, oval, or diamond boxes), qualified by attributes of situations (bold type), to form 22 emotions grouped into six families (italic type).

of these sources of value. The most obvious of these sources are goals, including what we have called "active pursuit goals" and "interest goals" (Ortony, et al., 1988, pp. 39–44). However, goals are not the only kinds of value underlying emotions. Emotions are also driven by standards and by tastes. For example, moral outrage concerns not goals but standards, and beauty concerns neither goals nor standards, but tastes. When works of art or pieces of music move us, it is not because they further our goals, but because we find them (and similarly with a variety of more mundane pleasures) satisfying in themselves. In the final analysis, we simply find them appealing. Which of the three kinds of value is involved in a given emotional episode depends on the kind of situation and the focus of one's attention. Depending on the situation, one can attend to the outcomes of events, the actions of agents, the attributes of objects, or some combination of these.

We believe that these three domains of attention are comprehensive, covering anything to which one can attend. Appraisals can therefore concern the *outcomes of events* evaluated as *desirable* (or not) in terms of goals, the *actions of agents* evaluated as *praiseworthy or blameworthy* relative to one or another kind of standard, or the *attributes of objects* evaluated as *appealing* (or not) as a function of one's tastes. These three sources of evaluation yield three kinds of affect that contribute to the distinctiveness of various classes of emotion, namely, being *pleased or displeased* about event outcomes, *approving or disapproving* of the actions of agents, and *liking or disliking* (the attributes of) objects.

The idea that there are different sources of value has been, we believe, a missing piece in the emotion puzzle in most theories of emotion. Being displeased about an event outcome is quite different in experience and implication than disapproving of an action that led to the outcome. And, being displeased about an outcome while disapproving of the action that gave rise to it is different from disliking the person who committed that action. In everyday life, one might feel all of these things in a jumble and perhaps be at a loss to know exactly what one was feeling other than generally negative. One benefit of talking to someone else about how one feels is that one must make some basic distinctions in order to communicate, distinctions that may help one disentangle the various strands of feeling.

Specific emotions are particular forms of these affective reactions. Whether one responds to an outcome with sadness or fear, for example, depends on whether one attends to a known outcome (sadness) or a prospective outcome (fear), and whether one feels sadness or pity depends on whether the undesirable outcome is one's own (sadness) or another's (pity). These qualifying conditions are sometimes referred to as *appraisal dimensions*, but that seems to us a misnomer. They are not dimensions of evaluation but perceived situational qualifications on evaluations. One appraises something by reference to some source of value, although often not consciously. The qualifying conditions serve to specify the precise object being appraised (Clore & Ortony, 2008).

With this introduction to the OCC account of emotions as a background, in the remainder of this chapter we discuss issues relating to the four questions that were raised by the editors (roughly):

1. Are emotions psychological events constructed from more basic ingredients?
2. If there are such ingredients, which combinations of them are emotions and which are not?
3. Is there variability across and within emotions and people(s)?
4. What sort of evidence can support constructionist (and our own) accounts?

Are Emotions Constructed from Elements?

The question of whether emotions are psychological events constructed from more basic elements has two major parts. The first concerns whether emotions are events as opposed, presumably, to states. We discuss this aspect of the question in the next main section. What we discuss here is the implicit part of the question having to do with what the elements might be. There are several kinds of answers to this, depending on the perspective one takes. As will become apparent as we proceed, there are many ways to cut the pie, but for now we focus on one of the most widely held views, namely, that there exists a small set of privileged emotions, the "basic" or "primary" emotions, which constitutes the foundation of the emotion system.

Could Basic Emotions Be the Elements?

There are many variants of the basic emotion view, but the general idea is that a few emotions—typically, happiness, sadness, fear, disgust, anger, and surprise—have evolved as tightly organized, biological programs for mobilizing adaptive action and, when triggered by distinctive stimuli, they preempt attention and elicit stereotypical feelings, facial expressions, and action tendencies. Most proponents of this position claim that since similar reactions can be seen in not only animals but also quite elemental organisms, these emotions are primitive automatic reactions to eliciting stimuli that are specific to particular species. And since human facial expressions of these emotions are alleged to be recognized the world over, the corresponding emotions are assumed to be basic and universal.

The basic emotions view has been criticized on several grounds (e.g., Ortony & Turner, 1990). For example, there is no plausible account of how proposed basic emotions relate to the other, "nonbasic," emotions. Another objection is that there is no agreed-upon criterion for deciding which emotions are basic and why, which explains the wide range of basic emotions that have been proposed. For many decades, a favorite criterion of "basicness" has been the universality of associated unique facial expressions (e.g., Ekman, Friesen, & Ellsworth, 1982). However, recent evidence (e.g., Jack, Garrod, Yu, Caldara, & Schyns, 2012) challenges the universality criterion, because even though Westerners do indeed have common mental representations of the facial expressions associated with the six "basic" emotions, Easterners do not. A second, more general problem with the universality criterion is that of a double dissociation: on the one hand, some alleged basic emotions (e.g., Izard, 1977, lists both guilt and shame) are not associated with any universally recognizable facial expressions; on the other hand, some universally recognizable facial expressions are associated with conditions whose status as emotions can be challenged, with surprise being a good example.

As we have already indicated, emotions are quintessentially about evaluation—about goodness or badness. The problem with surprise is that even if we acknowledge that it has a universally recognizable facial expression, surprise is not about the goodness or badness of something. One can have an affectively neutral surprise—something unexpected happens, and one does not care. It is, of course, true that one can have a pleasant or unpleasant surprise, but then it is the pleasant or unpleasantness that makes it emotional, not the surprise itself. Thus, contrary to many of our colleagues and to accepted wisdom in emotion theory, our view is that despite its important and undeniable contribution to emotional intensity (which makes it a good candidate for a constituent of emotions), because surprise is not inherently good or bad, it is not itself an emotion, let alone a basic emotion. It violates the principle we mentioned at the outset, namely, that where there is no evaluation, there is no emotion.

The basic emotions view is part of a long tradition in psychology of attempting to frame explanations solely in bottom-up terms (Clore & Ortony, 2008). We believe, however, that cognitive, social, linguistic, and cultural factors (e.g., Jack et al., 2012) must be seen not merely as domains in which emotions are expressed but as formative parts of emotions. If so, solely bottom-up views will not suffice. We now know that higher processes are not simply the flowering of low-level processes. They also regulate what happens at early stages of processing (e.g., Phelps, Ling, & Carrasco, 2006; Ochsner & Gross, 2005), and such processes are iterative and constructive over time (Cunningham & Zelazo, 2007). Nevertheless, in spite of the various difficulties confronting the basic emotion view, and in spite of the skepticism expressed by several theorists (e.g., Barrett, 2006a), a recent special issue of *Emotion Review* devoted to basic emotions indicates that the idea is still alive and well. However, partly, but not just for the kinds of reasons discussed earlier, we see no prospect of basic emotions serving as the elements out of which all (other) emotions are constructed. Basic emotions cannot serve the constructionist enterprise.

Given our reservations about the whole idea of basic emotions, and therefore about their candidacy as the building blocks of all other emotions, might not emotions have other, "nonbasic" emotions as constituents? Leaving aside the fact that this would have no explanatory value because it leads to an infinite regress, what raises this possibility is the fact that an emotion can sometimes be the object of another emotion. For example, one might feel ashamed (or even angry) that one had been angry. However, most of the time, emotions do not have other emotions as their objects, and even when they do, being the object of an emotion is not the same thing as being a constituent of an emotion. In fact, more often than not, it is not a "whole" emotion that is the object, but the fact that one outwardly expressed or revealed an emotion. Furthermore, there are constraints on which emotions can be the object of other emotions—a topic that to the best of our knowledge has not been seriously studied. In any event, the fact that an emotion can sometimes be the object of another emotion does not invalidate our claim that emotions do not have other emotions as constituents.

At first blush, our denial that some of the fundamental constituents of emotions are themselves emotions might seem problematic, because in OCC we had discussed a class of emotions that we characterize as "compound emotions." These involve an amalgam of the eliciting conditions of two other emotions. But, again, we did not claim that these compound emotions have emotions as *constituents*. Our claim was, and is, that these emotions, which can be roughly characterized using the words *gratitude, anger, gratification*, and *remorse*, are actually the emotions that arise from the conjunction of two kinds of eliciting conditions, not the mixing of two distinct emotions wherein one emotion has the other emotion as a constituent.

Constructionism

Although ours is an appraisal approach, we are certainly committed to the idea that emotions are emergent interactions of various (non-emotional) constituents, and this we see as the hallmark of the constructionist view of emotions (e.g., Gross & Barrett, 2011). Thus, from our perspective, the two views are perfectly compatible. However, Gendron and Barrett (2009) distinguish between a constructionist view, which they embrace, and an appraisal view, which they do not. One explanation for why they see the two views as being at odds with each other is that they view appraisal theories as characterizing the *causes* of emotions, which to them implies that emotions exist as *entities*—entities that can be triggered or activated by the appraisals that precede them. We share their reluctance to embrace this position, but we are nevertheless comfortable with the appraisal label, because our version of appraisal theory does not assume that appraisals are causal antecedents of emotions but that appraisals are constituents of emotions (Clore & Ortony, 2008). Instead of viewing emotions as tightly organized, evolved modules, as do basic emotion theorists, we, like Barrett, Russell, and their colleagues (e.g., Barrett, 2009; Barrett, Wilson-Mendenhall, & Barsalou, Chapter 4, this volume; Russell, 2003; Chapter 8, this volume) subscribe to a componential constructionist view. And while we are happy to consider ours to be an appraisal theory, we note that Russell (and Barrett, too, notwithstanding her rejection of it by implication) is in fact committed to the appraisal theory idea, at least insofar as it holds that specific emotions can be distinguished from each other on the basis of the psychological situations in which they arise.

We have argued that our appraisal view is quite compatible with a psychological construction approach to emotion. However, just as there are many variants of the basic emotions view and many variants of appraisal theories, so too are there many variants of constructionist approaches. In order to assess more carefully the relationship between the two approaches, we have chosen to take Russell's (2003) seminal article "Core Affect and the Psychological Construction of Emotion" as a paradigmatic example of the constructionist approach. The gist of Russell's version of the constructionist approach is that affective conditions of all kinds (see Clore, Ortony & Foss, 1987; Ortony, Clore & Foss, 1987) are rooted in simple feelings of pleasure and displeasure. This "valence" dimension, when crossed with an "activation" dimension (ranging from excited to sleepy) yields a space that Russell refers to as "core affect"—a consciously accessible neuropsychological feeling state.

What makes Russell's view one of psychological construction of (specific) emotions is the fact that additional ingredients need to be entered into the mix. In the case of a "full-fledged" emotion, Russell identifies these additional ingredients as *perception of affective quality, attribution to the object* (of the emotion), *appraisal, action, emotional meta-experience,* and *emotion regulation.* One might argue about whether this is overkill—about whether emotion regulation, for example, is an ingredient of a prototypical emotion—but the general idea that in addition to core affect, emotions have constituents that are not themselves emotional or affective is one that we share. In fact, although we have never proposed an analysis of core affect that comes close to the level of detail that Russell provided, we have nevertheless championed a similar idea in several places. For example, in Ortony et al. (1988, p. 20, emphasis added), we wrote, "The particular words 'pleased' and 'displeased' represent the best we can do to find . . . English words that refer (only) to the *undifferentiated affective reactions.*" Similarly, Ortony and Turner (1990), in their critique of basic emotions, observed that specific emotions are best thought of as specializations of more amorphous affective states resulting from the involvement of different combinations of elements that are not themselves emotions. And more recently, Ortony, Norman, and Revelle (2005) argued that full-fledged emotions are cognitively elaborated and interpreted feelings, and that at rock bottom, these feelings comprise simple unelaborated affect, which they called "proto-affect," and which is restricted to the here and now.

Finally, to see the similarity between Russell's elements and our own view, we should mention that we have in various places (e.g., Clore & Ortony, 2000; Ortony, 2008) proposed a general model in which a typical emotion is an affective condition having four major components—an interpretive–cognitive, a motivational–behavioral, a somatic, and a subjective–experiential component. The cognitive component involves representations (sometimes consciously accessible and sometimes not) of the emotional meaning and personal significance of emotion-relevant situations. The motivational–behavioral component involves desires and inclinations to act (or not) relating to the interpretations of such situations. The somatic component concerns autonomic and central nervous system activity and their visceral and musculoskeletal effects, including changes in body-centered feelings (Damasio, 1994), as well as the neurochemical and neuroanatomical processes involved in emotions. And finally, the subjective–experiential component involves the subjective feelings of emotion—a component that is probably especially elaborate in humans, generally involving an awareness of an amalgam of feelings, beliefs, desires, and bodily sensations, as well as efforts to label the emotion. We refer to these four as components rather than as effects of emotion, because we consider emotion to emerge from these separate reactions to psychologically important situations rather than being caused by (or causing) them (Clore & Ortony, 2008).

Thus, it seems to us that we have long held the essence of the psychological construction view, namely, that emotions are made up of, or are the emergent result of (Coan, 2010; Coan & Gonzalez, Chapter 9, this volume) the interaction of various non-emotion components. To be sure, Russell has his constituents and we have ours, but they are not entirely mutually exclusive. For example, Russell proposes an action component, which in spirit is similar to our motivational–behavioral component, and his emotional meta-experience is in many ways similar to our subjective–experiential component. On the other hand, Russell seems to view appraisal theories as subscribing to some sort of temporal sequencing of events. For example, he claims that appraisal theories often take appraisal to be a "cognitive computation that occurs after the antecedent and before the emotion" (Russell, 2003, p. 161). Our view is that the emotion is the *ongoing interaction* of its constituents rather than a process that unfolds in a particular temporal order.

As we said earlier, there are many ways in which one can cut the pie—the OCC model cuts it one way and our four-components view cuts it another (and in the next section we reveal yet another). Nevertheless, provided that it is always the same pie, each way of cutting it is as legitimate as any other, just as is the perspective of each proverbial blind man describing the proverbial elephant. In summary, we should reiterate that notwithstanding some minor concerns, we are in substantial agreement with the psychological construction view advocated by Barrett and Russell and colleagues. In fact, we consider our own position to exemplify that view.

Constituent Combinations

Emotions versus Non-Emotions

If we ask which combinations of constituents are emotions and which are not, we are essentially addressing the question of what are the boundary conditions of emotions. The need to do this should be obvious, but in our case it is particularly important, because of our claim that some purported emotions, such as surprise, are not emotions at all, let alone basic ones. A theory of emotion, and indeed of emotion constituents, that does not (need to) include a state such as surprise in its coverage is likely to differ in important ways from a theory that does. This being the case, if we are to address the question of the relation between element combinations and emotions, it would seem wise to have some idea about how to distinguish emotions from non-emotions, which amounts to asking the age-old question (James, 1884) "What is an emotion?"

An early project of ours (Clore & Ortony, 1988; Clore et al., 1987; Ortony et al., 1987) involved using both theoretical and empirical methods to examine the referential status of some 500 English affective terms that had appeared in discussions of emotions in much of the then extant literature (e.g., Averill, 1975; Bush, 1973; Dahl & Stengel, 1978; Russell, 1980). Troubled by the fact that many of the terms in such discussions seemed not to refer to emotions at all, we sought to determine which words in what we called the "affective lexicon" were examples of emotions (e.g., *afraid, angry, happy*) and which were not (e.g., *tearful, sleepy*), and why. Furthermore, we were leery about committing ourselves to the view that all words in our corpus referred to states, so we chose to think in terms of the less constrained superordinate concept of *conditions*, some of which (e.g., *confident, exasperated, gratified*) are easily seen as states, whereas others (e.g., *attractive, despicable*) are not. The results of our efforts led us to conclude that good examples of emotion terms all refer to internal mental as opposed to physical (e.g., *breathless, jittery*) or external (e.g., *ridiculous, alone*) conditions. Of the mental conditions, some, such as *interested* and *perplexed*, that we referred to as cognitive conditions, and others, such as *argumentative, careful,* and *submissive,* that we called cognitive-behavioral conditions, we deemed to be devoid of any significant affect. This left us with three main groups of conditions that had clear affective content: affective-behavioral conditions (e.g., *cheerful*), affective-cognitive conditions (e.g., *encouraged*), and affective states (e.g., *grateful, disappointed*). Of these, it seemed clear that the best emotion terms shared a primary focus on affect or evaluation, rather than on cognition or behavior[2]—they were the "pure" affective states, and the best examples of emotions. A focus on affect means that as opposed to being simply evaluative in one way or another, the focus is on different kinds of goodness and badness.

While we concluded that good examples of emotion are states that focus primarily on affect, with less-good examples being tinged with cognition or behavior, there are three other important affective conditions—moods, attitudes, and temperaments—that can be differentiated from emotions and each other in terms of two sets of constraints (see Figure 13.2). Specifically, moods are object-diffuse, undifferentiated affective states (e.g., Clore & Ortony, 2000; Ortony et al., 2005)—they are not cognitively elaborated, and they lack a salient object. Affective conditions become mood-like to the extent that they are about things in general rather than about whatever might have been their original cause. So emotions tend to have salient objects, and moods do not, but both are relatively short-lived. By contrast, attitudes and temperaments are generally much more enduring. But like emotions, attitudes have specific objects, whereas temperaments, like moods, are not about anything in particular and hence have broad rather than targeted effects. It is interesting to note (although beyond the scope of this chapter) that many emotion words (e.g., *happy, angry, sad*) refer not only to emotional states but also to traits (which contribute to temperament) and to moods.

	Affective Conditions	
	States (temporary conditions)	Dispositions (enduring conditions)
Object Salient (i.e., intentional)	**Emotions**	**Attitudes**
Object Diffuse (i.e., nonintentional)	**Moods**	**Temperament**

FIGURE 13.2. The temporal and object constraints on four affective conditions. Note: The sense of *intentionality* in this figure refers to the notion of *aboutness* (i.e., the object that the mental condition is about).

Where Does Affect Come From?

Given our view that the foundation of emotions is not other emotions, we have to deal with the question of where affect comes from. It has to come from somewhere. Our basic answer is that the source of affect is always one of the three kinds of value identified in OCC, namely, goals, standards, and tastes. These three taken together are reminiscent of what Nico Frijda (e.g., 1986) refers to as "concerns," although he believes (personal communication, August 22, 2011) that the notion is "one of the worst elaborated and investigated notions that we have." On the other hand, he goes on to say that concerns are "what others describe as 'major goals,' as 'values,' as 'instincts,' or 'needs.'" So we are quite willing to refer to our goals, standards, and tastes, as concerns. As we go about our daily lives, many, but not all, of the experiences we encounter touch our concerns, some directly and some indirectly, some powerfully and some weakly. We might see a parent inappropriately smacking his or her child and feel a little uncomfortable. Why? Perhaps because what we see conflicts with our standards about decent and reasonable ways to treat children. We might get caught in an unexpected downpour and get soaked to the skin on a cool and windy day, and this might cause us to feel irritated and upset because our latent desire (goal) to stay comfortable is thwarted. Depending on who we are, and the details of the two situations just described, the intensities of the emotional responses to these situations are likely to be different, but both are emotional responses.

Central to the OCC model is the idea that these different kinds of value subserve different classes of emotions. Each source of value, when engaged, often leads rapidly and automatically to one of the three corresponding kinds of undifferentiated affect, because it is already part of our perception and comprehension of what we experience. Just as when we perceive one line in the Müller–Lyer illusion as being longer than the other, we see it *as* being longer—directly and immediately—and thus directly perceive what, in a sense, is an already (mis)interpreted reality, so too the affective reaction to a personally relevant object can be simple, direct, and immediate. So, for example, consider how one might react to the taste of rancid butter. It is quite simple; if it tastes rancid—spit it out! We do not have to taste it as bad and subsequently elaborate it as a rancid bad (even though that is indeed possible). We taste it *as* rancid, and experience disgust immediately and without inference (see, e.g., Zajonc, 1980). Something's tasting rancid is a particular way of that thing tasting bad. One might say that it is directly perceived as elaborated badness.

As with tastes, goals and standards can participate in emotions directly. We are not saying that it is impossible to get into a particular emotional state by doing a great deal of cognitive work first, but we are saying that undifferentiated affect routinely finds itself elaborated by ongoing perceptual and cognitive processes. We express it in this rather awkward way in an attempt to avoid the implication that we are talking about sequential processing. To repeat, when we speak of undifferentiated affect being cognitively (and perceptually) elaborated, we do not mean that the elaboration follows (although sometimes it can); we mean that the undifferentiated affect is augmented with details. To understand what we have in mind, imagine a color picture of a rustic scene. If we were to describe it as a picture of a rustic scene elaborated with color (clumsy, but not incorrect), we would not mean that first there was a picture that was subsequently colored; we would mean that the color was *part of* the picture. This is the sense of "elaborated" that we have in mind when we speak of elaborated undifferentiated affect. Another way of putting all of this is to say that different emotions are different and more or less detailed ways of feeling good or bad. Fear, shame, and disappointment are simply different ways of feeling bad, and pride, joy, and relief are different ways of feeling good.

Whereas we locate the sources of affect in the three kinds of values, Russell (2003), grappling with this problem in the context of tastes, came to a rather different conclusion. His position is that what he calls affective quality (valence) is *inherent in the object*. Affective quality is, he wrote, "a property of the thing perceived. It is the garden that is lovely, the stench that is offensive, and the tune that is joyous" (p. 157). We, on the other hand, view the perception of the smell and taste as rapid forms of appraisal. It cannot be that the badness of the smell is inherent in the object—the odor it emits can be, but its badness cannot, because its badness presupposes a perceiver. It must somehow have been evaluated—appraised. Russell's view is that the perception of affective quality is a "cold" process, whereas we view it as simply a matter of the degree to which the object is evaluated or appraised as being positive or negative. To use an analogy, a joke is not intrinsically funny. To be funny, a joke has to be perceived as such by someone. Similarly, a foul taste is not intrinsically foul. It is foul to those who dislike it, but not to those who do not. Infants dislike bitter tastes; many adults do not. The bitterness is not intrinsically negative.

Are Emotions States or Events?

In discussing our work on the affective lexicon, we were careful to talk of "conditions" rather than "states," even though our conclusion about genuine emotion terms was that they referred to (purely) affective *states*. Given the linguistic perspective that we were taking in that work, characterizing emotions as states seems to us to be a perfectly defensible position, but from the psychological, experiential perspective, we perhaps need to be a little careful in this regard, even though in everyday language we generally talk about emotions as states. The problem is that *state* implies a static entity, which in turn makes it easier to think in terms of stable constituents. It is true that thinking of emotions as states does indeed capture some aspects of emotion, but only at the cost of failing to capture others, the most important of which is the fact that emotions change over time (Frijda, Ortony, Sonnemans & Clore, 1992), not only with respect to their intensity, but also, concomitantly, in the role and nature of their facets. This fact tends to get lost if we conceptualize emotions as states. Consider a case of anger in which a person has been annoyed by someone but over time grows less angry. In this case, the motivation somehow to harm the offending person diminishes, and the accompanying somatic aspects of the emotion change. This suggests that there is utility in thinking of emotions as mental *events*. It may still make sense to think of them as states, but before explaining why we think this is so, it is perhaps worth considering what it means to construe emotions as events (see also Barrett, 2006b).

We like to think of emotions as one thinks of earthquakes. In the case of an earthquake, there is some initiating event—the movement of tectonic plates of sufficient significance to have some measurable consequences. In the case of an emotion, the initiating event is the construal of something in one's world of sufficient significance to have perceptible (affective) consequences.[3] The earthquake itself might last only a few seconds, but we do not think of it as a state. Apart from its magnitude, it has various (other) facets—changes in geological and geographical morphology; changes in the behavior of animals, before, during, and after the movement of the plates; and implications for lives and property. And finally, earthquakes usually have aftershocks, which, in the case of emotions, are equivalent to emotion-initiating events having emotional consequences after a period of quiescence. Presumably we do not need to spell out further the parallels in order to make the case that it is easy to think of emotions as events unfolding in time.

There are two clear advantages of not losing sight of the time course of emotions. First, it encourages serious attention to the sources of changes in emotional intensity. This is an issue we took very seriously in the OCC model, where we devoted an entire chapter to an analysis of the variables that can influence intensity. Many of these variables (e.g., arousal, unexpectedness, proximity) are also candidates, albeit again from a different perspective, for constituents of emotions. A second advantage of taking the dynamic quality of emotions into account is that it allows us to better understand the effects of emotions on behavior. An emotion involves responses to some situation in the world perceived to be relevant to the experiencer's concerns. The rise time of these reactions can be fast or slow; the experienced feelings may persist for a long time or a short time, even while changing from moment to moment; and they can dissipate quickly or slowly. And, importantly, the effect on the behavior of the experiencer or on others interacting with the experiencer will be influenced by where the emotion is in its temporal trajectory at the moment a decision is made or an action is taken. Imagine a woman becoming increasingly frustrated with her uncooperative employee. The employee, seeing this, might well refrain from defending herself, because she believes that to do so would probably make matters worse. On the other hand, if the employee views her boss as calming down, she might be more willing to risk putting forward her explanation or defense. In such situations, the employee is taking into account her (possibly implicit) beliefs about whether the anger of her boss is waxing or waning, and using this information to make a decision about what to say or do, and when and how. Thinking of the emotion only as a stable uniform state would not help us understand how it might contribute to decision making in this way. All this means that if one is trying to model the effects of emotion on behavior, the model should take into account the effect of timing on behavior, including the point in, and the recent history of, the temporal course of the emotion—that is, whether the emotion is waxing, waning, or relatively stable.

So, when we think of emotions as states, we need to remember that we are restricting ourselves to a relatively stable portion of an emotional event. Of course, we can always talk meaningfully about an emotional state if we think in terms of a momentary snapshot of an event in much the same way as a single frame in a film strip is a representation of a frozen moment, although, as we have just seen, the danger here is that the "snapshot" loses the temporal context. In any event, whichever way one looks at it, it is worth bearing in mind that when we talk of emotional states, the "whole thing" is not static; it changes over time (cf. Cunningham & Zelazo, 2007). Sometimes this can be important, since it has implications for behavior.

Another Analogy

We mentioned earlier that there are many ways to cut the emotion pie, and have subsequently discussed various kinds of constituents as we moved from one perspective to another. In the context of the OCC model, we have touched on the issue from both the structural and the intensity perspectives. From the former we get a more course-grained view of constituents than we get when we consider intensity. The broader, structural perspective gives us one of the three kinds of value, augmented by cognitive and perceptual constituents that represent details of the psychological situation, such as whether a standards-violating action is construed as being one's own or another's. Meanwhile, thinking of candidate constituents from the point of view of intensity variables gives us more specific candidates to explore. But then we also discussed our four-components view in which, under normal circumstances, every emotion is undifferentiated affect augmented with not only perception and cognition but also three other interacting components (somatic, behavioral–motivational, and subjective–experiential). And from a linguistic perspective we again saw a distinction between pure affect and cognition and behavior. This perspective allows us to see how the different components get reflected and emphasized or deemphasized in language. None of these different perspectives are at odds with one another; they merely *are* different perspectives, and whichever perspective we take, we generally arrive at the same point, namely, that different components are constantly interacting with each other to give the emergent subjective experience of an emotion—the way it feels—but this, too, we regard as a component, because it can feed back into the entire system and change it. For us, it is these interactions that constitute the process of element "combination."

Traditionally emotion has been viewed as an entity that *causes* the various emotional indicators such as expressions, feelings, and thoughts. However, the failure to find much coherence among them (e.g., Barrett, 2006a; Lang, 1968; Mauss & Robinson, 2009) suggests that this view is inadequate. Our view is that the most profitable way of thinking about the relation between emotions and their various manifestations is to adopt the kind of syndrome approach that is used to think about diseases. In the case of a disease, multiple events *constitute* the disease, rather than the disease existing separately and causing its symptoms. Similarly, an important psychological event occasions multiple reactions, which together constitute the emotion; the emotion has no separate existence. It all boils down to whether one focuses on some biopsychological representation of a situation as the emotion, which then causes other manifestations or, alternatively, whether one focuses, as we do, on the psychological situation itself, to which many subsystems respond and jointly constitute the emotion. Thus, the question is whether an important situation causes emotions, which then causes symptoms of that emotion, or whether an important situation causes multiple representations of the importance of that situation, which jointly constitute the emotion. On this latter view—our view—rather than a threat causing an emotion, which in turn causes threat-related thoughts, threat-related feelings, and threat-related physiology, to perceive something as a threat is to have some complex of threat-related thoughts, feelings, and physiology, the co-occurrence of which constitutes fear (Clore & Ortony, 2008).

Emotion Variability

In contrast to the basic emotions view, we assume that of the infinite number of emotions, none are basic in the sense of being the basis of all others.[4] In our view, emotions are representations of the value and urgency of significant psychological situations. Such representations are multimodal, potentially involving experience, expression, cognition, action, and other affective representations. The reactions that comprise emotions play an important role in regulating perception, thought, and behavior, all helping the individual to cope with or otherwise manage the situation represented.

Unlike the traditional view, ours locates the major constancies that distinguish one emotion from another in the kind of psychological situation that each represents, rather than in the feelings, expressions, thoughts, and actions that might be involved. Threats of loss are marked by fear-like states, and in that we see no variation. Thus, in the OCC account, fear-like reactions involve being *displeased at the prospect of an undesirable event* (Ortony et al., 1988). How one reacts to such prospects should vary with the precise nature of the event deemed undesirable. Fearing that one's savings will be wiped out in a serious economic recession will elicit different thoughts, feelings, and actions than fearing injury from a bear in the woods. We, of course, are a species for whom worrying about losing life savings is a possibility, whereas for other species it is not. From our perspective, what this means in terms of emotion variability is that which emotions can be experienced by a species (or by an individual for that matter) depends on what situations can be perceived as being psychologically important; in the particular case of fear (or anxiety),[5] it depends on what counts as the prospect of an undesirable event.

Presumably, organisms with similar biology represent common problems in similar ways. Just as the eye of the frog is adapted to its unique mode of feeding, so the approach and avoidance tendencies of different species are adapted to the relation between their basic biologies and the different kinds of stimuli likely to be encountered in their environments. Unlike the dung beetle, humans are repelled by rather than attracted to bodily waste. But attraction and repulsion are presumably basic dimensions of motivation for all behaving organisms, and the things that are attractive are usually also the stimuli that afford a species sustenance and safety as opposed to depletion and danger. Addressing animal emotions, LeDoux (2012) has recently proposed that a more fruitful strategy than trying to find human emotions in animals would be to look in humans for the basic survival circuits of animals that contribute to distinctively human emotions. In the process, he proposes an approach to emotion that is compatible with a constructionist view.

Although the similarity or variability in emotions across organisms (and people) lies in the kinds of situations that different species (and individuals within species) find psychologically significant, there are, of course, some universals among the kinds of situations with which living creatures must cope, including things such as threat, competition, access to resources, access to mates, group inclusion, nurturance of young, and so on. These are elements of the kinds of situations that elicit approach–avoidance motivation, affective reactions, and emotions. It is the obstacles and opportunities relative to these kinds of important situations that are universal and stable in affective reactions and emotions. There is, however, considerable variability across species, cultures, and individuals in how they respond to them.

For some creatures, important stimuli are innately "valued" in that they are reliably approached or avoided (e.g., amoebas approach light). As organisms become more complex, they exhibit fewer such tropisms or built-in evaluations. Despite the fact that human adults everywhere tend to respond negatively to snakes and spiders, neither humans nor other primates fear them innately (LoBue & DeLoache, 2008; Mineka, Davidson, Cook, & Keir, 1984). Accordingly, there is variation across individuals and groups in what humans find good and bad. Such variation is apparent both in reactions to stimuli that are concrete (e.g., whether dogs, cockroaches, snails, or pigs are good to eat) and to those that are abstract (e.g., what is considered holy, heretical, or blasphemous). There is, then, some variation among cultures and individual humans in the stimuli that elicit particular emotional reactions.

At another level, however, we expect all instances of a particular emotion type, such as fear, to be similar. The appraisal theorists of the 1980s sought to capture those similarities by writing elicitation rules for each of the common emotions (e.g., Ortony et al, 1988; Roseman, 1984; Smith & Ellsworth, 1985). There is some disagreement about whether such elicitation conditions are best thought of as "causes" (e.g., Roseman, 1984) or characterizations of emotions (Ortony et al., 1988). In the OCC model of emotion, for example, we specify the eliciting conditions of fear as *the prospect of an undesirable event*, and the emotion type, fear, as *displeasure at the prospect of an undesirable event*. These statements might suggest that perception of threat comes first and that fear then emerges as one becomes displeased, but as indicated earlier, we see no substantive difference between the perception of a threat with its different components and the emotion of fear. To us, it seems reasonable to say that something akin to the prospect of an undesirable event outcome (or the detection of threat) is a part of what we mean by fear, rather than a separable cause of fear. In any case, OCC is an account of the *structure* of emotions, not the *process* of emotion elicitation.

In a related way, and to return to our disease analogy, *amoebic dysentery* refers to the presence of a pathogen and its attendant bodily symptoms, not to either the pathogen or the symptoms by themselves. *Disease* can be defined as a change away from a normal state of health to an abnormal state in which health is diminished. Both normality and health, like emotions, are emergent conditions. Health is not some "thing" that can be caused by or that can cause other things. It is not an agent or an entity but an emergent condition. If the major biological systems are functioning in the normal range and a person experiences no symptoms and shows no signs of disease, he or she is healthy. But if he or she develops a fever, digestive problems, and particular amoebas are detected in the blood, then the person is no longer healthy—he or she has amoebic dysentery. Did that cause the loss of health? No. Rather than being a separate entity that might cause the loss of health, the fact of dysentery *is* the loss of health. And so it is with emotions; when someone with a furrowed brow reports feeling tense and having ruminative thoughts, that person is worried or afraid.

Emotion Specificity

In contrast to the idea that emotions such as fear, shame, and sadness have universal and fixed attributes, including distinctive expressions, feelings, cognitions, and behaviors, we assume that specific instances of these reactions are likely to be somewhat variable in their components and manifestations, not only across individuals but sometimes even within individuals. This conclusion follows from our view of emotions as situated affective reactions. They are situated in that each instance of a given emotion necessarily occurs in some particular situation at some particular point in time, so that however similar to other occurrences, each is nevertheless unique. Beyond its logical necessity, such a seemingly mundane claim about the particularity of emotions has important consequences.

As discussed earlier, moods are affective conditions with few cognitive, perceptual, or situational constraints. One feels positive or negative or irritable, but a mood is not necessarily about the situation in which one finds oneself, and sometimes it is not *about* much of anything. Specific emotions, on the other hand, have cognitive, perceptual, and (therefore) situational content. So emotions of sadness have to do with displeasure about undesirable event outcomes, whereas fear-like emotions involve displeasure over the prospect of an undesirable outcome, and disappointment is displeasure about the nonoccurrence of an anticipated desirable outcome, and so on. That is, each emotion can be thought of as an affective reaction (e.g., displeasure) occasioned by a different kind of situation. But more than that, each instance of an emotion type is situated, in that it has a specific object—it is about something; it is intentional (in the philosophical sense).

Because emotions are affective states occurring at specific times with specific objects, they can direct attention, thought, and action in ways that moods and other undifferentiated affective states cannot. So when one feels uneasy or anxious, one does not know exactly what to do. Full-fledged emotions, on the other hand, because they reflect the particulars of the situations in which they occur, motivate more specific thoughts and actions. Psychologists have never been terribly successful at specifying the motivations involved in specific emotions. Fear in general involves an inclination to withdraw or escape, but beyond that, not much can be said. But fear of one's investments losing value has motivational and behavioral implications that can be better specified. Emotions do not exist in the abstract. They occur in specific situations, at specific times, in people with specific

histories, expectations, desires, and so on. It is this limitless specificity that makes each emotion and each emotional moment different from
the next, and it is this difference that makes the specificity impactful and
consequential. So if we ask, "What does fear do to people?", our answer
is that it depends on who they are, where they are coming from, and of
what they are afraid. The important, impactful, consequential aspects of
emotion—the reason we care one way or the other about understanding
emotions—is that they are emergent from lives lived in situations in real
time, in moments that are rarely, if ever, repeated. And when the moment is
gone, and the ephemeral constituents of an emotion are gone, the emotion
is gone as well. With reference to the current question, such considerations
argue that instances of a given emotion type are likely to be quite varied,
especially in humans.

Theory Validation

Appraisal and Testability

One criterion for assessing the value of a theory is whether it is testable
and generates research. The claims of various appraisal theories, including
those of Frijda, Roseman, Scherer, and Smith and Ellsworth, have been
subjected to empirical tests. A common approach to testing such theories
has been to compute correlations between potentially important factors
and self-reported emotions. Much of this research, however, has been based
on emotion vignettes in which participants indicate how they think they
would respond under specified, imagined conditions or how they remember
(or misremember) past situations and their emotions. Such research can be
rightly criticized for saying more about people's concepts of various emotions than about the actual conditions for emotion elicitation. More fundamentally, however, one can ask questions about whether theories focused
on emotional appraisal really have much empirical content at all (Smedslund, 1991). The OCC account, for example, proposes eliciting conditions
of classes of emotion types that are essentially abstract but systematic statements of the necessary, but not necessarily sufficient, conditions for the
associated emotions to occur. Thus, the OCC account says that emotions
of, for example, the relief type involve being *pleased at the disconfirma-
tion of the prospect of an undesirable event*, which is a large part of what
is meant by the term *relief*. Therefore, one might complain that research
aimed at determining whether people really do report relief when they are
pleased that an anticipated bad outcome did not come to pass would be
as uninformative as research aimed at seeing whether all bachelors really
are unmarried. On the other hand, failures of predictions from appraisal
theories sometimes do lead to changes in emotion characterizations (e.g.,
Roseman, Antoniou, & Jose, 1996). Even formulations that are essentially

definitional can be shown to be inadequate by finding conditions that are seen as valid instances of a given emotion but that fall outside the characterization.

Having said this, we should mention that the OCC approach does make some genuine empirical claims. One large-scale attempt to test aspects of the account involved an examination of the emotions of fans of college basketball (Clore, Ortony, & Brand, 2006). We collected data from fans during a whole season before, during, and after games, asking a variety of questions about the quality of play, predictions about whether the team would win, and participants' specific emotions at the time of their occurrence. Data from wins and losses were analyzed separately, but both produced analyses of postgame emotions that clustered into three groups, including (goal-based) event-focused emotions, a separate set of (standards-based) emotions in response to the quality of play of the team, and (taste-based) emotions having to do with the degree of liking or disliking of the coach. The results were encouraging, since the theory specifies these three different sources of value based on these same categories of outcomes, actions, and objects. Moreover, the same result was obtained independently in both win and loss data.

Another problem is that adequate testing of appraisal theories is often limited by the need for research participants to understand and agree on the qualitative distinctions between such related states as resentment and anger, or sympathy and pity. One way around this limitation is to focus research on intensity, a quantitative rather than a qualitative aspect of emotion (Frijda et al., 1992). The OCC approach makes predictions about the variables that govern the intensity of emotions, in addition to the conditions that constitute them. It hypothesizes that emotions with a common set of cognitive and situational specifications should be governed by a common set of intensity variables. The theory therefore makes intensity predictions that allow quantitative comparisons that are inherently less ambiguous than the solely qualitative comparisons typical of many appraisal theories. For example, questions about *how much* anxiety or guilt is experienced in one situation compared to another are more empirically tractable than questions about whether the experience is one of anxiety or guilt.

Observations about emotional intensity can also provide a quantitative basis for assessing hypotheses about the structural relationships among different emotions. For example, suppose research designed to identify determinants of intensity finds that the intensity of anger is best predicted by people's perceptions of both the severity of a bad outcome and how much some agent was deemed responsible for that outcome. Finding that the intensity of anger is determined by both of these factors would support structural claims that typical cases of anger involve a joint focus on outcomes (appraised as undesirable) and actions (appraised as blameworthy). Hypotheses about emotional intensity therefore put some empirical meat on the theoretical bones of the OCC account. And, of course, evidence that different combinations of elements yield different emotions also supports a constructionist account of emotion.

Computational Modeling

Although the OCC model could serve as the basis for many predictions relating to element combinations and emotion intensity, disappointingly few have been examined in psychology. Instead, most of the "evidence" for the model comes from computer science. The cognitive revolution of the 1970s and 1980s broadened the horizons of psychologists, allowing them to examine the mental processes involved in thought and behavior. But even at the beginning, Herbert Simon (1967) argued that a cold cognitive approach would not be adequate. He noted that emotions play a pivotal role in regulating cognitive processing by altering one's processing agenda.

Subsequently, Donald Norman (1981) proposed that 12 major challenges would have to be met for the new cognitive science to be a success, and he included emotion as one of those challenges. About this same time, we began working on the OCC model, and one of our goals was to develop an account of emotion that, at least in principle, would be implementable on a computer. The idea was not to have computers feel emotions, of course, but for intelligent computational agents to be able to reason and make appropriate inferences about emotional situations (e.g., O'Rorke & Ortony, 1994).

In the intervening years, computer scientists have sought to develop "believable agents" (e.g., Ortony, 2003) that can display emotions and respond appropriately to the emotions of others. *Affective computing* (Picard, 2000) has become an umbrella term for these and other efforts to include emotion-relevant capabilities in artificially intelligent systems. The idea is to build computer systems that can recognize emotion in text, speech, and behavior, and to endow virtual characters with some emotional competence to help them interact with humans and other agents more successfully.

The field has now reached a point where emotion generation and recognition models are regularly used to enhance the emotional, social, and practical intelligence of autonomous virtual characters in all kinds of domains, but perhaps most notably in video games—a domain that now constitute a multibillion dollar industry.[6] To be effective, a working model of emotion must allow virtual agents to make plausible inferences about the emotions, desires, and intentions of others during social interactions. Many virtual agents have been fashioned not only to act but also to look somewhat life-like, and big increases in computing power have opened up new possibilities. Since emotions and their detection and expression are important in regulating decision, thought, actions, and interactions for real humans, they are also important for virtual humans and for human–computer interaction.

In conclusion, just as collecting theory-supporting data from psychological experiments cannot establish the veracity of a theory, neither can embedding a psychological theory in a computational model. However, embedding a theory into working models can be a strong test of a theory, and indeed this is a well-accepted principle in cognitive science. There are two general reasons why computational modeling of a theory like OCC is a powerful test. First, if the theory is precise and formalizable, it is at the very least coherent, and one test of whether a theory is precise and formalizable is that it can be implemented. Then, barring major weakness in these respects, failures offer the prospect of improving the theory, as has happened with OCC (e.g., Steunebrink, Dastani, & Meyer, 2009). Second, if the emotion-related behavior exhibited by a computational device or virtual agent in which a theory is embedded is plausible and consonant with people's intuitions, it is reasonable to conclude that at least in some important respects, and at some reasonable level of description, the theory is doing a good job of accounting for (and predicting) behavior. In this respect we believe that the OCC model has been a success. It has clearly resonated with computer scientists, and it is by far the most cited psychological work in the field of affective computing. As Bartneck and Lyons (2009) put it:

> the OCC model . . . has established itself as the standard model for emotion synthesis. A large number of studies [have] employed the OCC model to generate emotions. . . . Many developers of [embodied] characters believe that this model will be all they ever need to add emotions to their character (pp. 36–37).

And indeed, the OCC model has been used by hundreds of researchers in affective computing and in hundreds of applications ranging from modeling students' emotions while they learn (e.g., Katsionis & Virvou, 2005) to simulating agents in agent-based combat scenarios (Van Dyke Parunak, Bisson, Brueckner, Matthews, & Sauter, 2006), to giving emotional comfort to victims of cyberbullying (van der Zwaan, Dignum, & Jonker, 2010), to sentiment analysis in text (e.g., Shaikh, Prendinger, & Ishizuka, 2009). Its widespread adoption and apparent success in computational modeling contexts leads us to believe that, at least in some respects, the OCC model is on the right track.

ACKNOWLEDGMENTS

The authors acknowledge support from National Institutes of Health Grant No. MH 50074 and National Science Foundation Grant No. BCS-1252079 to Gerald Clore.

NOTES

1. The reason we speak of emotion "types" is that we think it important to acknowledge differences between various tokens of the same emotion type. For example, the fear or anxiety one might experience at thinking one might have made a bad investment is likely to be qualitatively (as well as quantitatively) different from the fear or anxiety one might experience when anticipating a biopsy result that might portend cancer. Nevertheless, both are tokens of the type "fear."

2. The three groups are roughly isomorphic with the classical trilogy of affection, conation, and cognition (e.g., Hilgard, 1980).

3. This raises the question of perceptible to whom (e.g., when a person observes that another is angry without the other acknowledging or even recognizing his or her anger). This is a complicated issue. Unfortunately, a proper discussion of it is beyond the scope of this chapter.

4. In fact, we would be willing to ascribe some sort of special, "basic" status to the two forms, one positive the other negative, of what we have referred to as undifferentiated affect (for a detailed discussion, see Ortony, Norman, & Revelle, 2005).

5. Although OCC makes no distinction between fear and anxiety (and at the level of granularity of being displeased at the prospect of an undesirable event, justifiably so), we think it important to note that from a biological perspective there are good reasons to believe that they are distinct (e.g., Gray & McNaughton, 2000). They have distinct neural substrates and are modulated by distinct classes of drugs (McNaughton & Corr, 2004).

6. According to the Entertainment Software Association website (*www. theesa.com*), consumers spent almost $20.77 billion on video games, hardware, and accessories in 2012.

REFERENCES

Averill, J. R. (1975). A semantic atlas of emotion concepts. *JSAS Catalog of Selected Documents in Psychology, 5*, 330 (Manuscript 421).

Barrett, L. F. (2009). The future of psychology: Connecting mind to brain. *Perspectives on Psychological Science, 4(4)*, 326–339.

Barrett, L. F. (2006a). Emotions as natural kinds? *Perspectives on Psychological Science, 1*, 28–58.

Barrett, L. F. (2006b). Solving the emotion paradox: Categorization and the experience of emotion. *Personality and Social Psychology Review, 10(1)*, 20–46.

Bartneck, C., & Lyons, M. J. (2009). Facial expression analysis, modeling and synthesis: Overcoming the limitations of artificial intelligence with the art of the soluble. In J. Vallverdu & D. Casacuberta (Eds.), *Handbook of research on synthetic emotions and sociable robotics: New applications in affective computing and artificial intelligence* (pp. 33–53). Hershey, PA: IGI Global.

Bush, L. E. (1973). Individual differences multidimensional scaling of adjectives denoting feelings. *Journal of Personality and Social Psychology, 35*, 50–57.

Clore, G. L., & Ortony, A. (1988). The semantics of the affective lexicon. In V. Hamilton, G. H. Bower, & N. H. Frijda (Eds.), *Cognitive perspectives on emotion and motivation* (pp. 367–397). Dordrecht, The Netherlands: Kluwer.

Clore, G. L., & Ortony, A. (2000). Cognition in emotion: Always, sometimes, or never? In L. Nadel, R. Lane, & G. L. Ahern (Eds.), *The cognitive neuroscience of emotion* (pp. 24–61). New York: Oxford University Press.

Clore, G. L., & Ortony, A. (2008). Appraisal theories: How cognition shapes affect into emotion. In M. Lewis, J. M. Haviland-Jones, & L. F. Barrett (Eds.), *Handbook of emotions* (3rd ed., pp. 628–642). New York: Guilford Press.

Clore, G. L., Ortony, A., & Brand, S. (2006). *The joy of victory and the agony of defeat: The emotions of sports fans.* Unpublished manuscript, University of Virginia, Charlottesville, VA.

Clore, G. L., Ortony, A., & Foss, M. A. (1987). The psychological foundations of the affective lexicon. *Journal of Personality and Social Psychology, 53,* 751–766.

Coan, J. A. (2010). Emergent ghosts of the emotion machine. *Emotion Review, 2,* 274–285.

Cunningham, W. A., & Zelazo, P. D. (2007). Attitudes and evaluations: A social cognitive neuroscience perspective. *Trends in Cognitive Science, 11,* 97–104.

Dahl, H., & Stengel, B. (1978). A classification of emotion words: A modification and partial test of de Rivera's decision theory of emotion. *Psychoanalysis and Contemporary Thought, 1,* 261–312.

Damasio, A. R. (1994). *Descartes' error: Emotion, reason, and the human brain.* New York: Avon Books.

Ekman, P., Friesen, W. V., & Ellsworth, P. (1982). What emotion categories or dimensions can observers judge from facial behavior? In P. Ekman (Ed.), *Emotion in the human face* (pp. 39–55). New York: Cambridge University Press.

Frijda, N. H. (1986). *The emotions.* Cambridge, UK: Cambridge University Press.

Frijda, N. H., Ortony, A., Sonnemans, J., & Clore, G. (1992). The complexity of intensity: Issues concerning the structure of emotion intensity. *Review of Personality and Social Psychology, 13,* 60–89.

Gendron, M., & Barrett, L. F. (2009). Reconstructing the past: A century of ideas about emotion in psychology. *Emotion Review, 1,* 1–24.

Gray, J., & McNaughton, N. (2000). *The neuropsychology of anxiety.* Oxford, UK: Oxford University Press.

Gross, J. J., & Barrett, L. F. (2011). Emotion generation and emotion regulation: One or two depends on your point of view. *Emotion Review, 3,* 8–16.

Hilgard, E. R. (1980). The trilogy of mind: Cognition, affection, and conation. *Journal of the History of the Behavioral Sciences, 16,* 107–117.

Izard, C. E. (1977). *Human emotions.* New York: Plenum Press.

Jack, R. E., Garrod, O. G. B., Yu, H., Caldara, R., & Schyns, P. G. (2012). Facial expressions of emotion are not culturally universal. *Proceedings of the National Academy of Sciences, 109,* 7241–7244.

James, W. (1884). What is an emotion? *Mind, 9,* 188–205.

Katsionis, G., & Virvou, M. (2005). Adapting OCC theory for affect perception in educational software. In *Proceedings of the 11th International Conference on Human–Computer Interaction,* Mahwah, NJ: Erlbaum.

Lang, P. J. (1968). Fear reduction and fear behavior: Problems in treating a construct. In J. M. Shlien (Ed.), *Research in psychotherapy* (Vol. 3, pp. 90–102). Washington, DC: American Psychological Association.

LeDoux, J. (2012). Rethinking the emotional brain. *Neuron, 73*, 653–676.

LoBue, V., & DeLoache, J. S. (2008). Detecting the snake in the grass: Attention to fear-relevant stimuli by adults and young children. *Psychological Science, 19*, 284–289.

Mauss, I. B., & Robinson, M. D. (2009). Measures of emotion: A review. *Cognition and Emotion, 23*, 209–237.

McNaughton, N., & Corr, P. J. (2004). A two-dimensional neuropsychology of defense: Fear/anxiety and defensive distance. *Neuroscience and Biobehavioral Reviews, 28*, 285–305.

Mineka, S., Davidson, M., Cook, M., & Keir, R. (1984). Observational conditioning of snake fear in rhesus monkeys. *Journal of Abnormal Psychology, 93*, 355–372.

Norman, D. A. (1981). Twelve issues for cognitive science. In D. A. Norman (Ed.), *Perspectives on cognitive science* (pp. 265–295). Hillsdale, NJ: Erlbaum.

Ochsner, K. N., & Gross, J. J. (2005). The cognitive control of emotion. *Trends in Cognitive Sciences, 9*, 242–249.

O'Rorke, P., & Ortony, A. (1994). Explaining emotions. *Cognitive Science, 18*, 283–323.

Ortony, A. (2003). On making believable emotional agents believable. In R. Trappl, P. Petta, & S. Payr (Eds.), *Emotions in humans and artifacts* (pp. 189–211). Cambridge, MA: MIT Press.

Ortony, A. (2008). Affect and emotions in intelligent agents: Why and how? In J. Tao & T. Tan (Eds.), *Affective information processing* (pp. 11–21). Berlin: Springer.

Ortony, A., Clore, G. L., & Collins, A. (1988). *The cognitive structure of emotions*. New York: Cambridge University Press.

Ortony, A., Clore, G. L., & Foss, M. A. (1987). The referential structure of the affective lexicon. *Cognitive Science, 11*, 341–364.

Ortony, A., Norman, D. A., & Revelle, W. (2005). Affect and proto-affect in effective functioning. In J. M. Fellous & M. A. Arbib (Eds.), *Who needs emotions: The brain meets the robot* (pp. 173–202). New York: Oxford University Press.

Ortony, A., & Turner, T. J. (1990). What's basic about basic emotions? *Psychological Review, 97*, 315–331.

Phelps, E. A., Ling, S., & Carrasco, M. (2006). Emotion facilitates perception and potentiates the perceptual benefits of attention. *Psychological Science, 17*, 292–299.

Picard, R. W. (2000). *Affective computing*. Cambridge, MA: MIT Press.

Roseman, I. J. (1984). Cognitive determinants of emotion: A structural theory. In P. Shaver (Ed.), *Review of personality and social psychology: Vol. 5. Emotions, relationships, and health* (pp. 11–36). Beverly Hills, CA: Sage.

Roseman, I. J., Antoniou, A. A., & Jose, P. J. (1996). Appraisal determinants of emotions: Constructing a more accurate and comprehensive theory. *Cognition and Emotion, 10*, 241–277.

Russell, J. A. (1980). A circumplex model of affect. *Journal of Personality and Social Psychology, 39*, 1161–1178.

Russell, J. A. (2003). Core affect and the psychological construction of emotion. *Psychological Review, 110,* 145–172.

Shaikh, M. A. M., Prendinger, H., & Ishizuka, M. (2009). In J. Tao & T. Tan (Eds.), *Affective information processing.* (pp. 45–73). Berlin: Springer.

Simon, H. A. (1967). Motivational and emotional controls of cognition. *Psychological Review, 74,* 29–39.

Smedslund, J. (1991). The pseudoempirical in psychology and the case for psychologic. *Psychological Inquiry, 2,* 325–338.

Smith, C. A., & Ellsworth, P. C. (1985). Patterns of cognitive appraisal. *Journal of Personality and Social Psychology, 48,* 813–838.

Steunebrink, B. R., Dastani, M. M., & Meyer, J.-J. C. (2009). The OCC model revisited. In D. Reichardt (Ed.), *Proceedings of the 4th KI Workshop on Emotion and Computing: Current research and future impact* (pp. 40–47). Paderborn, Germany: Kuenstliche-intelligenz Society.

van der Zwaan, J., Dignum, V., & Jonker, C. (2010). Simulating peer support for victims of cyberbullying. In *Proceedings of the 22nd Benelux Conference on Artificial Intelligence* (pp. 1–8). Luxemburg: University of Luxembourg.

Van Dyke Parunak, H., Bisson, R., Brueckner, S., Matthews, R., & Sauter, J. (2006). A model of emotions for situated agents. In H. Nakashima, M. P. Wellman, G. Weiss, & P. Stone (Eds.), *Proceedings of the 5th International Joint Conference on Autonomous Agents and Multiagent Systems* (pp. 993–995). New York: ACM Digital Library.

Zajonc, R. (1980). Feelings and thinking: Preferences need no inferences. *American Psychologist, 35*(2), 151–175.

CHAPTER 14

Basic Emotions, Psychological Construction, and the Problem of Variability

ANDREA SCARANTINO

The most influential recent challenge to the scientific viability of Basic Emotion Theory (BET) comes from psychological constructionists, who have argued that, contrary to BET's claims, the empirical data do not support the existence of coordinated packages of biological markers—either in the body or in the brain—associated with candidate basic emotions such as anger, fear, happiness, disgust, and so forth (Russell, 2003; Barrett, 2006a, 2006b).

The take-home message of this chapter is that the empirical data undermine what I call *traditional BET* but are not fatal to BET as a research program. I will show how a *new BET* can be formulated so as to answer the constructionist critique (see also Scarantino, 2012a, 2012b, 2012c; Scarantino & Griffiths, 2011). Furthermore, I will highlight some challenges that psychological constructionists face in their quest to account for emotion episodes without invoking specialized emotion mechanisms.

Seven Commitments for Traditional BET

BET finds inspiration in Darwin's (1872) theory of emotional expressions.[1] In the 1960s, Darwin's evolutionary approach was embedded into a general theory of affects by Tomkins (1995), and powerfully articulated into modern-day BET by Ekman (1980, 1999), Izard (1977, 1992), Panksepp

1. *If emotions are psychological events constructed from more basic ingredients, then what are the key ingredients from which emotions are constructed? Are they specific to emotion or are they general ingredients of the mind? Which, if any, are specific to humans?*

According to the version of basic emotion theory I present in my contribution to this volume—the new BET—basic emotions are evolved programs that coordinate more basic ingredients such as facial muscle responses, autonomic blood flow, subjective experiences, respiratory and vocal changes, motor patterns, thoughts, memories, images, and so on. In this limited sense, the new BET is *compositionally constructionist*, because emotions are analyzed in terms of more elemental building blocks (programs, physiological changes, expressions, behaviors, etc.). I emphasize that the only building block specific to emotion is the program associated with each basic emotion. All building blocks elicited and coordinated by the program are instead also involved in non-emotional processes. For example, motor patterns and autonomic blood flow are involved not only in basic emotions but also in the non-emotional activity of doing push-ups. Some of the ingredients of human basic emotions are specific to humans, because they reflect capacities only humans have. Three ingredients of human basic emotions that are good candidates for being specific to humans are conceptual thoughts (e.g., "This is the third time I have been disrespected by my boss in front of my wife"), imaginings (e.g., to imagine hitting the boss without doing it), and at least some subjective experiences (e.g., the meta-experience of perceiving oneself as being angry at the boss). On the other hand, the basic emotion programs that elicit and coordinate emotional responses exist not only in humans but also (in homologous form) in related species. Finally, since I do not consider basic emotions to exhaust the domain of emotions, I am open to the possibility that there may be some nonbasic emotions that are exclusively human (e.g. regret).

2. *Which processes bring these ingredients together in the construction of an emotion? Which combinations are emotions and which are not (and how do we know)?*

According to the new BET, what brings the ingredients of a basic emotion together is an evolved and specialized basic emotion program. The program was selected to coordinate organismic resources to deal successfully with fundamental life tasks such as avoiding dangers, removing obstacles, coping with losses, and so on. In this view, what is distinctive about basic emotions is not the specific responses they involve but the programs that recruit such responses in a task-oriented and (often) context-dependent fashion.

There are two ways in which we can determine whether a certain combination of ingredients counts as an emotion or not. The first is through what I call the *Folk Emotion Test*. The test is passed by a certain configuration C of ingredients insofar as C is sufficiently similar to the prototype (or exemplar, or other suitable construct supported by psychologists of concepts) of

(continued)

a vernacular emotion such as *anger, fear, regret, guilt, shame, awe*, and so forth. Passing the Folk Emotion Test entails being an emotion in the ordinary sense of the term. The second is what I call the *Natural Emotion Test.* The test is passed by a certain configuration C of components insofar as C satisfies the condition of membership of a natural emotion kind, which is (roughly) a theoretically homogenous class of emotions about which a great many explanatory and predictive generalizations can be formulated in affective science. The account of basic emotions I offer in this chapter aims to individuate a combination of ingredients that passes the Natural Emotion Test. I have also argued that passing the Folk Emotion Test is not sufficient for passing the Natural Emotion Test. This is to say that a certain combination C of ingredients can qualify as fear, or anger, or happiness in the ordinary sense, without individuating a natural kind of emotion. This is due to the heterogeneity of folk emotion categories, which collect members that are arguably too different from one another for purposes of scientific investigation. For this reason, I have recommended that basic emotion theorists stop designating basic emotions using folk psychological emotion categories, which fail to capture natural kinds.

   3.   *How important is variability (across instances within an emotion category, and in the categories that exist across cultures)? Is this variance epiphenomenal or a thing to be explained? To the extent that it makes sense, it would be desirable to address issues such as universality and evolution.*

I have distinguished among three types of variability: variability across instances of a given folk emotion category, variability in the folk emotion categories that exist across cultures, and variability in the manifestation of a basic emotion. All forms of variability must be explained. But it is important not to confuse them. The variability we find within folk emotion categories such as "fear" or "anger" is a threat to their scientific status, because it stands in the way of formulating scientific generalizations that apply to all members of the category. The variability we find across cultures, instead, has no impact on the scientific status of folk emotion categories, because it does not affect the set of members such categories contain in any given language. The variability we find in the manifestation of a basic emotion, finally, has two main sources. The first is that basic emotions evolved to deal with fundamental life tasks that take on different forms, and require different responses on different occasions to be dealt with successfully. As a result, basic emotion programs need to be able to produce flexible responses. The second is the fact that basic emotions interact with other emotions and other mental states, which also leads their manifestations to differ from occasion to occasion. Because of these two sources of variability, the new BET holds that what is universal when it comes to basic emotions are first and foremost the evolved programs that run them. On this view, the program evolved to deal with dangers or the program evolved to remove obstacles are universals, in the sense that they are found in every culture and in related species in homologous form. But the specific

(continued)

manifestations of the activation of such programs are not necessarily universal. This marks a key difference with traditional BET, which has looked for universality in the actual bodily and neural changes associated with each basic emotion. Although some universal responses are going to be found in the (rare) occasions in which the elicitors of a basic emotion activate a rigid cascade of mandatory responses, most instances of basic emotions lack mandatory outputs and will only lead to irruptive and prioritized response tendencies whose actual manifestations are highly variable and context-sensitive.

   4. *What constitutes strong evidence to support a psychological construction to emotion? Point to or summarize empirical evidence that supports your model or outline what a key experiment would look like. What would falsify your model?*

I consider psychological constructionism to include both a positive program and a negative program. The negative program holds that there are no hardwired emotion mechanisms uniquely associated with anger, fear, happiness, sadness, disgust, and so forth that are causally responsible for coordinating patterns of tightly associated components with a one-to-one correspondence with the relevant folk emotion categories. I think this component of psychological constructionism is strongly supported by the empirical evidence on variability with respect to the neural circuitry, physiological changes, expressions, behaviors, and phenomenological changes associated with anger, fear, happiness, sadness, disgust, and so forth.

   The positive program of psychological constructionism would need to achieve two objectives in order to be fully supported: accounting for the relevant empirical data better than all competing models and providing a viable account of how emotion episodes come about without invoking specialized emotion mechanisms. I have argued in this chapter and in Scarantino (2012a) that, although both Russell's version and Barrett's version of psychological constructionism account for the empirical evidence better than traditional BET, they do not provide a viable account of how emotion episodes come to be.

   I have offered the new BET as an alternative model that combines insights from the constructionist camp with insights from traditional BET. The new BET, just like psychological constructionism, predicts that instances of folk emotion categories like anger, fear, happiness, sadness, and disgust, will not all manifest the same neurophysiological signature, nor will display high correlation between changes in physiology, expressions, behaviors, phenomenology, and so forth. In this sense, the new BET is compatible with the empirical data that falsify traditional BET.

   Unlike psychological constructionism, however, the new BET makes a further prediction, namely that we will find evidence for the existence of specialized emotion programs designed to solve evolutionary problems in a context-dependent and yet task-oriented fashion. The new BET is going to be empirically supported insofar as we can find evidence in three domains (conversely, absence of evidence in all such domains would falsify the new BET):

(continued)

(i) *Evidence of hard-wiredness*: Evidence that there are hardwired neural circuits designed to orchestrate solutions to evolutionary problems such as dealing with dangers, removing obstacles, expelling noxious substances, suffering losses, and so forth.

(ii) *Evidence of distinctness and continuity of responses*: Evidence that the presentation of focused/powerful/sudden/prototypical elicitors leads to a cascade of highly coordinated responses specific to distinct basic emotions, functional to the solution of a fundamental life task and continuous across cultures and species

(iii) *Evidence of distinctness and continuity of functional variants*: Evidence that the presentation of less focused/ powerful/sudden/prototypical elicitors leads to context-dependent yet task-oriented combinations of functional variants that are specific to distinct basic emotions and continuous across cultures and species

Although the bulk of recent empirical research has been aimed at either confirming or falsifying traditional BET, some of the evidence collected so far can be interpreted as supporting the new BET, and I predict that significantly more evidence in its favor will be forthcoming.

Re (i): We have evidence for the existence of hardwired circuits for orchestrating responses to the sorts of challenges basic emotions evolved to solve, including distinct circuits for responding to unconditioned threats and conditioned threats (Le Doux, 2012), distinct circuits for producing defensive aggression and predatory aggression (Moyer, 1976; Blanchard & Blanchard 2003), distinct circuits for responding to body-boundary violations and repulsive foods (Harrison, Gray, Giarnos, & Critchley 2010), and many others (see Panskepp, 1998 and LeDoux, 2012, for two alternative taxonomies of adaptive neural circuits shared across mammals). These circuits combine with learning and other forms of higher cognition to give rise to the full panoply of context-dependent manifestations of basic emotions.

Most of these circuits have been studied in rodents, but there are reasons to think that they are at least to some extent conserved across species and found in similar form in humans (Le Doux, 2012; Panskepp, 1998). This being said, it is an open question whether any phenomenological changes are associated with the activation of such circuits in non-human animals. What is quite clear is that multiple circuits can underlie solutions to the same evolutionary life task, which suggests the need for moving away not only from folk psychological categories (there is no neural circuit for fear, no neural circuit for anger, etc.), but also from simple basic emotion categories. (There are multiple circuits underlying basic fear, so we should distinguish between conditioned basic fear and unconditioned basic fear; there are multiple circuits underlying basic anger, so we should distinguish between defensive basic anger and offensive basic anger; and so forth.)

Re (ii) & (iii): The study of the evidence for distinctness has been set back by failure on the part of basic emotion theorists to acknowledge that basic

(continued)

emotion programs have two different modes of operation. When the basic emotion program is activated by elicitors that are "focused, powerful, sudden, and closely match prototypical antecedent conditions" (Levenson, 2011, p. 382), it coordinates a rigid cascade of facial, autonomic, behavioral, and phenomenological changes of the sort posited by traditional emotion theorists.

Testing for this hypothesis requires exposing individuals to elicitors such as loud sounds or deadly predators for basic fear; physical restraint or sudden pokes in the back for basic anger; dead insects in one's soup or feces for basic disgust; and so on. What the new BET predicts is that in such cases, and only in such cases, the basic emotion program will lead to a rigid cascade of responses that are specific to each basic emotion.

For basic fear, it is predicted for instance that exposure to a charging bear will lead humans to manifest autonomic changes such as increased heartbeats, increased myocardial contractility, vasoconstriction, and electrodermal activity (Kreibig, 2010); expressions such as eyes and mouth open, lips retracted, and eyebrows raised (Matsumoto et al., 2008); behaviors such as freezing and then running away and unpleasant feelings. These responses are expected to be found in different cultures and across species, but they are not expected to be found in all manifestations of basic fear, let alone in manifestations of fear that are not basic.

The best evidence we have for continuity of responses across cultures and species concerns facial expressions. There is evidence that the kinds of "exaggerated"[2] facial responses associated with basic emotions in prototypical cases are recognized beyond chance by perceivers from different cultures (Ekman, 1972; but see Russell, 1994 for worries about the methods used), involve similar facial muscles across cultures (Ekman, 1972; Matsumoto & Willingham, 2006), are displayed by children born blind (Matsumoto & Willingham, 2009), and have homologous expressions in non-human primates (Chevalier-Skolnikoff, 1973; Waller et al., 2006).

The mistake of traditional basic emotion theorists has been to suggest that the "exaggerated" expressions associated with basic emotions in the presence of focused/powerful/ sudden/prototypical elicitors are universally found whenever "fear" or "anger" or "disgust" are activated. This prediction has been widely and rightly debunked by psychological constructionists, who have demonstrated that the facial expressions associated with fear, anger, disgust, and so forth vary with cultures, are perceived differently depending on context, and are often not present at all in fear, anger, disgust, and so forth (see Russell, Chapter 8, this volume).

As noted by Levenson (2011, p. 382), the sorts of elicitors used in social science experiments "are typically mild, gradual in onset, diffuse, and do not closely match prototypes." When the basic emotion program is activated by elicitors that are less focused/powerful/ sudden/prototypical, we should expect it to coordinate a flexible, yet task-oriented, combination of facial, autonomic, behavioral, and phenomenological changes.

(continued)

In this case, there will be a range of what I have called *functional variants* (i.e., different ways in which facial, behavioral, autonomic, and phenomenal changes can be manifested while preserving the task-oriented nature of the response). What psychological constructionists have in my view not fully appreciated is that the variability characteristic of basic emotions often involves functional equivalents. For instance, it is true that we can respond to dangers by running away from a bear, freezing when seeing a snake, shooting through a closed door toward an intruder, and by calling a doctor when feeling gravely ill, but these are all functional variants of avoidance behaviors.

So, although it is true that basic emotions will involve different behaviors, and with them different patterns of expressions, autonomic changes, and feelings, basic emotions can still be associated with distinct patterns of functional variants that will be continuous across cultures and species. Further support of the new BET will come from studies specifically designed to unveil the functional variants associated with the same basic emotion, namely the sets of facial expressions, sets of autonomic changes, sets of behaviors and sets of phenomenological changes that tend to be associated with the activation of a given basic emotion program in different contexts.

Central empirical challenges for future basic emotion theory will include figuring out which contextual cues determine which specific functional variants are instantiated, what patterns of mutual change functional variants display, how such patterns are related to the notion of emotional intensity for basic emotions, and how basic emotions, nonbasic emotions and core affect are related.

(1982, 1998), Levenson (1988, 1992), and many others. Individual authors differ on several dimensions of analysis, but they share a number of commitments that define BET as a research program.[3] I present the following seven commitments as lying at the heart of *traditional BET*, the version of BET most prominently associated with Ekman and his colleagues:

• TB1: *Basic emotions are evolutionary adaptations, selected for because they are efficient solutions to fundamental life tasks.* As Ekman and Cordaro (2011, p. 364) put it, "Each basic emotion prompts us in a direction that, in the course of our evolution, has done better than other solutions in recurring circumstances that are relevant to our goals." The proposal is that basic emotions were selected over evolutionary time because they are efficient solutions to fundamental life tasks such as dealing with dangers, removing obstacles, suffering losses, being frustrated, and so on (cf. Tooby & Cosmides, 2000; Ekman, 1999).

• TB2: *Basic emotions are associated with programs.* Ekman, following Tomkins, assumed that basic emotions are managed by *affect programs* that control when the emotions are elicited and how they unfold. Other researchers speak of basic emotion *systems* (Panskepp & Watt, 2011) or basic emotion *mechanisms* (Levenson, 2011). Despite these terminological differences, these accounts all agree that basic emotion programs–systems–mechanisms are causally responsible for the coordination of organismic resources toward the goal of efficiently dealing with an evolutionarily relevant emotion-specific life task.

• TB3: *Basic emotions are associated with emotion-specific hardwired neural circuits.* Basic emotion theorists generally assume that basic emotions have a one-to-one correspondence with hardwired neural circuits. Levenson (2011, p. 382) points out that "the central organizing mechanism would have to be initially hard-wired in the nervous system in at least a primitive form." A hardwired circuit is one that is "built in the nervous system" (p. 382), inherited, present at birth, and homologous to the brain circuits present in evolutionarily related species. Ekman and Cordaro (2011, p. 366) mention "the central brain mechanisms that are organizing and directing our emotional responses." Izard (2011, p. 375) argues that "each of the small set of emotions . . . I have called 'basic' . . . have dedicated . . . neural systems." Panskepp (1998) has explored basic emotion networks in mammalian brains in great detail, arguing that they are evolutionarily old, subcortical, and capable of being stimulated chemically and electrically in ways that directly result in emotional responses.

• TB4: *Basic emotion programs are elicited by automatic appraisals, and generate automatic and mandatory responses.* On the input side, it is assumed that basic emotion programs are activated by automatic appraisals.[4] The automatic appraisal mechanism scans the environment for "prototypical situations that have profound implications for the organism's immediate well-being and long-term survival" (Levenson, 2011, p. 381), activating a basic emotion program when such situations are found. Each basic emotion will be activated by a distinctive appraisal, which aims to detect cues reliably associated with the life task the emotion evolved to solve.[5]

On the output side, it is assumed that the activation of a basic emotion program leads to a suite of automatic and mandatory responses. As Ekman and Cordaro (2011, p. 366) put it, as soon as the basic emotion program is activated a

cascade of changes (without our choice or immediate awareness) occurs in split seconds in: the emotional signals in the face and voice; preset actions; learned actions; the autonomic nervous system activity that regulates our body; the regulatory patterns that continuously modify our behavior; the retrieval of relevant memories and expectations; and how we interpret what is happening within us and in the world.[6]

• TB5: *Basic emotions are associated with emotion-specific responses.* The mandatory nature of the responses associated with basic emotion programs means that each basic emotion is associated with a distinctive *pattern of responses* (or components). Basic emotion theorists further assume that each component of the pattern is *emotion-specific.* In other words, it is generally presupposed that each response associated with a basic emotion corresponds *one-to-one* with that emotion.

Tomkins (1995, p. 58) initially argued that affect programs control "facial muscle responses, autonomic blood flow, respiratory, and vocal responses," suggesting that "these correlated sets of [distinctive] responses will define the number and specific types of primary affects." Contemporary basic emotion theorists have expanded the set of emotion-specific responses beyond expressions and autonomic bodily changes to include, among others, instrumental behaviors, subjective experiences, thoughts, memories, and images.

Even though there is a mandatory core to the responses associated with basic emotions, basic emotion theorists acknowledge that such responses can be partially regulated. The prime example of regulation is constituted by culturally specific *display rules* that affect whether the automated signals in the face and body are quickly inhibited or allowed to unfold without interference (Ekman & Friesen, 1969).

• TB6: *Basic emotions are pancultural, present across species, and emerge early in development.* Since basic emotions are evolutionary adaptations, basic emotion theorists expect to find them in different human cultures and in homologous form in related nonhuman species. Additionally, it is expected that basic emotions will emerge early in development, prior to the development of sophisticated cognitive capacities. Some have argued that most basic emotions emerge by the ninth month of life in human infants (Campos, Barrett, Lamb, Goldsmith, & Stenberg, 1983; see also Lewis, 2007).

The bulk of the evidence for evolutionary continuity across cultures and species pertains to facial expressions (Matsumoto, Keltner, Shiota, O'Sullivan, & Frank, 2008). Darwin suggested that emotional expressions were pancultural, but added that they did not evolve for their communicative function. Ekman (1999) proposed instead that the communicative function of emotional expressions is crucial to their evolutionary origin. As he put it, "I believe it was central to the evolution of emotions that they inform conspecifics, without choice or consideration, about what is occurring" (p. 47). This has turned the assumption of emotion-specific facial expressions into a non-negotiable tenet for traditional basic emotion theorists.

• TB7: *Basic emotions are designated by folk psychological emotion categories such as anger, fear, happiness, disgust, and so forth.* Although contemporary basic emotion theorists disagree to some extent on which specific emotions are basic, the lists they propose show significant overlap. On pretty much everyone's list we find *anger* and *fear*. *Happiness, sadness*, and *disgust* are also widely invoked as examples of basic emotions (Ekman & Cordaro, 2011; Levenson, 2011). More idiosyncratic examples include *surprise* (Ekman & Cordaro, 2011; Levenson, 2011) and *interest* (Izard, 2011). Several more instances are judged by various authors to be candidate basic emotions for which we are likely to find empirical evidence in the future (e.g., *contempt, guilt, shame, amusement, pride, embarrassment*, and *relief*).

The Problem of Variability

The seven commitments introduced in the previous section lead to a number of empirical predictions. The viability of traditional BET hinges on whether such predictions are supported by evidence. Here, I focus on emotions that are basic on most theorists' lists, and on the two predictions that have elicited the lion's share of empirical work:

> *Prediction 1*: There should be hardwired neural networks with a one-to-one correspondence to anger, fear, happiness, sadness, disgust, and so forth.
>
> *Prediction 2*: There should be coordinated packages of responses with a one-to-one correspondence to anger, fear, happiness, sadness, disgust, and so forth.

Even though basic emotion theorists are convinced that the evidence supports both predictions, psychological constructionists such as Russell (2003), Barrett (2006a, 2006b) and Lindquist, Wager, Kober, Bliss-Moreau, and Barrett (2012) have made a strong case to the contrary. They have published several meta-analyses of the empirical literature and have concluded that they support the following two theses, which are incompatible with traditional BET:

> *No one-to-one correspondence* (NOC) *thesis*: There is no one-to-one correspondence between anger, fear, happiness, sadness, and so forth, and any neurobiological, physiological, expressive, behavioral, or phenomenological responses.
>
> *Low coordination* (LC) *thesis*: There is low coordination between neurobiological, physiological, expressive, behavioral, or phenomenological responses among instances of anger, fear, happiness, sadness, and so forth.

Basic emotion theorists have responded to NOC and LC in a variety of ways. They have either reasserted their original position despite the contrary evidence (e.g., Ekman & Cordaro, 2011) or added minor qualifications to their original accounts to accommodate the contrary evidence (e.g., Izard, 2007, 2011), or invoked specific empirical studies that are compatible with traditional BET (e.g., Panskepp & Watt, 2011) or published alternative meta-analyses that seem more favorable to traditional BET (e.g., Kreibig, 2010; Stephens, Christie, & Friedmana, 2010; Lench, Flores, & Bench, 2011; but see Lindquist, Siegel, Quigley, & Bararett, 2013). I have argued elsewhere that none of these strategies is likely to succeed (Scarantino, 2009, 2012a, 2012b, 2012c).

The core problem is that Predictions 1 and 2 are *a priori* unreasonable. There is no good reason to expect hardwired neural networks with a one-to-one correspondence to anger, fear, happiness, sadness, disgust, and so forth, or packages of highly coordinated responses with a one-to-one correspondence to anger, fear, happiness, sadness, disgust, and so forth. On the contrary, variability should be expected with respect to the folk categories of anger, fear, happiness, and so on, for at least three reasons: (1) because of how such categories are formed in natural languages, (2) because of the flexibility required for basic emotions to deal successfully with life tasks, and (3) because basic emotions interact with other mental states.

Acknowledging these three sources of variability will lead to what I call the *new BET*, an updated version of BET that acknowledges the constructionist critique while preserving the notion that basic emotions are specialized and evolved programs for dealing with fundamental life tasks. This modification of BET is required in order to account for the empirical data, and I argue that it is in keeping with how scientific theories should be modified to accommodate anomalies.

From Variability to Psychological Constructionism

Compositional Constructionism versus Psychological Constructionism

Psychological constructionists have interpreted the evidence for variability as supporting the following thesis:

> *No programs thesis* (NPT): There are no hardwired programs associated with anger, fear, happiness, sadness, disgust, and so forth, that are causally responsible for coordinating patterns of emotion-specific responses.

Since NPT is incompatible with traditional BET, psychological constructionists have suggested that we should give up on BET all together, and take the constructionist alternative seriously. The orienting thought of psychological constructionism is the assumption that the scientific understanding of psychological phenomena requires breaking them up into their most primitive components. These are what Russell (2003, p. 146) has called "elemental—but still psychological—building blocks."

In an article on the history of psychological constructionism, Gendron and Barrett (2009) have traced its origins back to Spencer (1855), and suggested that prior to the 20th century the approach "was most clearly articulated by William James and Wilhelm Wundt" (p. 319). Here I focus on James, singled out by Mandler (1990, p. 180) as the proponent of "the first constructionist psychology, attempting to understand the processes that generate and construct behavior and conscious experiences." Focusing on James's version of constructionism allows me to distinguish between two notions of "construction" that have often been conflated.

James famously argued that emotions were "constructed" by means of two building blocks: perception and bodily changes. Furthermore, he suggested that the perception of these bodily changes follows *directly* the perception of some exciting fact. This contradicts common sense, according to which "the mental perception of some fact excites the mental affection called the emotion, and that this latter state of mind gives rise to the bodily expression" (James 1890, p. 449).

In James's account, there is no *psychic entity* that mediates between the mental perception of the exciting fact and the bodily expression, in the sense that "*the bodily changes follow directly the* PERCEPTION *of the exciting fact*" (p. 449) and "*our feeling of the same changes as they occur* IS *the emotion*" (p. 449, emphasis and capitalizations in original).

James's approach expresses a methodological position I call *compositional constructionism*:

> A theory is *compositionally constructionist* with respect
> to emotion episodes if and only if such episodes are analyzed
> into building blocks.

James's theory is compositionally constructionist because it takes emotion episodes to be feeling episodes analyzed in terms of perception and bodily changes. Basic emotion theory is also compositionally constructionist, because basic emotions are analyzed in terms of physiological, expressive, behavioral, and phenomenological building blocks coordinated by basic emotion programs.

To qualify properly as *psychologically constructionist*, I submit, a model of emotions must do more than break emotions apart into building blocks: It must also hold that the building blocks are not specific to emotions, and that there are no mechanisms specific to emotions that bring such building blocks together into an emotion episode. When both conditions apply, the occurrence of an emotion episode can be explained in terms of non-emotional processes.

Basic emotion theory is clearly not psychologically constructionist in the sense just described, because an underlying affect program is assumed to coordinate the physiological, expressive, behavioral, and phenomenological building blocks into which emotions are analyzed.

My view is that James's theory is also not psychologically constructionist. Although he did not consider perception and bodily changes to be specific to emotions, he did posit the existence of emotion-specific mechanisms that couple the perception of an exciting fact with the occurrence of the bodily changes whose perception constitutes the emotion. This interpretation is admittedly contentious (see Gendron & Barrett, 2009, for an alternative interpretation), but I think it is backed up by ample textual evidence. Consider the following excerpt:

> The love of man for woman, or of the human mother for her babe, our wrath at snakes and our fear of precipices, may all be described similarly, as instances of the way in which peculiarly conformed pieces of the world's furniture will fatally call forth most particular mental and bodily reactions, in advance of, and often in direct opposition to, the verdict of our deliberate reason concerning them. (James 1890, p.191)

In this passage, James appears to be arguing that emotion mechanisms independent of "our deliberate reason" are automatically activated by "peculiarly conformed pieces of the world's furniture" and mandatorily—"fatally"—cause the bodily reactions whose perception gives rise to the feelings of love or wrath or fear. This interpretation is further bolstered by the fact that James draws an analogy between the way pieces of the world's furniture "call forth" bodily reactions and the way *keys* open *locks*: "Every living creature is . . . a sort of lock, whose wards and springs presuppose special forms of key" (James 1890, p. 192).

For example, the lock associated with delight makes it so that "no woman can see a handsome little naked baby [a key for delight] without delight," and the lock associated with fear makes it so that "in advance of all experience of elephants no child can but be frightened if he suddenly finds one trumpeting and charging upon him [a key for fear]" (James 1890, p. 192). In this picture, which I find much closer to basic emotion theory than to psychological constructionism, there exist causally powerful mechanisms specific to emotions, whose job is to "call forth" the specific bodily reactions whose perception amounts to love, wrath, and fear.

If so, we should not mistake James's opposition to the idea that there is a "psychic entity" mediating between pieces of the world furniture and bodily reactions for an opposition to the idea that there is a specialized "causal entity" mediating between pieces of the world furniture and bodily reactions.[7] It is precisely the existence of this specialized causal entity that psychological constructionists deny, suggesting instead that episodes of love of man for woman, or wrath at snakes or fear of precipices, can be explained without invoking specialized emotion mechanisms. As I argue below, the viability of psychological constructionism hinges on how convincing these alternative explanations turn out to be for making sense of emotion episodes.

Two Varieties of Psychological Constructionism

Several influential psychological constructionists have emphasized the importance of one primitive in particular, namely *core affect*, which is defined as a blend of hedonic and arousal values and hailed as "the most basic building block of emotional life" (Barrett 2006a, p. 48). Core affect is ubiquitous, because one is always in a state characterized by some degree of pleasure ranging from extreme unpleasantness (e.g., agony) to extreme pleasantness (e.g., ecstasy), and by some degree of arousal ranging from extreme deactivation (e.g., sleep) to extreme activation (e.g., frantic excitement).

I want to introduce a critical but often neglected difference between varieties of psychological constructionism that hinges on how an emotion episode is supposed to be constructed out of core affect. The difference concerns the role played by *conceptualization*:

> *Nonconceptualist Psychological Constructionism* (NCPC): Episodes of anger, fear, happiness, sadness, disgust, and so forth, occur independently of conceptualization, but the meta-experiences of anger, fear, happiness, disgust, and so forth, require conceptualization of an underlying state of core affect.

> *Conceptualist Psychological Constructionism* (CPC): Episodes of anger, fear, happiness, sadness, disgust, and so forth, require conceptualization of an underlying state of core affect in order to come about.

NCPC is the position held by Russell (2003, 2012), and CPC is the position held by Barrett (2006a, 2006b, 2012). Whereas Russell thinks that conceptualization affects the perception of oneself as having a certain emotion (the meta-experience of the emotion) but not whether the emotion occurs, Barrett considers conceptualization necessary to generate an emotion episode in the first place.[8] Let us consider the two models in turn.

Russell's Nonconceptualist Psychological Constructionism

Psychological construction is for Russell (2012, p. 82) "an umbrella term for three sets of processes, those that produce: (a) the [emotion] components, (b) associations among these components, and (c) the categorization of the pattern of components as a specific emotion." The components of discrete emotions include the familiar ones invoked by basic emotion theorists (appraisals, expressions, autonomic changes, instrumental actions, subjective experiences) plus some new ones: the perception of affective quality of an antecedent event (i.e., whether the antecedent event is pleasant–unpleasant and arousing–not arousing), the change in core affect resulting from this perception, the attribution of this change to some antecedent event (e.g., the event of encountering a charging elephant), meta-experience (the experience of categorizing oneself as afraid or angry or happy, etc.), and regulation (the deliberate attempt to self-regulate that follows the categorization of oneself as having a certain emotion).

Russell points out that the emotion components associated with fear, anger, happiness, and so on, do not correlate to the extent that basic emotion theorists have predicted, but he acknowledges that they correlate to some extent. In fact, whether a discrete emotion episode is instantiated hinges on the extent to which such components correlate. If they correlate sufficiently to match the mental script (or prototype) for some folk emotion category *E*, an episode of *E* is instantiated (whether or not anyone categorizes the episode as *E*) (Fehr & Russell, 1984).

Russell's model explains the variability within folk emotion categories in terms of the fact that several different combinations of components can match the script associated with each folk emotion category. For example, there will be cases of fear that include facial signals and cases that do not, cases of fear that include autonomic bodily changes and cases that do not, and so on. Furthermore, when a given component is instantiated, variability in the way it is instantiated will be the norm. Among instances of fear associated with physical actions, some will involve running, whereas others will involve hiding, shooting, climbing trees, making phone calls, and an open range of other possible actions.

In the rare cases in which all or most components are instantiated, the instance of a folk emotion category *E* will become *prototypical*. Most members of folk emotion categories will be nonprototypical members, instantiated by virtue of a fairly weak correlation among components. Finally, when the components are neither sufficiently many for clear membership nor sufficiently few for clear nonmembership, instances will become borderline cases of emotion.

The central challenge for NCPC is to explain what underlies the correlations among components of fear, anger, and so on, in both prototypical and nonprototypical cases. Three possibilities must be considered. The first is that there is a unique emotion mechanism or program associated with each folk emotion category *E* that is causally responsible for bringing about the components that instantiate *E*. The second is that multiple emotion mechanisms associated with each folk emotion category *E* are causally responsible for bringing about the components that instantiate *E*. In such case, different instances of *E* will be caused by different emotion mechanisms. The third possibility is that there are no emotion mechanisms at all, and that the components instantiating folk emotion categories are brought together by non-emotional means.

Traditional BET favors the *unique emotion mechanism* assumption, but I have argued that this assumption is at odds with the empirical data. Russell favors the *no emotion mechanisms* assumption, and proposes three causes other than emotion mechanisms why the emotion components correlate: "(a) features in the environment have a correlational structure, which then creates correlations among components, (b) one component can influence another, and (c) two components are correlated when they are both influenced by the same central mechanism such as attention" (Russell, 2012, p. 83).

I have considered these alternative explanations elsewhere and argued that they do not successfully explain why the components correlate to the (limited) extent that they do (Scarantino, 2012a). My proposal is that a better explanation for the existing correlations among components is the presence of *multiple causal emotion mechanisms* associated with the same folk emotion category.

In his reply, Russell (2012b) has pointed out that my proposal is largely speculative, in that I have not provided details on what these multiple causal mechanisms are, and on how they are supposed to work. This is a fair criticism. In the next section, I start providing some of the missing details, illustrating how the new BET can put theoretical flesh around the multiple emotion mechanisms assumption.

The third leg of Russell's constructionism is the idea that the categorization of the pattern of components that instantiates a specific emotion generates a *meta-experience* of emotion. This is the experience associated with categorizing oneself under a certain folk emotion category (e.g., the experience associated with categorizing oneself as "angry" or "afraid"). Russell (2012, p. 105) is clear that "emotional episodes can occur unaccompanied by an Emotional Meta-Experience." This is the case for infants and animals, on the assumption that they do not possess folk emotion concepts. It is also the case for adult human beings who are deeply engrossed in an emotion episode and lack the attentional resources required to categorize themselves under an emotion concept.

Finally, based on Russell's theory, emotion categorizations can be mistaken. For example, an episode of fear may be instantiated by virtue of the fact that enough fear components have co-occurred to match the fear script, but the fearful person may wrongly categorize him- or herself as "angry." Russell (2012, p. 105) gives the example of alexithymics, namely diseased patients whose defining feature is their inability to categorize correctly the emotions they are undergoing.

Barrett's Conceptualist Psychological Constructionism

Russell's proposal differs from Barrett's (2006a, 2206b) CPC, according to which concept use is constitutive of emotion episodes. Whereas Russell endorses a prototype theory of concepts, Barrett endorses Barsalou's (1999) theory of concepts, according to which concepts are *goal-related* (we conceptually represent things in order to do things with them) and *situated* (things are not represented in isolation but in a setting that will make inferences about what do to with them more effective).

A defining feature of Barsalou's theory is that concepts are not amodal collections of features either classically or prototypically organized but rather multimodal integrations of modality-specific memory traces—perceptual symbols—stored in long-term memory and "organized into a simulator that allows the cognitive system to construct specific simulations of an entity or event" (Barsalou 1999, p. 586). The fact that perceptual symbols are organized into a simulator is one of the elements distinguishing Barsalou's theory from a straightforward exemplar theory of concepts, in which memory traces of encounters are not integrated into a unified representation.

Perceptual symbols in a simulator span every experiential modality in which previous encounters with instances of the category have occurred, including sensory experience, motor experience, and emotional experience. For instance, the simulator for CAR will include memories of how cars looks and sound, memories of the actions involved in interacting with cars, and memories of the emotions elicited by cars.

Simulators produce simulations in working memory, namely activations of a subset of the information stored in the simulator in the form of a partial reenactment that may be conscious or unconscious. Every simulation counts as a specific *conceptualization* of a given *concept*, which according to Barsalou's (1999) theory is the integrated collection of multimodal memory instances of a certain category organized into a simulator.

When objects and events are perceived, they are categorized as members of a certain category just in case the simulator associated with such category produces a simulation that "fits" the perceived object or event. The same simulator can produce many distinct simulations depending on context, which accounts for the variability that characterizes the instances of most lexical concepts, whose members share nothing more than family resemblances.

Once a categorization has taken place, the simulator for the categorized object or event is updated with a new memory of an encounter with a category instance. Finally, producing the categorization activates inferences and possibly bodily states that help interact with the category instance in the circumstances at hand. Which inferences and bodily states are activated will depend on the specific simulation triggered and on the situational demands of the context.

Barrett (2006a, 2006b) puts Barsalou's theory of concepts at the core of her own *conceptual act theory* (CAT) of emotions, the most careful and detailed proposal to emerge so far from the CPC camp. CAT's central thesis is that emotions are *situated conceptualizations* (cf. Wilson-Mendenhall, Barrett, Simmons, & Barsalou, 2011). This is to say that "categorizing the ebb and flow of core affect into a discrete experience of emotion corresponds to the colloquial idea of 'having an emotion" (Barrett 2006a, p. 49). What is being claimed here is not that conceptualizing oneself under an emotion concept E produces an emotional meta-experience of E (NCPC), but, more strongly, that it produces emotion E (CPC). To put it in slogan form, no conceptualization, no emotion.

Consider an episode of fear. According to Barrett and her colleagues, "*fear* cannot be understood independently of an agent conceptualizing his [sic]- or herself in a particular situation" (Wilson-Mendenhall et al., 2011, p. 1108). How so? In a nutshell, a fear conceptualization is a simulation produced by the FEAR simulator. As we have seen, this is an integrated, multimodal collection of perceptual, motoric, and affective memories of fear experiences. Barrett's proposal is that producing a fear conceptualization of an underlying state of core affect *is* having fear.

The causal role that basic emotion theorists give to *affect programs* and that Russell gives to a heterogeneous variety of *non-emotional factors* (e.g., the correlation of features in the environment, the causal connections among components, and the presence of non-emotional mechanisms such as attention) is in Barrett's theory given to *situated conceptualizations* of folk emotion concepts:

> Although a person is always in some state of core affect . . . a situated conceptualization has the capacity to shift core affect toward a state typically experienced during emotion episodes for a particular kind of situation. Along with core affect, the situated conceptualization produces related changes in bodily states, such as muscle tension and visceral activity. Additionally, the situated conceptualization may initiate relevant actions that are typically associated with the emotion in this situation, with core affect and bodily states often motivating and energizing these actions. Finally, the situated conceptualization may produce perceptual construals of the current situation, biasing and distorting perception toward typical experiences associated with the respective type of situation. (Wilson-Mendenhall et al., 2011, p. 1109)

This passage makes it clear that the physiological, expressive, behavioral, and phenomenological components commonly associated with fear (muscle tension, visceral activity, avoidance actions, perceptual changes, etc.) are assumed to be "produced" by a *conceptual act*, namely a situated FEAR simulation. The variability of instances of folk emotion categories is explained by the variability of context-dependent simulations associated with the same folk emotion category.

Consider the difference between the fear one may undergo when lost in the woods at night and the fear one may undergo when realizing that one's work presentation is not ready (Wilson-Mendenhall et al., 2011). These two instances of fear will presumably differ in terms of the components associated with them at the level of physiological changes, expressions, behaviors, and phenomenology, as well as at the neural level. Barrett thinks that they do because two different FEAR simulations have produced them.

CAT is remarkably original and thought provoking, but it is also potentially problematic on a number of fronts. Here, I briefly introduce three conceptual challenges for CAT, in the spirit of fostering further discussion:

1. *How do we transition from a world without the FEAR concept to a world with the FEAR concept?* An obvious requirement for producing a fear conceptualization is having a FEAR concept, which according to Barrett's theory is an integrated, multimodal set of memories of fear experiences. The problem is that CAT holds that every fear experience presupposes an act of conceptualization, which is to say that it presupposes having a FEAR concept in the first place. This makes a mystery of how we ever transition from a world without a FEAR concept to a world with a FEAR concept. The formation of the FEAR concept according to Barrett's theory requires that someone experiences fear (no one can have memories of fear without someone having had fear experiences), but experiences of fear simply cannot happen according to CAT in a world where no one has the FEAR concept. So how is the FEAR concept supposed to emerge?

2. *What exactly is being categorized as fear if fear does not exist prior to the categorization?* In standard cases of categorization—say, the categorization of a car under the CAR concept—the concept user compares a perceived instance X with a situated CAR simulation, and categorizes X as a car if the simulation "fits" X. Importantly, whether or not X is a car does not hinge on whether it is categorized as such: cars are not situated CAR conceptualizations.

Barrett's claim is that things are different when it comes to emotions. An instance of fear is supposed to occur *by virtue of* a fear simulation. This creates a puzzle, namely that it is hard to see how there could be a fit between a perceived instance X and a FEAR simulation if X is not fear until it has been categorized as such. Analogously, if something became a car by virtue of being categorized as such, there could not be a fit between a perceived instance X and a CAR simulation, because X would not be a CAR until so categorized.

Another way to put the problem is that if what is causally responsible for the activation of the components associated with fear is a FEAR simulation, as Barrett argues, there are no components to be "fitted" by the FEAR simulation, because such components are not present until a satisfactory fit has been provided. But what could possibly ground such fit then?

Note that a fear categorization is not an evaluation that fear "fits" the circumstances at hand (e.g., the circumstances of being in the forest all alone at night or being unprepared for a work presentation). This sort of evaluation can certainly occur prior to the fear components being in place, and it is what basic emotion theorists call an *appraisal* of danger. Rather, a fear categorization aims to determine whether a FEAR simulation "fits" a perceived event sequence already under way in the circumstances at hand. How is this latter evaluation going to take place if the fear components have yet to be produced?

3. *How can a fear categorization be necessary and sufficient for having fear?* CAT holds that categorizing an underlying state of core affect as fear is *necessary* for having fear. It follows that no humans who lack the FEAR concept, no infants, and no animals can have fear.[9] The problem with this position is that creatures without the relevant concepts appear perfectly capable of manifesting the combinations of components we associate with fear.

Consider a patient with alexithymia who systematically misapplies the FEAR concept, an infant, and a dog. Suppose that they are suddenly thrown into a cage with an elephant that starts trumpeting and charging. My prediction is that, just like James suggested, all three creatures would automatically and mandatorily manifest the prototypical components of fear at the level of physiology, expressions, behavior and phenomenology, with the exception of the *meta-experience* of fear. Since such creatures by assumption lack the ability to correctly apply the FEAR concept, they cannot have the experience associated with categorizing themselves under such a concept.

CAT goes well beyond this claim, and commits us to saying that even though we perceive them as being afraid, these creatures are *not* truly afraid. As Barrett (2012, p. 420) puts it with respect to anger, "if some people do not have a concept of anger, then [a] constellation [of components such as a scowl, blood pressure increase, and a feeling of offense] will never exist as anger for those people (i.e., it is not that they are truly angry and don't know it)." This position is unpersuasive.

First, it is unclear why such creatures would not be truly angry or afraid if they fitted, respectively, the ANGER and the FEAR simulations of creatures endowed with the relevant concepts. When we travel to another country where no one has the ROSE concept and find in a garden something that fits our ROSE simulation, we correctly conclude that we have encountered a rose abroad, even though the locals do not know it. Why would things work any differently for emotion concepts?

Second, it is unclear why CAT assumes that situated categorizations are necessary for bringing about the components of anger or fear, if creatures that lack the ability to engage in such categorizations can still manifest such components. This calls into question the causal role allegedly played by conceptual acts in producing the constellations of components associated with discrete emotions.[10]

CAT also holds that categorizing an underlying state of core affect as fear is *sufficient* for having fear. This proposal is also hard to swallow, because it would seem to prevent the possibility of categorization errors. According to CAT, emotion concepts are such that emoters cannot apply them wrongly to their own emotions. For example, if the alexithymic patient in the elephant example categorized him- or herself under the ANGER concept while manifesting all the components of fear, we would presumably not conclude that he or she is angry rather than afraid, contrary to CAT. Any good account of emotion episodes should allow for the possibility of introspective error concerning which emotions one is having, and it is unclear how CAT can account for that.

Although I have raised some challenges for CAT, I want to emphasize that I do not deny the important role that categorizations play in affecting the unfolding of an emotion episode. Among other things, the ability to self-categorize as being angry or afraid will have an impact on the experience associated with the emotion episode, on whether and how a memory of the episode is formed, and on whether and how the emotion episode is regulated over time.[11]

From Variability to a New BET

As Barrett (2009, p. 1290) puts it, "[d]uring the late nineteenth century . . . and mid-twentieth century . . . many psychological constructionist models of emotion were proposed, all of them inspired by the observation of variability in emotional responding and the failure of basic emotion approaches to account for this variability."

This quotation usefully emphasizes that a primary motivation for constructionist proposals is the conviction that BET does not have the resources to account for variability. We must also note that worries about the variability of the bodily changes associated with emotions were the primary motivators for two of the revolutions in affective science of the 20th century, namely the *behaviorist revolution* and the *cognitivist revolution*. Behaviorists like Skinner (1953) argued that "[i]n spite of extensive research it has not been possible to show that each emotion is distinguished by a particular pattern of responses of glands and smooth muscles" (pp. 160–161), a view Cannon (1929) had influentially attacked. Skinner had the same worry about facial expressions of emotions, as he said that "it has not been possible to specify given sets of expressive responses as characteristic of particular emotion" (1953, p. 161).

The cognitivist model of emotions proposed by Schacter and Singer (1962) was also driven by the view that "the variety of emotion, mood, and feeling states are by no means matched by an equal variety of visceral patterns" (p. 379). The absence of physiological differentiation raised the question of what distinguished from one another emotions associated with undistinguishable physiological changes. This led Schachter and Singer (1962) "to suggest that cognitive factors may be major determinants of emotional states" (p. 379).

These quotes reveal how accounting for variability has historically been a central challenge for models of emotions, and one that basic emotion theory needs to successfully address in order to stay competitive. According to Barrett (2009), basic emotion models assume that "observed variability in emotional responding is the result of epiphenomenal social factors, like display rules or other regulation processes that mask or inhibit prepotent, stereotyped responses" (p. 1288). Additionally, basic emotion theorists often "explain the variability away as error or failure of experimental design" (p. 1288).

Regulation processes and experimental error do have a role to play, but I agree with Barrett that they fall short of explaining the massive amount of variability we find associated with basic emotions. Unlike Barrett, however, I am convinced that BET has the resources to account for variability. In what follows, I distinguish between three sources of variability—concept-dependent, context-dependent, and interaction-dependent variability—and explain how taking them into account can lead to a promising new version of BET.

Concept-Dependent Variability

As we have seen, the standard lists of basic emotions provided by basic emotion theorists comprise folk psychological categories such as *anger, fear, happiness, sadness, disgust*, and so on. This terminological choice reveals the conviction that all the items we call *anger, fear, happiness*, and so forth, in English are basic emotions. The assumption then is that all members of these folk emotion categories evolved to solve fundamental life tasks, are implemented by an emotion-specific neural program, involve a highly coordinated set of emotion-specific responses, and so on.[12]

Since the empirical evidence has been unfavorable to this hypothesis, psychological constructionists have concluded that the folk emotion categories used by basic emotion theorists to designate basic emotions fail to designate *natural kinds*. A natural kind is (roughly) a theoretically homogenous class of items about which a great many explanatory and predictive generalizations can be formulated in a certain scientific discipline (cf. Boyd, 1999; Scarantino, 2012c).

I have emphasized (Scarantino, 2012c) that the assumption that folk emotion categories designate natural kinds is typical not only of BET but also of the great majority of theories of discrete emotions. The problem is that no theory has so far been able to unveil the scientifically interesting explanatory and predictive generalizations that are true of all members of any folk emotion category. For every candidate generalization at the level of bodily changes, neural circuits, origins, current function, and development, we seem to be able to find members of any given folk psychological category *E* to which the generalization applies and members to which it does not apply.

One interpretation of this failure is that emotion theorists have not been sufficiently ingenious so far. The other interpretation, which both psychological constructionists and I favor, is that folk emotion categories are highly heterogeneous, to the point that *no* scientifically interesting generalizations are likely to apply to all of their instances. If this is so, a fundamental rethinking of the categories on which affective science relies is in order.

The methodological approach I recommend differs from the one championed by psychological constructionists. Whereas psychological constructionists have rejected the view that there are specialized emotion mechanisms causally responsible for the coordination of physiological, expressive, behavioral, and phenomenological responses, I think the search for such mechanisms is exactly the way to go, provided that we stop assuming that there is a *unique* specialized emotion mechanism associated with each folk emotion category.[13] Rather, a *multiplicity* of such mechanisms should be expected to correspond with anger, fear, disgust, and so on.

Whereas traditional BET assumes that all items included in the folk categories of *anger, fear, happiness*, and so forth, share an emotion-specific neural program or an emotion-specific package of coordinated responses, the new BET rejects this assumption, proposing instead that only a subset of the members of the folk categories of *anger, fear, happiness*, and so forth, are basic.[14] The transition from traditional BET to the new BET is modeled after similar transitions that have occurred in other scientific domains over time. For example, whereas the initial assumption in memory science was that the folk psychological category of *memory* designates a unique information-retention mechanism, it is now commonly acknowledged "that memory can be divided into multiple forms or systems–collections of processes that operate on different kinds of information and according to different rules" (Schacter, 2004, p. 644). The received view currently is that multiple memory systems exist, are activated by distinct tasks, and differ on a number of important theoretical dimensions (e.g., duration, storage modality, capacity, neural underpinnings).[15]

This has led to the proliferation of a fine-grained non-folk psychological taxonomy, which distinguishes, for instance, between *long-term memory* and *short-term memory* (a.k.a. *working memory*), and between varieties of each (e.g., *declarative long-term memory* and *procedural long-term memory*). Note that the idea that memory is not a theoretically homogeneous category "was hardly acknowledged until a window was opened into the normal operations of the mind through the study of cognitive losses suffered by brain-damaged patients" (Rosenbaum et al., 2005, p. 990). This evidence conclusively showed that brain damage can impair some forms of memory but not others, eventually leading to the now "widely accepted idea of multiple memory systems" (p. 990).

My view is that the time has come for emotion science to undergo a similar transition. The empirical data on neural circuitry, phenomenology, physiology, expressions, and behavior should lead us to take seriously the idea of multiple emotion systems, multiple anger systems, multiple fear systems, multiple disgust systems, and so on (Scarantino, 2012c). Just as the fact that the folk psychological category of "memory" is not a natural kind is compatible with the existence of natural kinds of memory (e.g., procedural long-term memory), the fact that the folk psychological categories of *anger, fear, disgust, happiness* and so forth do not designate natural kinds is compatible with the existence of natural kinds of anger, natural kinds of fear, natural kinds of disgust, natural kinds of happiness, and so forth. Emotion scientists will have to find out how many of these there are, what defines them, and what scientifically interesting explanatory and predictive generalizations are true of them.

The new BET I outline in what follows offers an account of *some* of the natural kinds into which folk emotion categories should split. Contrary to traditional BET, the new BET does not aim to capture what *all* emotions or *all* angers or *all* fears are like, but only what some relevant subsets of such folk categories are like. I propose that we initially designate such subcategories as *basic anger, basic fear, basic disgust, basic happiness*, and so on, in order to emphasize that the predictive and explanatory generalizations formulated by the new BET are not meant to apply to all members of the folk emotion categories (as I will argue below, there are reasons to further refine the basic emotions taxonomy). This once again replicates the model of memory studies, in which scientifically interesting generalizations are taken to apply only to instances of theoretically motivated subcategories such as *short-term memory* or *long-term memory*, rather than to the folk psychological category of *memory* writ large.

I conclude by discussing a different type of variability that has no impact on the natural kind status of folk emotion categories. It is a well-known fact that various cultures differ in terms of the folk emotion categories their languages contain. For example, the superordinate category of *emotion* is absent from several languages. Some languages also use subordinate categories that English lacks and lack subordinate categories we commonly use. Some lexical categories, finally, are hard to translate between cultures, because they capture a combination of components not labeled lexically in another culture (cf. Russell, 1991; Mesquita & Frjida, 1992; Mesquita, 2003).

What are we to make of this *linguistic* variability? Russell (2012a) and others have considered it a reason to conclude that folk emotion categories in English are scientifically unsuitable. While I agree with the conclusion, I disagree with the rationale. What matters for the scientific suitability of an emotion category is whether it designates a theoretically homogeneous category for the explanatory and predictive purposes of affective science (i.e., a natural kind). The fact that other cultures lack a category equivalent to, say, "fear" does not affect whether "fear" designates a natural kind. This is because it does not affect the extension of the category in English, and it is this extension alone that determines whether the explanatory and predictive generalizations that substantiate natural kind status can be formulated about instances of fear.

Russell (2012b, p. 286) has replied that "it would be pure coincidence if English got it right, and all languages that categorize emotions differently got it wrong" when it comes to parsing the affective domain into suitable scientific categories. It would indeed be a pure coincidence, and we should definitely not expect that all folk emotion categories in English are scientifically suitable, whereas all non-English folk emotion categories are scientifically unsuitable. This reply, however, does not address my point that whether a folk emotion category *E*—in English or in any another language—captures a scientifically suitable category is independent of what folk emotion categories exist in other languages. This is because what determines whether a category *E* is scientifically suitable in any given language hinges on what is contained in *E*, and is entirely unaffected by whether categories lexically equivalent to *E* exist in other languages.

What we should expect is rather that every natural language "got it wrong" when it comes to the scientific suitability of its folk emotion categories (give or take a few possible exceptions). Since natural languages do not generate folk psychological categories with the intent of capturing homogeneous domains of scientific investigation, the discovery for such domains, in English as in every other language, generally requires substantial linguistic refinement.

Context-Dependent Variability

A second important reason why variability should be expected is not due to the fact that folk emotion categories have theoretically heterogeneous extensions, but to a central commitment of BET, namely that basic emotions evolved to deal efficiently with fundamental life tasks, such as dealing with danger, fighting, suffering losses, being frustrated, and so forth. What basic emotion theorists have neglected (with a few exceptions) is that, in many cases, what such tasks require is not a rigid cascade of responses but a set of flexible response *tendencies* that are adaptable to the context at hand.

The key difference between traditional BET and the new BET is that the latter, unlike the former, allows basic emotions to have highly flexible manifestations. More precisely, the new BET draws a distinction between two types of activations of a basic emotion program/mechanism: output-rigid activations and output-flexible activations. Whereas output-rigid activations involve *mandatory responses* to stimuli, just as traditional basic emotion theorists have posited, output-flexible activations only involve *irruptive* and *prioritized* response *tendencies* to stimuli (Frjida 1986, 2007).

The first thing to emphasize with respect to output-rigid activations is that different theorists have interpreted the rigidity of the output in different ways. Some output-rigid basic emotions are *unconditioned reflexes*. The unconditioned fear reflex, automatically elicited in a variety of species by, among other things, sudden loss of support and loud sounds, is an example of an output-rigid basic emotion. Some basic emotion theorists have suggested that unconditioned reflexes are the *only* emotions truly deserving of the qualifier "basic." According to Panskepp and Watt (2011, p. 388, emphasis in original), "*basic emotions* can only exist clearly at primary-process levels, namely before learning and higher order thoughts add rich developmental and cultural complexities." Panskepp (2012, p. 32) describes *primary-process levels* as "intrinsic (unconditioned) neuropsychological functions of the brain, responsive initially to only limited sets of environmental events (i.e., unconditional stimuli)."[16]

Other basic emotion theorists have been more inclusive with what they count as basic emotions. Izard (2011), for instance, has proposed that both conditioned and unconditioned reflexes qualify as basic or, as he put it, "first-order emotions." Once higher cognition rather than learning enters the picture, however, a basic emotion is turned into what Izard (2011, p. 372) calls an *emotion schema*: "Emotion schemas always involve interactions among emotion feelings [i.e., basic emotions] and higher order cognition—thoughts, strategies, and goals that complement and guide responding to the emotion experience."

Ekman's view is even more liberal, in that the intervention of both learning and higher order cognition is compatible with the basic status of an emotion. Ekman and Cordaro (2011, p. 367) considers basic emotions to be *open programs* in Mayr's (1974) sense, namely sets of instructions that allow for additional input from experience during the lifetime of the individual. However, according to Ekman's view, basic emotions are also output-rigid. This is because the open programs associated with basic emotions generate what Ekman has characterized as "inescapable" changes in facial signals, in the autonomic nervous system, in preset and learned actions, and in other emotion components.

The responses are inescapable (or mandatory) in the following sense: "Once set into motion through automatic appraising, the instructions in the affect programs run until they have been executed; that is, they cannot be interrupted" (Ekman & Cordaro, 2011, p. 367). Different components will be uninterruptible for different periods. For facial signals, the period lasts less than a second, after which emoters can deliberately affect their facial expressions. On the other hand, "[t]he changes in our respiration, perspiration, and cardiac activity . . . have a longer time line, some stretching out to 10 or 15 seconds" (p. 367) during which they cannot be interrupted.

The assumption that basic emotions are rigid on the output side has led traditional BET to posit the presence of a pattern of highly coordinated components associated one-to-one with each basic emotion. But there is no good reason to form such an expectation, if we consider the fact that basic emotions evolved to deal with fundamental life tasks that take on different forms and require different adaptive responses. According to the new BET, the rigidity of the output is the exception rather than the rule for basic emotions.

Consider the task of avoiding dangers. Dangers differ in terms of how serious they are, in terms of how distant they are, and in terms of the responses required to avoid them. Some dangers are relatively negligible and quite distant (e.g., a big dog barking in the distance while tied to its owner's leash), and they demand nothing more than orienting and getting ready for unspecified actions if the danger increases. Some dangers are significant and imminent (e.g., being run over by a car), and they demand very specific and reflex-like actions (e.g., immediately jumping away from the car's trajectory).

Some dangers are also significant and fairly imminent (e.g., being attacked by an unleashed dog charging from a faraway distance), but they can be dealt with successfully by a nonspecific range of actions that requires some degree of planning and bodily control (e.g., finding a tree and climbing it, getting a long stick and keeping the dog at bay with it, reaching for a gun and shooting the dog with it).

This is to say that, in order to serve its evolutionary function, a basic emotion that evolved to deal with danger needs occasionally to work as an output-rigid program (the suddenly looming object case), but most of the time as an output-flexible program. Output-flexible basic emotions are best understood as *irruptive* and *prioritized* response *tendencies*.

The response tendencies are *irruptive* in the sense that they are automatically activated by the appraisal system, and they are *prioritized* in the sense that they manifest what Frjida (1986) has labeled *control precedence*.

Response tendencies with control precedence endow a specific task/goal (e.g., avoiding a serious and imminent danger) with precedence over other possible tasks/goals of the organism, and exercise control over all organismic resources, until such task/goal is fulfilled (or its pursuit is inhibited). Frjida (1986, p. 78) suggests that action tendencies with control precedence "clamor for attention and for execution": They "tend to persist in the face of interruptions," they "tend to interrupt other ongoing programs and actions" and they "tend to preempt the information-processing facilities."

Crucially, these prioritized action tendencies are flexibly manifested depending on the context, leading to high variability in the actual responses associated with any output-flexible basic emotion. Furthermore, different instances differ in terms of the degree of control precedence of their associated action tendencies, leading to more or less *intense* instances of the same basic emotion, which affect both the responses associated with the emotion and their degree of coordination.

Generally speaking, the higher the control precedence, the higher the intensity, and the more highly correlated the manifestations of a basic emotion will be. What holds the manifestations of an output-flexible basic emotion together is that they all share the same abstract life task (e.g., avoiding a danger, dealing with a loss, reacting to a frustration) and pursue such a task with (some degree of) control precedence.

Finally, the new BET gives up on the assumption that a unique neural circuit must underlie all instances of an emotion evolved to solve a given fundamental life task T. For instance, some evolutionary solutions to task T will rely on circuitry N_1 and others will rely on circuitry N_2. This is to say that not only there are instances of what we call "fear" in ordinary English that do not share neural circuitry with "basic fear" (this is what concept-dependent variability alone leads us to expect), but also that "basic fear," understood as an evolutionary solution to the fundamental life task of avoiding dangers, is likely to be too coarse-grained a category for purposes of neural investigation. Neurobiologists should adopt LeDoux's (2012) most recent "one emotion at a time" methodology, according to which neural circuits are studied one at a time within well-controlled behavioral tasks, without assuming that a single neural circuit will correspond to all instances of emotions with same adaptive function.[17]

I emphasize that we should expect differences at the level of neural circuitry not only between output-rigid and output-flexible solutions to life task T, but also between varieties of output-rigid and varieties of output-flexible solutions to life task T. For example, there is evidence that the neural circuit for *unconditioned basic fear* is different from the neural circuit for *conditioned basic fear*, even though both are instances of output-rigid basic fear.[18] The new BET expects that similarly fine-grained distinctions will apply to the neural circuitry associated with other basic emotions.

Interaction-Dependent Variability

A third important reason why variability should be expected is due to the fact that basic emotions interact with other mental states in ways that affect their manifestations. Roseman (2011) has provided some useful examples of this sort of variability.[19] The primary source of interaction-dependent variability is due to the interaction between *basic emotions* and *regulation* (Gross, 1998). Levenson (1999, 2011) has offered a compelling account of such interaction in terms of what he calls a *two-system design*, according to which the manifestations of basic emotions result from the interaction between a *core system* "designed early in evolution to cope effectively with a few very basic, ubiquitous problems" and a *control system* "more recently evolved . . . [and] . . . designed to influence the actions of the core system" (Levenson, 1999, p. 483). The job of the control system is to rely on learning and higher cognition to affect both what stimuli activate the core system and what responses the core system produces.

It is through regulation that individual and cultural variables affect the manifestation of basic emotions. The learning history of the individual, and his or her cognitive capacities and personality traits, affect both the input and the output sides of the core system. For example, social rules about what is appropriate or inappropriate in the affective domain have a significant effect on how basic emotions are manifested. Display rules about facial expressions have been especially prominent in the debate on basic emotions (Ekman 1972), but a great many other social rules also likely affect how basic emotions are manifested.

Another source of interaction-dependent variability is connected to the "occurrence of multiple emotions in response to the same event" (Roseman, 2011, p. 435). For example, if my basic fear interacts with my basic anger, as it may happen when a menacing adolescent in a parking lot viciously insults me for no good reason, the manifestations of both emotions will be affected. Another source of interaction-dependent variability is connected to what Roseman (p. 436) called "other motivational, cognitive, and situational determinants," which may include "physical activity, eating, and sleep deprivation" and "can alter physiological responses that are also affected in emotion (such as heart rate, cortisol secretion, and serotonin levels)."

This list of potentially interacting mental states is not exhaustive, but it does point to the fact that the new BET should ideally make its predictions about the bodily and neural changes associated with basic emotions sensitive to which other mental states are activated while the basic emotion is under way. This is because the same basic emotion can lead to different manifestations depending on what it is co-occurring with it. This problem is pressing for output-flexible basic emotions, which unlike output-rigid basic emotions may be significantly influenced by co-occurring mental states.

A central area of future research for the new BET concerns the interaction between basic emotions and core affect. Even though I have challenged some of the proposals of psychological constructionists, I am in agreement on the importance of core affect as a building block for our emotional lives. What is important in the context of the new BET is to understand how core affect is influenced by the activation of basic emotion programs, and what role changes in core affect play in either facilitating or impeding the functioning of basic emotions.

The New BET Defended

The new BET replaces the seven original commitments of traditional BET with the following six commitments:

- NB1: *Basic emotions are evolutionary adaptations, selected for because they are efficient solutions to fundamental life tasks.*

- NB2: *Basic emotions are associated with programs.*

- NB3: *Basic emotions are associated with hardwired neural circuits, but such circuits do not correspond one-to-one with any folk psychological emotion category.*

- NB4: *Basic emotion programs are elicited by automatic appraisals and can be either output-rigid or output-flexible. Output-rigid activations are associated with automatic and mandatory responses, whereas output-flexible activations are associated with automatically elicited response tendencies with control precedence that lead to context-dependent responses. Both mandatory and context-dependent responses are oriented toward solving a specific fundamental life task.*

- NB5: *Basic emotions are pancultural, present across species and emerge early in development.*

- NB6: *Basic emotions are not designated by folk psychological emotion categories such as anger, fear, happiness, and so forth, but by theoretically motivated subcategories such as unconditioned basic fear, conditioned basic fear, body-boundary violation basic disgust, core ingestive basic disgust, defensive basic anger, and so forth.*

The core idea at the heart of the new BET is that basic emotions are programs evolutionarily selected to provide generalized solutions to recurrent evolutionary problems by coordinating, in a highly context-dependent yet task-oriented way, clusters of biological markers driven by hardwired neural programs. The new BET differs from the traditional BET in a number of important respects. First, it is no longer assumed that there is a one-to-one correspondence between neural circuits and folk psychological categories such as anger, fear, disgust, and so on. Hardwired neural circuits are only expected to be found at a much finer grain of analysis (e.g., the unconditioned basic fear circuit).

Second, it is no longer assumed that the output of basic emotions must necessarily be a rigid cascade of mandatory responses. This will only be expected for eliciting stimuli that are "focused, powerful, sudden, and closely match prototypical antecedent conditions" (Levenson, 2011, p. 382). In the general case, each basic emotion will be associated with prioritized response tendencies geared toward solving a specific fundamental life task in a context-dependent way. This will lead to a range of what I call *functional variants* (i.e., different ways in which facial, behavioral, autonomic, and phenomenal changes can be manifested while preserving the task-oriented nature of the responses).[20]

Third, the folk psychological taxonomy on which basic emotion theorists traditionally rely is replaced with a theoretically motivated taxonomy that aims to track bodily and neural differences that exist between basic emotions. This non-folk psychological taxonomy aims to collect emotions into subcategories about which scientifically interesting explanatory and predictive generalizations can be formulated (i.e., natural kinds of emotions; Scarantino, 2012c).

The main advantage of the new BET is that it is compatible with the empirical data on variability that psychological constructionists have so aptly used against traditional BET. This is not surprising, because the new BET introduces a number of changes specifically designed to accommodate the empirical challenges faced by traditional BET. This fact can, in principle, be used against it. A critic may object that the new BET differs so significantly from the traditional BET that describing the former as a version of the latter is a bit like describing Darwin's theory of natural selection as the new creationism.[21] Relatedly, a critic may suggest that failure to abandon basic emotion theory after the empirical data have refuted it amounts to turning basic emotion theory into an article of faith rather than a scientific theory.

My reply is that the transition from traditional BET to the new BET is in keeping with how scientific theories should be modified over time to solve the empirical anomalies they inevitably face. The relation between the new BET and traditional BET, I suggest, is the relation between two different versions of the same research program, whereas the relation between Darwinism and creationism is the relation between two distinct research programs (one of which, incidentally, is not scientific). Whereas it is sleight of hand to use the same label for two distinct research programs, it is both legitimate and advisable to use the same label for two different versions of the same research program.

The idea that the units of scientific progress are *research programs* has been influentially defended by philosopher of science Lakatos, who was responding to Popper's (1959) view that science proceeds through a cycle of conjectures and refutations. As Kuhn (1962) convincingly argued in light of the history of science, the idea that scientists abandon scientific theories as soon as they find empirical facts that falsify them is entirely unrealistic. It fails to acknowledge that all scientific theories are born refuted or falsified, in the sense that they face a number of empirical facts that contradict the theory's predictions.

Lakatos's view was that scientific theories are best understood as *research programs* rather than collections of easily falsifiable declarative statements. Lakatos distinguished two main parts of a research program: a nonrevisable *hard core* and a revisable *protective belt*. The hard core of a research program is a set of commitments that are essential to the research program, in the sense that abandoning them amounts to giving up on the research program as a whole. For example, the three laws of motion and the law of gravitation constituted the hard core of the research program of Newtonian physics in the 19th century. These commitments were eventually abandoned in the transition from Newtonian to relativistic physics in the 20th century.

Newtonian physics, however, faced a number of empirical anomalies even in its heyday. Three especially stubborn ones concerned the orbit of the terrestrial moon, the perihelion of Mercury, and the orbit of Uranus, none of which fit the motions predicted by Newton's laws. This is why research programs need a *protective belt*, namely a set of auxiliary hypotheses whose job is to protect the hard core from refutation in the face of anomalies.

As stated by Lakatos (1970, p. 133), "[i]t is this protective belt of auxiliary hypotheses which has to bear the brunt of tests and get adjusted and re-adjusted, or even completely replaced, to defend the thus-hardened core." The auxiliary hypotheses that Newtonian physicists modified over time concerned atmospheric refraction, the propagation of light, the number of planets in the solar system, and other hypotheses changed to "digest anomalies and even turn them into positive evidence" (Lakatos, 1998, p. 24).

Unlike Kuhn (1962), Lakatos (1970) emphasized that sticking with a research program is not always rational. He thought that scientific standards are upheld only when researchers stick with a *progressive* research program, whereas they are violated when they stick with a *degenerative* research program. A progressive research program is one in which earlier versions of the program are replaced by later versions that predict more facts and have their predictions confirmed. A research program whose protective belt is exclusively devoted to protecting the hard core from refutation, without making any new observationally confirmed predictions, would instead be degenerative.

Lakatos exemplified the difference by contrasting Newtonian physics with Marxism. Whereas Newtonian physicists replaced old auxiliary hypotheses with new ones that ultimately increased the predictive power of the theory, Marxism "lagged behind the facts and has been running fast to catch up with them" (Lakatos, 1998, p. 25), ultimately turning into a pseudoscience.

I suggest that the replacement of traditional BET with the new BET involves changes in the protective belt of the research program, while leaving the hard core intact. I take the hard core to be constituted by the following commitments: basic emotions are evolutionary adaptations; they are associated with programs and with hardwired neural circuits (although not circuits corresponding one-to-one to folk emotion categories); and they are pancultural, present across species, and emerge early in development.

The remaining commitments of traditional BET I take to belong to the protective belt. I have proposed the modification of two auxiliary hypotheses in particular: I have argued that evolved emotion programs can also be output-flexible rather than just output-rigid and that basic emotions should not be designated by theoretically heterogeneous folk psychological categories like anger, fear, disgust, and so forth.

Only time will tell if the research program of basic emotion theory continues to be progressive or becomes degenerative. If it becomes degenerative, sticking with it will indeed turn basic emotion theory into a pseudoscience. What I have argued in this chapter is that we are not there yet. Not only has the BET research program been progressive so far, but the empirical evidence that contradicts traditional BET can be accounted for with plausible modifications that lead to a new BET while leaving the hard core of the research program intact.

I want to emphasize in conclusion that the changes I have recommended are not unprecedented within basic emotion theory itself. A good example of the rejection of folk psychological emotion categories by a basic emotion theorist is offered by Panskepp (2012, p. 33), who has "pointedly chosen not to use vernacular terms for primary-process [a.k.a. basic] emotional systems" in order "to avoid part–whole confusions." As an alternative, Panskepp (2012) favors using capitalized versions of ordinary lowercase English emotion terms such as SEEKING, RAGE, and FEAR (see Scarantino, 2012c, for further discussion).

The view that basic emotion programs can have flexible outputs is also present, although far from prominent, within basic emotion theory. As early as 1990, Nesse argued that "far more useful than fixed patterns of response are patterns and regulatory mechanisms that adjust to the needs of the current environment" (Nesse, 1990, p. 280).[22]

In his more recent work, Levenson (2011) has stated that basic emotions may be less "deterministic" in their connection to emotional responses than commonly assumed: "The influence of basic emotions on behaviors and thoughts becomes most deterministic under those conditions in which antecedent conditions closely match prototypical elicitors. . . . When these conditions are *not* met, the plasticity and flexibility of the emotion system becomes more ascendant" (p. 382). This is precisely the idea I have defended in this chapter, in which I have suggested that flexibility should be expected if basic emotions are to fulfill their evolutionary functions, because of the differences that exist in the way the same fundamental tasks are instantiated in different circumstances.

Roseman (2011, p. 435), whose work I acknowledge as an inspiration for this chapter, has also argued that most of the "action tendencies hypothesized to be characteristic of emotions . . . are not fixed action patterns, but complex and flexible action programs", and correctly emphasized that "a contingent relationship between an emotion and a behavioral or physiological response is *very* different from an absence of relationship" (p. 436).

Finally, in their summary of contemporary basic emotion theory, Tracy and Randles (2011, p. 400) have suggested that "as individuals develop higher level cognitive and social capacities that allow for emotion regulation, these causal effects [of basic emotions on responses] become probabilistic, merely increasing the likelihood of emotion-congruent behavior."

What these quotes reveal is that there already is a minority position in basic emotion theory that demands changes along the lines I have recommended. I hope that the general framework I have offered here will turn this minority position into the majority view, leading to a version of BET that is informed and ultimately strengthened by the insights emerging from the critique of psychological constructionists.

Conclusion

Psychological constructionists have done a real service to affective science by bringing to center stage the variability of neural circuitry and physiological, behavioral, expressive, and phenomenological responses associated with anger, fear, disgust, and so on. As they have forcefully argued, this variability is incompatible with basic emotion theory as traditionally understood (traditional BET).

Constructionists have used the evidence for variability to support an entirely new approach to the scientific study of emotional phenomena. A defining tenet of psychological constructionism is the idea that emotion episodes can be explained without invoking specialized emotion mechanisms.

I have distinguished between two varieties of psychological constructionism, a nonconceptualist one (Russell) and a conceptualist one (Barrett), and presented some challenges for both (see also Scarantino, 2012a).

The take-home message of my chapter is that basic emotion theory can only survive the constructionist critiques if it introduces substantive rather than merely cosmetic changes. In particular, the new BET I have introduced gives up on two of the defining tenets of traditional BET: the idea that basic emotions correspond neatly with folk emotion categories, and the idea that their outputs must comprise mandatory and emotion-specific responses.

The payoff of this transformation is that the new BET is compatible with the empirical evidence that there are no signatures in the brain or body with a one-to-one correspondence with anger, fear, disgust, and so forth. Finally, I have argued that this transformation is not a sleight of hand but is instead a scientifically warranted attempt to preserve the hard core of the basic emotion research program by changing its protective belt.

Although I have defended basic emotion theory from the constructionist critique, I do not consider basic emotions as defined by the new BET to be the building blocks of all other emotional phenomena,[23] nor do I consider them theoretically more important than nonbasic emotions. Finally, I am convinced that core affect is an important building block of our emotional life, just as psychological constructionists have argued. So my ecumenical conclusion is that the new BET and psychological constructionism should engage in a cooperative venture for mutual advantage and explore which aspects of our emotional life involve changes in core affect, changes in basic emotions, and coordinated changes in both.

ACKNOWLEDGMENTS

I want to thank Jim Russell and Lisa Barrett for their meticulous commentary on the first draft of this chapter. I hope that trying to respond to their objections and requests for clarification has made the chapter better. The errors, of course, remain all mine. I also want to thank Luc Faucher for his helpful feedback on a previous draft.

NOTES

1. What BET has in common with Darwin (1872) is the idea that emotions are reliably expressed in the face, voice, and posture. Darwin's understanding of the evolutionary origins of emotional expressions, however, differed from the one endorsed by basic emotion theorists. In particular, whereas BET theorists assume that expressions are adaptations for purposes of communication, Darwin thought that expressions emerged as vestigial by-products of adaptive actions (principle of serviceable associated habits) or morphological opposites of vestigial by-products

(principle of antithesis) or direct effects of nervous excitation (principle of direct action of the nervous system).

2. The facial expressions used are "exaggerated" in a literal sense, in the sense that they are often faked by actors who overemphasize the expression.

3. In this chapter, by *basic emotion* I mean "biologically basic emotion." As clarified by Ortony and Turner (1990), there are at least two other notions of basicness: *conceptual basicness* and *psychological basicness*. I have discussed how they differ from the notion of *biological basicness* in Scarantino and Griffiths (2011).

4. Automatic processes are understood as processes that use limited cognitive resources, are quick, effortless, unattended to, and do not require volitional control (Shiffrin & Schneider, 1977). Most basic emotion theorists accept that there are exceptions to the rule that basic emotions are elicited by appraisals. Nonstandard cases of elicitation include direct stimulation of the brain, facial feedback, and drugs (Izard, 1993).

5. The idea that an organism's appraisal of the circumstances plays a key causal and differentiating role is at the heart of so-called "appraisal" theories of emotion. Appraisal theories, however, are committed neither to the automaticity of appraisal nor to the idea that what appraisals elicit are evolutionarily evolved affect programs. See Scherer, Schorr, and Johnstone (2001) for an informative collection of articles on appraisal theories.

6. Many basic emotion theorists also assume that these responses are short-lived, in the sense that they last "not hours or days" but "more in the realm of minutes and seconds" (Ekman, 1999, p. 54).

7. Since James thought that emotions are perceptions of bodily changes and that perception and bodily changes are not specific to emotions, he concluded that there are no "separate and special centres" in the brain that function as the "brain-seat" of emotions. On this view, "the emotional brain-processes not only resemble the ordinary sensorial brain-processes, but in very truth *are* nothing but such processes variously combined" (James, 1884, p. 188). At the same time, I have argued that James accepted that there are internal emotion mechanisms causally responsible for pairing "peculiarly conformed pieces of the world's furniture" with the "bodily reactions" whose perception is the emotion. From this, it follows that if we give up on James's narrow view that emotions are nothing but perceptions of bodily changes, and think of emotions more broadly as the mechanisms (the locks) that lead to bodily changes in the presence of the right stimuli (the keys), then the "brain centres" of emotions become the brain centers associated with such causal mechanisms. James never explored the possibility that the "brain-seat" of emotions may be associated with causal mechanisms rather than feelings, but basic emotions theorists have done so with inconclusive results (for further discussion, see Lindquist et al., 2012; Scarantino, 2012b; Hamann, 2012). I will argue later in the chapter (p. 361) that finding the brain-seat of basic emotions requires replacing our folk psychological affective ontology with a theoretically motivated ontology that relies on more fine-grained subcategories (e.g., unconditioned basic fear).

8. Gross and Barrett (2011, p. 13) have also distinguished between two varieties of psychological constructionism: *elemental psychological constructionism*, which "ontologically reduce[s] emotion[s] to their more basic psychological

ingredients" and *emergent psychological constructionism*, which "view[s] emotions as being more than the sum of their parts." At first blush, Barrett's model of emotions is an emergent model, whereas Russell's is an elemental model. The distinction I have introduced is different, even though it also distinguishes Barrett's model from Russell's model. My distinction hinges not on whether emotions can be reduced to their building blocks, but on whether the instantiation of an emotion requires an act of conceptualization. Conceptualist varieties of psychological constructionism say yes, and nonconceptualist varieties say no. Furthermore, both elemental and emergent varieties of psychological constructionism differ from what I have called *compositional constructionism*. This is because both elemental and emergent psychologically constructionist models deny the existence of specialized emotion mechanisms, whereas compositional constructionism allows for the existence of specialized emotion mechanisms. All that compositional constructionism requires is that emotions be analyzed in terms of their building blocks, which may include specialized emotion mechanisms. As I have defined it, compositional constructionism is compatible with both *latent variable models of emotion* (Coan, 2010), which assume that "the measured indicators of emotion covary by virtue of some common executive, organizing neural circuit or network in the brain" (p. 274) (e.g., basic emotion theory), and with *emergent variable models of emotion*, which assume that "emotions do not cause, but rather are caused by, the measured indicators of emotion, assuming no executive neural circuit or network" (e.g., psychological constructionism; Coan, 2010, p. 274. Note the difference with Gross and Barrett's [2011] notion of emergence.). This is to say that all psychologically constructionist models are compositionally constructionist, but not all compositionally constructionist models are psychologically constructionist.

9. I am here assuming that conceptual capacities require cognitive resources that are unavailable to infants and animals, an assumption that Barrett (2012, p. 423) appears to share.

10. Note that neither problem affects NCPC, according to which the emotions are instantiated if the components match the relevant prototype (whether or not the emoters themselves know it), and causal factors other than categorization are causally responsible for bringing about the components.

11. Gross and Barrett (2011) have argued that the notion of regulation properly applies only to what they have called *emergent* varieties of psychological constructionism, according to which an emotion cannot be reduced to its component parts. Barrett's CAT is an example of an emergent model. See footnote 8 for further discussion of this distinction.

12. This is not to say that basic emotion theorists assume that every folk psychological emotion category designates a basic emotion. For instance, Ekman (1999) considered some folk emotion categories to designate *emotional plots* (e.g., jealousy, love), others to designate *moods* (e.g., irritability), and still others to designate *personality traits* (e.g., hostility).

13. Although psychological constructionists deny that there are specialized emotion mechanisms causally responsible for coordinating physiological, expressive, behavioral, and phenomenological responses, they neither deny that there

exist causal mechanisms other than emotions behind such responses, nor that emotions themselves have causal powers.

14. I complicate this "subset" picture a bit (Scarantino, 2012a), but for the purposes of this chapter, this formulation will do.

15. Even though important neural differences have been unveiled between memory systems (e.g., see chapters on memory in Gazzaniga [2004]), it is generally assumed that no memory system corresponds one-to-one to any brain region.

16. Panskepp (1998, 2012) has proposed that there are at least seven basic or *primary process emotions*: SEEKING, RAGE, FEAR, LUST, CARE, PANIC/GRIEF, and PLAY. *Secondary process emotions* emerge when classical and instrumental learning build on the unconditioned rewards and punishments associated with primary process emotions to enlarge the scope of stimuli that trigger emotions. *Tertiary process emotions*, finally, emerge when higher order cognitive processes such as thinking, ruminating, fantasizing, and so forth, interact with primary and secondary processes.

17. LeDoux (2012) assumes that basic emotion theory is committed to using folk psychological categories such as anger, fear, happiness, and so on, to designate basic emotions. Since such folk categories do not uniquely correspond to specific circuits in the brain and LeDoux wants to provide a brain-based taxonomy of affective phenomena, he rejects basic emotion theory. As an alternative, LeDoux offers an analysis of what he calls *survival circuits*, which are the "circuits involved in defense, maintenance of energy and nutritional supplies, fluid balance, thermoregulation, and reproduction" (p. 655). Although the terminology used by LeDoux differs from mine, what motivates his rejection of basic emotion theory is precisely what motivates my attempt to replace traditional BET with the new BET. Both proposals are responses to the realization that folk psychological categories are massively variable with respect to their neural circuitry, physiological changes, expressions, behaviors, and phenomenology. LeDoux's suggestion is to use neologisms (e.g., survival circuit) to capture affective phenomena that share neural circuitry, whereas my proposal is to follow the lead of memory studies and add qualifiers to folk categories (e.g., basic unconditioned fear) to capture affective phenomena that share neural circuitry, as well as physiological, expressive, behavioral, and phenomenological manifestations.

18. LeDoux (2012) uses a different terminology to draw the same distinction, differentiating between *defense reactions elicited by unconditioned threats* and *defense reactions elicited by conditioned threats*.

19. Roseman (2011) has also mentioned the role of action tendencies and emotional intensity in accounting for variability. I have discussed both topics under the heading of context-dependent variability.

20. Similarly, Roseman (2011, p. 441) has characterized the responses associated with basic emotions as a "functional behavior class".

21. I thank the volume editors for pressing me to consider this objection.

22. I thank Luc Faucher for pointing me to this quotation.

23. To use a distinction introduced in Scarantino and Griffiths (2011), I do

not consider emotions that are *biologically basic* to also be p*sychologically basic* (i.e., to be building blocks of all other emotions and affective phenomena).

REFERENCES

Barrett, L. F. (2006a). Are emotions natural kinds? *Perspectives on Psychological Science, 1*, 28–58.

Barrett, L. F. (2006b). Solving the emotion paradox: Categorization and the experience of emotion. *Personality and Social Psychology Review, 10*, 20–46.

Barrett, L. F. (2009). Variety is the spice of life: A psychological construction approach to understanding variability in emotion. *Cognition and Emotion, 23*, 1284–1306.

Barrett, L. F. (2012). Emotions are real. *Emotion, 12*, 413–429.

Barsalou, L. W. (1999). Perceptual symbol systems. *Behavioral and Brain Sciences. 22*, 577–660.

Blanchard, R. J., & Blanchard, D. C. (2003). What can animal aggression research tell us about human aggression? *Hormones and Behavior, 44*, 171–177.

Boyd, R. (1999). Kinds, complexity and multiple realization. *Philosophical Studies, 95*, 67–98.

Campos, J. J., Barrett, K. C., Lamb, M. E., Goldsmith, H. H., & Stenberg, C. (1983). Socioemotional development. In M. M. Haith & J. J. Campos (Eds.), *Handbook of child psychology: Vol. 2. Infancy and developmental psychobiology* (4th ed., pp. 783–915). New York: Wiley.

Cannon, W. (1929). *Bodily changes in pain, hunger, fear and rage*. New York, Appleton.

Chevalier-Skolnikoff, S. (1973). Facial expression of emotion in nonhuman primates. In P. Ekman (Ed.), *Darwin and facial expression* (pp. 11–89). New York: Academic Press.

Coan, J. A. (2010). Emergent ghosts of the emotion machine. *Emotion Review, 2*(3), 274–285.

Darwin, C. (1872). *The expressions of emotions in man and animals* (1st ed.). New York: Philosophical Library.

Ekman, P. (1972). Universals and cultural differences in facial expressions of emotion. In J. Cole (Ed.), *Nebraska Symposium on Motivation, 19*, 207–283.

Ekman, P. (1980). Biological and cultural contributions to body and facial movement in the expression of emotions. In A. O. Rorty (Ed.), *Explaining emotions* (pp. 73–102). Berkeley: University of California Press.

Ekman, P. (1999). Basic emotions. In T. Dalgleish & M. Power (Eds.), *Handbook of cognition and emotion* (pp. 45–60). Chichester, UK: Wiley.

Ekman, P., & Cordaro, D. (2011). What is meant by calling emotions basic? *Emotion Review, 3*(4), 364–370.

Ekman, P., & Friesen, W. V. (1969). The repertoire of nonverbal behaviour. *Semiotica, 1*(1), 86–88.

Fehr, B., & Russell, J. A. (1984). Concept of emotion viewed from a prototype perspective. *Journal of Experimental Psychology: General, 113*, 464–486.

Frijda, N. H. (1986). *The emotions*. Cambridge, UK: Cambridge University Press.

Frijda, N. H. (2007). *The laws of emotion*. Mahwah, NJ: Erlbaum.

Gazzaniga, M., (Ed.). (2004). *The cognitive neurosciences.* Cambridge, MA: MIT Press.

Gendron, M., & Barrett, L. F. (2009). Reconstructing the past: A century of ideas about emotion in psychology. *Emotion Review, 1,* 316–339.

Gross, J. J. (1998). The emerging field of emotion regulation: An integrative review. *Review of General Psychology, 2,* 271–299.

Gross, J. J., & Barrett, L. F. (2011). Emotion generation and emotion regulation: One or two depends on your point of view. *Emotion Review, 3*(1), 8–16.

Hamann, S. (2012). Mapping discrete and dimensional emotions onto the brain: Controversies and consensus. *Trends in Cognitive Sciences, 16*(9), 458–466.

Harrison, N. A., Gray, M. A., Giarnos, P. J., & Critchley, H. G. (2010). The embodiment of emotional feelings in the brain. *Journal of Neuroscience, 30,* 12878–12884.

Izard, C. E. (1977). *Human emotions.* New York: Plenum.

Izard, C. E. (1992). Basic emotions, relations amongst emotions and emotion–cognition relations. *Psychological Review, 99,* 561–565.

Izard, C. E. (1993). Four systems for emotion activation: cognitive and noncognitive processes. *Psychological Review, 100,* 68–90.

Izard, C. E. (2007). Basic emotions, natural kinds, emotion schemas, and a new paradigm. *Perspectives on Psychological Science, 2*(3), 260–275.

Izard, C. E. (2011). Cognition interactions—forms and functions of emotions: Matters of emotion. *Emotion Review, 3*(4), 371–378.

James, W. (1884). What is an emotion? *Mind, 9,* 188–205.

James, W. (1890). *The principles of psychology.* New York: Holt.

Kreibig, S. D. (2010). Autonomic nervous system activity in emotion: A review. *Biological Psychology, 84*(3), 394–421.

Kuhn, T. (1962). *The structure of scientific revolutions.* Chicago: University of Chicago Press.

Lakatos, I. (1970). Falsification and the methodology of scientific research programmes. In I. Lakatos & A. Musgrave (Eds.), *Criticism and the growth of knowledge* (pp. 91–195). Cambridge, UK: Cambridge University Press.

Lakatos, I. (1998). Science and pseudoscience. In M. Curd & J. A. Cover (Eds.), *Philosophy of science: The central issues* (pp. 20–26). New York: Norton.

LeDoux, J. (2012). Rethinking the emotional brain. *Neuron, 73,* 653–676.

Lench, H. C., Flores, S. A., & Bench, S. W. (2011). Discrete emotions predict changes in cognition, judgment, experience, behavior, and physiology: A meta-analysis of experimental emotion elicitations. *Psychological Bulletin, 137,* 834–855.

Levenson, R. W. (1988). Emotion and the autonomic nervous system: A prospectus for research on autonomic specificity. In H. L. Wagner (Ed.), *Social psychophysiology and emotion: Theory and clinical applications* (pp. 17–42). Chichester, UK: Wiley.

Levenson, R. W. (1992). Autonomic nervous system differences among emotions. *Psychological Science, 3,* 23–27.

Levenson, R. W. (1999). The intrapersonal functions of emotion. *Cognition and Emotion, 13,* 481–504.

Levenson, R. W. (2011). Basic emotion questions. *Emotion Review, 3*(4), 379–386.

Lewis, M. (2007). Self-conscious emotional development. In J. Tracy, R. Robins,

& J. P. Tangney (Eds.), *The self-conscious emotions: Theory and research* (pp. 134–152). New York: Guilford Press

Lindquist, K. A., Siegel, E. H., Quigley, K., & Barrett, L. F. (2013). The hundred years emotion war: Are emotions natural kinds or psychological constructions? Comment on Lench, Flores, and Bench (2011). *Psychological Bulletin, 139,* 255–263.

Lindquist, K. A., Wager, T. D., Kober, H., Bliss-Moreau, E., & Barrett, L. F. (2012). The brain basis of emotion: A meta-analytic review. *Behavioral and Brain Sciences, 35,* 161–162.

Mandler, G. (1990). William James and the construction of emotion. *Psychological Science, 1,* 179–180.

Matsumoto, D., Keltner, D., Shiota, M. N., O'Sullivan, M., & Frank, M. (2008). What's in a face?: Facial expressions as signals of discrete emotions. In M. Lewis, J. M. Haviland, & L. F. Barrett (Eds.), *Handbook of emotions* (3rd ed., pp. 211–234). New York: Guilford Press.

Matsumoto, D., & Willingham, B. (2006). The thrill of victory and the agony of defeat: Spontaneous expressions of medal winners at the 2004 Athens Olympic Games. *Journal of Personality and Social Psychology, 91*(3), 568–581.

Matsumoto, D., & Willingham, B. (2009). Spontaneous facial expressions of emotion of congenitally and non-congenitally blind individuals. *Journal of Personality and Social Psychology,, 96*(1), 1–10.

Mayr, E. (1974). Behavior programs and evolutionary strategies. *American Scientist, 62,* 650–659.

Mesquita, B. (2003). Emotions as dynamic cultural phenomena. In R. J. Davidson, K. Scherer, & H. H. Goldsmith (Eds.), *Handbook of affective sciences* (pp. 871–890). New York: Oxford University Press.

Mesquita, B., & Frijda, N. H. (1992). Cultural variations in emotions: A review. *Psychological Bulletin, 112,* 197–204.

Moyer, K. E. (1976). *The psychobiology of aggression.* New York: Harper & Row.

Nesse, R. (1990). Evolutionary explanations of emotions. *Human Nature, 1*(3), 261–289.

Ortony, A., & Turner, T. J. (1990). What's basic about basic emotions? *Psychological Review, 97,* 315–331.

Panksepp, J. (1982). Toward a general psychobiological theory of emotions. *Behavioral and Brain Sciences, 5,* 407–467.

Panksepp, J. (1998). *Affective neuroscience: The foundations of human and animal emotions.* New York: Oxford University Press.

Panskepp, J. (2012). In defence of multiple core affects. In P. Zachar & R. Ellis (Eds.), *Categorical versus dimensional models of affect: A seminar on the theories of Panskepp and Russell* (pp. 31–78). Amsterdam: Benjamins.

Panskepp, J., & Watt, D. (2011). What is basic about basic emotions?: Lasting lessons from affective neuroscience. *Emotion Review, 3*(4), 387–396.

Popper, K. (1959), *The logic of scientific discovery.* London: Hutchinson.

Roseman, I. J. (2011). Emotional behaviors, emotivational goals, emotion strategies: Multiple levels of organization integrate variable and consistent responses. *Emotion Review, 3,* 434–443.

Rosenbaum, R. S., Köhler, S., Schacter, D. L., Moscovitch, M., Westmacott, R.,

Black, S. E., et al. (2005). The case of K. C.: Contributions of a memory-impaired person to memory theory. *Neuropsychologia, 43*, 989–1021.

Russell, J. A. (1991). Culture and the categorization of emotions. *Psychological Bulletin, 110*, 426–450.

Russell, J. A. (1994). Is there universal recognition of emotion from facial expression?: A review of the cross-cultural studies. *Psychological Bulletin, 115*, 102–141.

Russell, J. A. (2003). Core affect and the psychological construction of emotion. *Psychological Review, 110*, 145–172.

Russell, J. A. (2012a). From a psychological constructionist perspective. In P. Zachar & R. Ellis (Eds.), *Categorical versus dimensional models of affect: A seminar on the theories of Panskepp and Russell* (pp. 79–118). Amsterdam: Benjamins.

Russell, J. A. (2012b). Final remarks. In P. Zachar & R. Ellis (Eds.), *Categorical versus dimensional models of affect: A seminar on the theories of Panskepp and Russell* (pp. 279–300). Amsterdam: Benjamins

Scarantino, A. (2009). Core affect and natural affective kinds. *Philosophy of Science, 76*, 940–957.

Scarantino, A. (2012a). Discrete emotions: From folk psychology to causal mechanisms. In P. Zachar & R. Ellis (Eds.), *Categorical versus dimensional models of affect: A seminar on the theories of Panskepp and Russell* (pp. 135–154). Amsterdam: Benjamins.

Scarantino, A. (2012b). Functional specialization does not require a one-to-one mapping between brain regions and emotions. *Behavioral and Brain Sciences, 35*, 161–162.

Scarantino, A. (2012c). How to define emotions scientifically. *Emotion Review, 4*(4), 358–368.

Scarantino, A., & Griffiths, P. (2011). Don't give up on basic emotions. *Emotion Review, 3*(4), 444–454.

Schachter, S., & Singer, J. E. (1962). Cognitive, social and physiological determinants of emotional state. *Psychological Review, 69*, 379–399.

Schacter, D. L. (2004). Introduction. In M. S. Gazzaniga (Ed.), *The cognitive neurosciences* (Vol. 3, pp. 643–645). Cambridge, MA: MIT Press.

Scherer, K. R., Schorr, A., & Johnstone, T. (2001). *Appraisal processes in emotion: Theory, methods, research.* New York: Oxford University Press.

Shiffrin, R. M., & Schneider, W. (1977). Controlled and automatic information processing: II. Perceptual learning, automatic attending, and a general theory. *Psychological Review, 84*, 127–190.

Skinner, B. F. (1953). *Science and human behavior.* New York, Macmillan.

Spencer, H. (1855). *Principles of psychology.* London: Longman, Brown, Green & Longmans.

Stephens, C. L., Christie, I. C., & Friedmana, B. H. (2010). Autonomic specificity of basic emotions: Evidence from pattern classification and cluster analysis. *Biological Psychiatry, 84*, 463–473.

Tomkins, S. S. (1995). *Exploring affect: The selected writings of Silvan S. Tomkins* (E. V. Demos, Ed.). Cambridge, UK: Cambridge University Press.

Tooby, J., & Cosmides, L. (2000). Evolutionary psychology and the emotions. In

M. Lewis & J. M. Haviland-Jones (Eds.), *Handbook of emotions* (2nd ed., pp. 91–116). New York: Guilford Press.

Tracy, J. L., & Randles, D. (2011). Four models of basic emotions: A review of Ekman and Cordaro, Izard, Levenson, and Panksepp and Watt. *Emotion Review, 3*(4), 397–405.

Waller, B. M., Vick, S.-J., Parr, L., Bard, K. A., Pasqualini, M. S., Gothard, K. M., et al. (2006). Intramuscular electrical stimulation of facial muscles in humans and chimpanzees: Duchenne revisited and extended. *Emotion, 6*(3), 367–382.

Wilson-Mendenhall, C. D., Barrett, L. F., Simmons, W. K., & Barsalou, L. (2011). Grounding emotion in situated conceptualization. *Neuropsychologia, 49,* 1105–1127.

CHAPTER 15

A Sociodynamic Perspective on the Construction of Emotion

MICHAEL BOIGER
BATJA MESQUITA

Emotions are powerful connections between our inner psyches and the outer world: Think of the last time you could not help brooding over a hurtful remark, spent hours discussing your worries and joys with a friend, or tried to appease someone by expressing your regret. Most psychological theories of emotion account for this social dimension by proposing that emotions can be elicited by social events. For example, according to psychological constructionist accounts of emotion, social events give rise to the psychological dynamics of meaning making that characterize emotion (e.g., Barrett, 2009a, 2009b; Gendron & Barrett, 2009; Gross & Barrett, 2011). In this chapter, we turn the process of emotion construction inside-out: Without denying the importance of individual processes in emotion construction, we explore a perspective of emotion construction that focuses on the role of social processes. Starting from the idea that emotion construction is a dynamically unfolding process, afforded and constrained by a complex social environment that is itself in motion, we discuss how the social dynamics of daily life shape, constrain, and define individuals' emotions across social contexts in a number of ways.

We discuss the sociodynamic construction of emotion for three social contexts that differ in scale and scope: moment-to moment interactions, developing and ongoing relationships, and sociocultural contexts (see also Boiger & Mesquita, 2012); for each context, we show how social realities afford the emotions that people experience—for example, by constraining the range of likely emotional reactions or highlighting certain emotional

1. *If emotions are psychological events constructed from more basic ingredients, then what are the key ingredients from which emotions are constructed? Are they specific to emotion or are they general ingredients of the mind? Which, if any, are specific to humans?*

We conceive of emotions as dynamic processes that unfold over time and are situated in interactions, relationships, and ultimately cultures. Rather than locating emotions exclusively "in the head" of individuals, we conceive of emotions as emerging dynamically from an individual's engagement in specific social contexts. What we call "emotion" is a collection of different constituents (e.g., cognitive, behavioral, physiological responses) that interact over time—both between people and their social contexts (our primary focus) and within people (not our primary focus, but consistent with our perspective). Only some of these constituents are specific to emotions; some, but not all of them are uniquely human.

2. *What brings these ingredients together in the construction of an emotion? Which combinations are emotions and which are not (and how do we know)?*

Emotions are constructed "in the moment" during ongoing interactions, they are afforded and constrained by the relationships in which they take place, and they depend on the pervasive cultural meanings and practices. Thus, in order to model emotions properly, they need to be contextualized within the interactions, relationships, and cultural contexts in which they emerge. Our perspective is agnostic with respect to the elements that make an interaction *uniquely* emotional. However, we would think that some urgency for acting on the part of one or both of the partners (with corresponding affect or appraisals of relevance) is a likely candidate.

3. *How important is variability (across instances within an emotion category, and in the categories that exist across cultures)? Is this variance epiphenomenal or a thing to be explained? To the extent that it makes sense, it would be desirable to address issues such as universality and evolution.*

Variability is key to our emotion model. We assume that emotions have primarily evolved to monitor and regulate the social world. Clearly, human beings needed the plasticity of emotions to adapt to their cultural and relational environment. Indeed, our review of the literature suggests that emotions are constructed in ways that are attuned to their cultural and relational environments. This construction is dependent on not only the prevalent concepts, meanings, or values but also the reinforcement contingencies that are in place. Thus, responses that are conducive to relational goal attainment are more likely to be "recruited" than responses that are not.

(continued)

---

4. *What constitutes strong evidence to support a psychological construction to emotion? Point to or summarize empirical evidence that supports your model or outline what a key experiment would look like. What would falsify your model?*

Some of the studies that have proven most difficult to publish provide in fact the best evidence for a constructivist view of emotions. These were qualitative interview studies with people from very different cultures (United States, Netherlands, Belgium, Japan, Surinamese immigrants in the Netherlands, Turkish immigrants in the Netherlands, and Mexican immigrants in the United States). Respondents reported certain types of emotional situations; examples of such situations were "being offended," "getting praise or admiration," and "being humiliated." For each type of relational plot, the typical course of emotional experience varied substantially across different cultures: The way respondents made sense of the situations, the most likely ways of acting, the ways in which others responded and the interactions that ensued, the development of relevant relationships, and the ways in which the emotions were shared with others all differed across cultures and relationships in systematic ways. The "mix" of emotions that people used to describe their experiences differed accordingly, and so did the duration and the lasting consequences of the emotional episode. While this research cannot rule out the existence of a priori emotions that are similar across cultures, it certainly suggests that the most important emotional episodes are constructed in very different ways across cultures. Our model would be falsified by the finding that an individual's emotional experience or expression is not dependent on the social context (i.e., interactions with others, relationships, cultural context). The evidence reviewed in this chapter strongly suggests that social context importantly shapes emotions.

---

meanings. We conclude the chapter by discussing how the psychological and sociodynamic construction of emotion are two sides of the same coin: One does not occur without the other and the full picture emerges only when both are taken into account. In doing so, we also show what can be gained from supplementing psychological construction with a sociodynamic perspective.

The Sociodynamic Construction of Emotion in Interactions, Relationships, and Cultures

At the smallest timescale, emotions in social settings emerge during *moment-to-moment interactions*: Which feelings surface and which behaviors are enacted depends on the ongoing interaction. Take, for instance, the emotions of Laura and Ann, two American women who are in a relationship. Ann calls home to say she will be home late tonight because there is an official function at work. Laura would have liked to spend some time with Ann, and after spending several days looking after her when Ann was home sick, Laura feels some entitlement. She responds to Ann's phone call by saying that it is irresponsible to work overtime after having been sick, and that Ann should take it easy. Ann feels trapped: She is behind on work and convinced it would look bad to skip an official function just after having taken sick leave. To top it off, she feels ill-understood by Laura. Ann is so frustrated that she snaps at Laura for paternalizing and hangs up quickly. Laura in turn feels taken for granted, and underappreciated.

The example illustrates the dynamic nature of most of our emotions in daily life: Emotions are processes that expand over time and are shaped by ongoing interactions. Our view that emotions derive their shape and meaning from interactions with others differs from existing psychological models of emotion. Both traditional cognitive (e.g., Lazarus, 1991; Smith & Ellsworth, 1985) and newer psychological constructivist approaches (e.g., Barrett, 2009a, 2009b; Gendron & Barrett, 2009; Gross & Barrett, 2011) propose that emotions are the results of individual meaning making, but they largely remain agnostic about the sources of meaning making (but see, e.g., Wilson-Mendenhall, Barrett, Simmons, & Barsalou, 2011). We propose that much of the meaning making occurs "in the moment," and is social and iterative in nature. Over the course of an interaction, one person's emotions are not only reactions to a previous event, but they also serve as strategic bids and stimuli for the further development of the interaction (Solomon, 2003). Individual meaning making is never a one-time process and does not occur in a social vacuum; rather, it is a social process through which people continuously integrate environmental information and, in doing so, update their emotional interpretations. The development of Laura's anger depends not only on her initial interpretation of Ann's action (the phone call) but also on her perception of Ann's ensuing emotional reactions—for example, on whether Ann responds to Laura's disappointment with anger, surprise, or indifference. Laura may experience her anger differently if Ann reacts aggressively than if she reacts with astonishment or breaks down in tears—the former may turn the developing conflict into a threat for Laura, while a more cooperative stance on Ann's part may render the conflict into a challenge (cf. Blascovich & Mendes, 2000). Figure 15.1 represents this dynamic interactive process of momentary emotion constructions between Ann and Laura from time 1 to time 2.

Emotion construction at any one point in time is constrained by the *ongoing or developing relationship* in which it takes place. The same interaction will give rise to different emotions depending on whether the relationship is, for example, strained or satisfying. Both the current relationship quality and future expectations for the relationship affect what emotions ensue. Anger in the context of a deteriorating relationship may be elicited more readily, feel different (e.g., come with hurt feelings, Leary & Leder,

2009), and have more far-reaching repercussions than anger in the context of a flourishing relationship. In the hypothetical scenario described earlier, Ann may have more readily responded with anger if her relationship with Laura was already strained. This readiness to experience anger in a strained relationship may occur because emotional interactions between partners have become rigid (e.g., anger always being reciprocated with anger in a strained relationship), or because existing relationship expectations (e.g., "Laura always does as she pleases; she never respects my feelings") may constrict the range of possible interpretations of the other person's action. In comparison, in a flourishing relationship, both partners may respond with warmth and understanding during a conflict of interests. Given different relationship frames, the interaction between Ann and Laura may have been one of escalated anger, hurt, and even fear of abandonment or, alternatively, one in which disappointment was met by reassurance, loving understanding, and gratitude. Figure 15.1 displays the relationship as a dotted frame that affords and constrains emotional interactions at any particular point in time. In turn, the combined ongoing emotions between Laura and Ann also define the quality of their relationship over time.

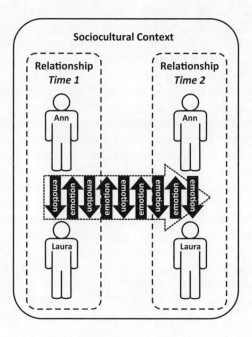

FIGURE 15.1. Emotion as a dynamic ongoing process that is constructed in the context of interactions, relationships, and culture. Adapted from Boiger and Mesquita (2012). Copyright 2012 by the International Society for Research on Emotion and SAGE. Adapted by permission.

Finally, the construction of emotion depends on the larger *sociocultural context*. Sociocultural contexts differ with respect to their normative and habitual interactions and relationships; emotions that are likely to be constructed differ accordingly. By highlighting certain constructions of the world as desirable, normative, or real, a person's cultural background can be said to limit the range of likely emotion interpretations. For example, anger-like emotions are more common in cultures that emphasize individual autonomy than in cultures that emphasize harmony and interdependence (e.g., Markus & Kitayama, 1991). Cultural differences in the construction of emotions may originate in the shared cultural concerns and ideas (e.g., the concern for autonomy), as well as in the common practices or reinforcement structures found in a given sociocultural environment (e.g., highlighting a first-person perspective when reminiscing about emotional events; Wang, 2001; see also Boiger, Mesquita, Uchida, & Barrett, 2013). For instance, in cultures valuing autonomy and self-promotion, the expression of anger may be welcome, because this emotion allows individuals to express their desires and to make necessary adjustments to their relationships (Averill, 1982). In comparison, in cultural contexts that value relational interdependence and self-effacement, the expression of anger may be discouraged and perceived as immature and childish (Azuma, 1984; White & LeVine, 1986). Accordingly, people will tend to ignore expressions of anger (Briggs, 1970), and anger will be less likely to escalate. In our example of Ann and Laura, American cultural values emphasizing the importance of autonomy may increase the likelihood of experiencing anger compared, for example, to Japanese cultural values emphasizing the maintenance of harmony and adjustment to others. Figure 15.1 depicts the cultural context as the pervasive background against which the social dynamics of emotion construction unfold.

In summary, we take the construction of emotion to be an iterative and ongoing process that emerges from interactions within relationships, which derive their shape and meaning from the prevailing ideas and practices of the larger sociocultural context. At different times, and in different contexts, the resulting emotions will be different. The nature of anger, for instance, will depend on the relationships one has with the target of anger; on the target being responsive or defensive, embarrassed, or full of contempt; and on whether the culture is self-promoting or self-effacing. While emotions are constrained by previous experience, sociocultural understandings, and practices, the construction of emotion is thought to be a continuous process that takes place during each emotional episode again and anew.

Caveats

Before we start discussing the empirical evidence for the sociodynamic construction of emotion, a few words of caution are in order. First, common (English-language) discourse on emotion—in everyday life and in emotion theory alike—favors a perspective of bounded, individual construction. For example, one "has" an emotion, one "feels" anger, or something "makes" a person happy. Emotions are "elicited," "experienced," and "expressed." All of these terms foreground individual experience and describe emotions as unitary, bounded events. It is much less common to speak of emotions as unfolding in interactions with others or of emotional meanings being negotiated or situated in the world. It is hard to conceptualize the sociodynamic construction of emotion properly, because these ideas are a departure from common discourse; however, the literatures on situated cognition, systems theory, and social constructionism have provided valuable guidance.

Second, we propose that emotions are *afforded* by social contexts; our use of the term *affordance* needs some explanation. Much like the original proposition by Gibson (1979), we see affordances as *opportunities for action*. Just as a street affords walking on (and not drinking from) and a cup affords drinking from (and not walking on), we argue that certain social contexts afford some emotions (and not others). For example, whereas a slap on the head during a heated debate between drunk friends may afford anger, a slap on the head by a stranger on a crowded New York street may afford fear; the same slap may afford shame in a woman smoking in a public Korean context, where norm-inconsistent behavior may be pointed out this way (Specht, 2010). This does *not* mean that social contexts mechanically elicit emotions; rather, social contexts constitute constraints to the range of likely (and functional) emotional responses. Which emotion surfaces is neither determined solely by the context nor by an individual's psychological tendencies, but by the organismic interplay of the two. In this view, contextual affordances and psychological processes are intertwined and co-constructed (see also Kitayama, Markus, Matsumoto, & Norasakkunkit, 1997).

Third, while a sociodynamic approach to emotion construction suggests that the optimal level of analysis would be interpersonal interactions over time (see, e.g., Butler, 2011), very few studies have taken these interactions as their focus. The result is that the extant literature only provides partial evidence for the processes of interest. Some studies show, for example, that others are important sources of information when making sense of emotional situations; however, they focus on short, one-time transactions. Those studies that investigated emotional dynamics between people over longer timeframes often fell short of a more detailed account of the emotions involved. We point to these inconsistencies where possible and show how, taken together, the evidence of several studies across multiple social contexts is nonetheless consistent with the view of emotions as sociodynamic constructions.

Emotions Derive Their Shape from Moment-to-Moment Interactions

At the smallest timescale of moment-to-moment interactions, others' (emotional) behavior may shape our emotions. Emotional affordances during interactions refer to the range of likely emotions during a *particular interaction*; emotional affordances may take a direct route (e.g., through emotion contagion between interaction partners) or a more indirect route (e.g., through the activation of conceptual meanings). The available research, which has mainly focused on short interactions (usually a single transaction) between people, indicates that emotions may develop quite differently depending on the input of others. Given that the sociodynamic construction of emotion is evident even within a single transaction, we expect that over longer interactions the course of emotions will be considerably shaped by others' (emotional) behavior.

In one study, undergraduates who were selected to be either high or low on social anxiety participated in a "getting to know you" task (Heerey & Kring, 2007). Participants were assigned to either nonanxious dyads, in which both interaction partners were low on social anxiety, or mixed dyads, in which one interaction partner was low and the other was high on social anxiety. During the interaction, anxious participants displayed more socially disengaging behaviors such as talking about themselves or reciprocating genuine smiles with polite smiles. Not surprisingly, nonanxious participants interacting with anxious partners were the only participants who did not report an increase in positive affect as a result of the interaction. Instead, the social anxiety of their interaction partners appears to have shaped their own emotional behaviors: The nonanxious participants in mixed dyads displayed, among other behaviors, an increase in fidgeting. Fidgeting, a behavioral sign of anxiety, tended to be initiated by the socially anxious partner and transmitted to the nonanxious partner. While it is unclear from this study whether the interaction with anxious participants afforded particular meanings ("There has to be something anxiety-provoking about this interaction if the other person is acting that nervously"), or whether it shaped the nonanxious participants' behavior via a more direct route (e.g., by emotion contagion; Hatfield, Cacioppo, & Rapson, 1994), this study illustrates how, over the course of an interaction, the emotions of one partner are shaped by the emotions of another person. Moreover, the anxiety that one person experiences concurrently with another person's anxiety may escalate (e.g., via positive feedback loops, Butler, 2011) and may have different psychological and social ramifications than anxiety with a different etiology—ramifications that remain undetected if emotions are studied solely at the level of isolated individual events.

That others' emotions do afford particular meanings and indeed guide people when making sense of a situation has been convincingly demonstrated in a study by Parkinson and Simons (2009). In this study, participants reported their emotions when making important decisions during a 2-week period. Each time participants were about to make an important decision, they indicated their level of anxiety, excitement, and their appraisal of the situation. They also indicated the level of anxiety and excitement that they perceived in others while making the decision. Whenever possible, the other person who was present also indicated to what extent he or she felt anxious and excited. The results showed that participants felt more anxious or excited when the other person also felt anxious or excited. Moreover, the other person's emotion served as information for the participant's appraisal of the situation: Participants referenced other people's emotions when evaluating the situation, and consequently experienced similar emotions; this was even the case when participants themselves were not consciously aware of the other person's feelings. Even though the original emotion-eliciting event (namely, the need to make a decision) remained the same, the participants' emotional reactions (and appraisals) were based on how others responded emotionally. Over the course of a longer interaction, the emotions of interacting partners may then mutually influence and constrain each other: For example, when one partner's anxiety is repeatedly met by another person's anxiety, the resulting emotions in both partners will differ from those in a scenario in which one person's anxiety does not get reciprocated. In the former case, both partners will increasingly reinforce appraisals of risk and helplessness, thereby justifying intense feelings of anxiety; in the latter case, anxiety may persist but not cycle out of control.

Over and above the actions and emotions of any one partner, objective features of the interaction may also function as sources for meaning making. For example, synchronic interactions with others are more likely to elicit feelings of compassion. In a recent study (Valdesolo & DeSteno, 2011), participants were instructed to tap out beats they heard through headphones. They were accompanied by a confederate who tapped along either synchronously or asynchronously. The confederates were then sent to fulfill an unpleasant task, and the participants were asked whether they wanted to help the confederates or not. Participants who had previously participated in the synchronous tapping interactions were more likely to feel compassion toward the confederate and offered their assistance for longer periods of time. This effect of synchrony on compassion was not due to the participants' increased liking of the confederates, but to the participants' appraisal of the confederates as being more similar to them. Engaging in something as simple as a synchronous tapping task must have shaped participants' appraisal of the event toward adopting a more compassionate stance.

There is also some anecdotal evidence that acting out emotions on the stage is more authentic when actors let themselves be guided by the ongoing interaction. In one school of acting, actors practice responding to each other during rapid cycles of spontaneous interactions (Meisner & Longwell, 1987). During these exercises, they are instructed to observe any (emotional) changes in their interaction partners and to respond to them spontaneously. With increasing proficiency, actors learn to respond to each other quickly, while remaining in the moment of the interaction. In many ways, these effortful exercises seem to mirror the playful emotional interactions of infants and caregivers, allowing actors to gain some awareness of (and, possibly, control over) the intricate social dynamics of emotional exchange. In contrast to traditional approaches such as method acting (Chekhov, 1953), in which actors are trained to reenact emotions based on their autobiographical memories, the result is described as a performance of actors who live "truthfully under imaginary circumstances" (Meisner & Longwell, 1987, p. 15). It appears that even on the stage, emotions that emerge from the spontaneous integration of available social information may be perceived as more authentic than those that are first conceived in actors' heads and then put into action.

Finally, a range of studies indicates that emotions serve as intentional and strategic bids in ongoing interactions. Which emotions ensue depends not only on past events but also future projections of what may be achieved in the interaction (Solomon, 2003). For example, anger is more likely if there is a prospect of getting what one wants; in situations where goals cannot be effectively reinstated, sadness is the more likely experience (Stein, Trabasso, & Liwag, 1993). Along similar lines, people tend to express more embarrassment when they assume that doing so may help to reinstate their social standing. In one experiment, participants felt less embarrassment after singing an embarrassing song when they thought that the experimenter already knew how they felt (Leary, Landel, & Patton, 1996). According to the authors, embarrassment served as a signal through which participants attempted to repair their social image; in situations where the experimenter was already aware of their feelings, the emotion lost its strategic function and was therefore not experienced. Neither finding can be explained solely by the eliciting event, but both become clear when the participant's social intentions and the extent to which they can be fulfilled in the social situation are taken into account.

In summary, there is support for the idea that emotions derive their shape from moment-to-moment interactions. New acquaintances quickly pick up the emotional behavior of their interaction partners; people rely on others' emotional reactions when evaluating ambiguous situations; synchronous interactions cause people to experience more compassion toward each other; and actors practice to respond spontaneously to interactions on the stage in order to perform authentic emotions. Finally, emotions are shaped by not only the previous events in the interaction but also the (desirable) course that the interaction takes.

Emotions Are Grounded in Ongoing Relationships

Emotional experience and expression at one particular moment in the social interaction are always contextualized by ongoing relationships with others. Ties with close others may constrain the range of likely emotions (i.e., afford particular emotions), and influence how and when these emotions are experienced. Emotional affordances in relationships refer to the range of emotions that are likely to occur within a *particular relationship:* The accumulated relational history of shared interactions constrains what is likely during any one interaction. Moreover, as people share emotions with each other, their relational patterns may change accordingly. Evidence for the relational grounding of emotions is fairly extensive, especially in the domain of marital relationships.

One of the most compelling examples of the ways in which emotions are grounded in relationships is the case of emotional convergence over time. In a series of studies, Anderson, Keltner, and John (2003) have demonstrated that that the emotions of same-sex roommates and heterosexual couples become more similar over time. In these studies, emotions were measured both by self-reports and facial coding, and they were elicited in a number of different ways (conversations about pleasant or unpleasant topics, emotion-eliciting tasks, watching emotion-eliciting movies). Participants' average levels of positive and negative emotions were more similar after 6 or 9 months than at the beginning. Moreover, emotional convergence did not depend on emotional contagion: Roommates who had not known each other prior to living together responded to emotion-eliciting movies with similar emotions, even when they were watching the movies in separate rooms. Living in the same space appears to have led to similarity in emotional reactivity in a relatively short time. One possible explanation may be that people in a relationship come to share certain rather stable expectations toward their world, causing them to respond to events in emotionally similar ways (there is some evidence that friends appraise certain situations in more similar ways than do strangers; Bruder, Dosmukhambetova, Nerb, & Manstead, 2012). Whatever the exact mechanism at play, the case of emotional convergence constitutes a strong point for the idea that sharing a relationship with someone has an impact on the kinds of emotions that people are likely to experience.

Romantic partners also develop synchronized emotional time–dynamics, with each partner's emotions covarying with the other (for a review, see Butler, 2011). Whereas the convergence literature focuses on mean levels of positive and negative emotions at one moment in time, research on emotional time–dynamics focus on covariation over time. For example, Butner, Diamond, and Hicks (2007) asked married or cohabitating heterosexual couples to complete measures of positive and negative affect for 21 days. The positive and negative affect of partners covaried on a daily basis beyond how positively or negatively partners had rated inter-actions with each other. Because this emotional synchrony was found even when controlling for each partner's interpretation of his or her interactions with the other, it appears that romantic partners develop mutual dependen-cies in their emotional lives that go beyond what can be explained through momentary constructions. The crucial point here is that being in a relation-ship restricted the range of emotions that partners were likely to experience on any one day: If one partner felt miserable, so did the other.

Evidence for emotional synchrony between partners has been found for not only self-reported emotions but also physiological parameters known to be associated with emotions. In their research on marital interac-tions, Levenson and Gottman (1983) observed that physiological patterns of partners become linked during emotionally intense interactions. In this study, several physiological parameters, such as heart rate and skin conduc-tance, were measured while couples discussed two topics—one neutral, the other highly conflictual. During the conflict discussion, partners' patterns of physiological responses were more interrelated than during the neutral discussion; moreover, physiological linkage was higher for couples with lower marital satisfaction. Recently, Saxbe and Repetti (2010) replicated this finding with real-life experience sampling. Repeated measurement of salivary cortisol levels throughout the day covaried between marital part-ners; again, couples with low marital satisfaction experienced more physi-ological linkage. In instable and strained relationships, negative affect and the associated physiological changes appear to be transmitted easily (while positive affect remains unaffected, e.g., Levenson & Gottman, 1983; see also Larson & Almeida, 1999), possibly reinforcing established patterns and leading to a further destabilization of the relationship. It is conceivable that partners pick up each others' physiological states unconsciously, for instance, through mimicry (e.g., Hatfield et al., 1994), social chemosig-nals (e.g., McClintock, 2002, as cited in Saxbe & Repetti, 2010), or touch (Coan, Schaefer, & Davidson, 2006).

As relationships expand over longer periods of time, close others may become an important basis for regulating biological rhythms—even though these functions may only become evident once the relationship with them is disrupted. For example, some theories of bereavement (Hofer, 1984; Sbarra & Hazan, 2008) argue that the profound emotional impact of losing a partner can, at least partially, be understood from the partners' role in keeping physiological and psychological functions in homeostasis. Accord-ing to Hofer (1984), interactions between partners may serve as a form of social entrainment for each partner's biological rhythms. Upon the death of a partner, these coregulatory processes are disrupted. Consequently, the surviving partner's biological rhythms become desynchronized, which would account for some of the psychological manifestations of grief. In sup-port of this claim, Hofer reviews evidence that jet lag—which, he proposes, resembles grief in terms of a decrease in appetite, vigilance, and overall well-being—is exacerbated for individuals who cannot engage in social interactions after moving to a new time zone (Klein & Wegman, 1974, as cited in Hofer, 1984). Grief and the associated physiological changes appear to depend on social processes that transcend individual minds and that are not entirely comprehended without taking the (disruption of) relationships with close others into account. Approaching bereavement as a disruption of socially regulated homeostasis has practical implications: For example, interventions for prolonged grief may be more successful if they not only target individual cognitive schemas but also ascertain regular social interactions with close others who may fulfill, at least partially, the regulatory function of the lost partner.

Understanding emotions as grounded in relationships implies that emotions are not only shaped by relational bonds but that, over time, they also shape the relationships in which they occur. For example, the accumulated experience and expression of negative emotions such as contempt may lead to a faster parting of the ways. In their longitudinal study of marital interaction and satisfaction, Gottman and Levenson (2000) predicted with 93% accuracy the development of heterosexual couples' relationships based on short emotional interactions. Couples who displayed more negative emotions such as contempt during a 15-minute discussion of conflictual topics were substantially more likely to be divorced 7 years later. The prevalence of positive emotionality in the relationship, however, appeared to have a safe-guarding function, preventing the escalation of negative exchanges during disagreements.

One positive emotion that appears to play an important role for relationship building and maintenance is gratitude (see also Fredrickson, 2001). Feeling gratitude helps establish new relationships (Algoe, Haidt, & Gable, 2008) and advances the short-term development of established romantic relationships (Algoe, Gable, & Maisel, 2010). But in the long term, gratitude also has maintenance effects on relationships: Four years into their marriage, marital partners who experienced more gratitude toward their partners (measured repeatedly since the beginning of their marriage) were found to be more motivated to engage in relationship maintenance behaviors; these maintenance behaviors were positively perceived by their partners, who in turn were more likely to also experience gratitude (Kubacka, Finkenauer, Rusbult, & Keijsers, 2011). Similarly, expressing gratitude at one point in time led partners to feel more mutual responsibility and generosity at a later time (Lambert, Clark, Durtschi, Fincham, & Graham, 2010).

In summary, emotions are grounded in people's relationships with others: On the one hand, people who share a relationship—from marital relationships to roommates in college—become emotionally attuned to each other. Emotional attunement seems to occur in terms of both direct,

proximal effects that partners have on each other (e.g., emotional covariation, physiological linkage) and overall tendencies to respond emotionally
to certain situations (e.g., emotional convergence). Moreover, the extent
to which people in a relationship become emotionally attuned depends on
the quality of the relationship and is reflected in not only emotional self-
report and observed behavior but also physiological patterns. On the other
hand, both negative emotions (e.g., contempt) and positive emotions (e.g.,
gratitude) are closely linked to the development of relationships, such that
negative emotions lead to a deterioration of the relationship, whereas positive emotions help to form and maintain relationships.

Emotions Depend on Cultural Values and Practices

In each cultural context, certain values and practices in terms of how to
act as a person and how to relate to others are emphasized or prescribed.
These cultural values constitute the rather persistent and pervasive meaning system against which people appraise what is happening around them.
For example, when the dominant cultural values emphasize the importance
of living up to social expectations, failure to do so in one's relationships
will likely elicit shame; shame in those cultural contexts may be a common
emotional experience. Beyond making certain values or meanings salient,
cultural contexts also differ in the practices in which people commonly
engage; these practices afford certain emotions by structuring the ecol-
ogy of daily situations and relationships that people encounter. For example, elaborate politeness rituals decrease the likelihood of experiencing
anger-eliciting situations; classroom routines that allow for the collective
monitoring of norm-inconsistent behavior (e.g., communal self-criticism,
or *hansei*, in Japanese classrooms; Lewis, 1995) render the experience of
shame-eliciting situations more common. Affordances in cultural contexts
refer to the range of emotions that are likely when engaging in a *particular
cultural context*; these affordances are kept in place through socialization
and social reward contingencies.

Cultural contexts highlight different ways to make sense of the world,
which, consequently, affords different emotional experiences. For example,
whereas European Americans tend to believe that the world is a controllable place (Mesquita & Ellsworth, 2001; Morling, Kitayama, & Miyamoto,
2002; Weisz, Rothbaum, & Blackburn, 1984), participants from India
and Tahiti do not show this tendency (Miller, Bersoff, & Harwood, 1990;
Savani, Morris, Naidu, Kumar, & Berlia, 2011). Appraising something as
within one's control is an important aspect of anger and frustration (Frijda,
Kuipers, & Ter Schure, 1989; Kuppens, Van Mechelen, Smits, & De Boeck,
2003; Stein et al., 1993): Experiencing anger implies that one's goals are
blocked, but that this situation is controllable and can be changed. If people
interpret the world through the lens of their cultural values, one would

consequently expect differences in the frequency and intensity of anger and frustration between European Americans, on the one hand, and Indians and Tahitians, on the other. Indeed, Roseman, Dhawan, Rettek, Naidu, and Thapa (1995) found that American, as compared to Indian students reported higher overall intensities of anger when remembering autobiographical events, and anger intensity was fully mediated by an appraisal of the event as being inconsistent with one's goals. A similar observation was made by anthropologist Robert Levy (1978, p. 288), who argued that the Tahitian's "common sense that individuals have very limited control over nature and over the behavior of others" is related to the near absence of anger in Tahitian culture. According to Levy, a world that is seen as unpredictable and uncontrollable might be "cognitively less frustrating than . . . realities in which almost anything is possible to individuals" (p. 226).

Cultural contexts also differ in terms of the practices in which people commonly engage and which may afford different emotional experiences. For example, people tend to seek out activities that elicit culturally "ideal" affect (Tsai, 2007). Whereas North Americans prefer active individual activities (e.g., running or rollerblading), up-beat music, and stimulants (e.g., amphetamines, cocaine), East Asians are more drawn to passive and collective activities (e.g., sightseeing, picnicking), calmer music, and sedatives (e.g., opiates) (Tsai, 2007). North American activities foreground high-activation positive emotions (e.g., excitement); East Asian activities facilitate low-arousal positive states (e.g., calm, relaxed). In our own research (Boiger et al., 2013) we found that people also encounter more interpersonal interactions in their culture that are associated with culturally desirable emotions (i.e., anger in the United States, shame in Japan). While interactions that afford strong feelings of anger appear to be promoted in the United States, these interactions are avoided Japan. The opposite picture emerges for shame: Interactions associated with stronger feelings of shame are promoted in Japan and avoided in the United States. These findings may explain why previous researchers have found that socially disengaging emotions (e.g., anger) are more salient in Americans' daily lives, whereas socially engaging emotions (e.g., shame) prevail in Japan (Kitayama, Markus, & Kurokawa, 2000; Kitayama, Mesquita, & Karasawa, 2006): People's environments appear to be structured in ways that give them more opportunities to experience the respective emotions.

Compared to the momentary constructions in social interactions and the patterns created within relationships, we assume that cultural values and practices are rather stable affordances in the construction of emotion. However, even at the level of culture, the construction of emotion is dynamic and not a simple one-time business. A particular case in point is emotional acculturation, that is, the tendency of migrants to adjust their emotional patterns to those of their culture of settlement. In one study, De Leersnyder, Mesquita, and Kim (2011) compared the emotional patterns of Turkish immigrants in Belgium and those of Korean immigrants in the United States with the average emotional patterns of their respective cultures of settlement. Participants, relative to emotional events from their own lives, reported to what extent they had felt each of 20 different emotions. The authors calculated the degree of emotional acculturation for each immigrant by comparing his or her individual profile with the average profiles of the respective host culture. The more time immigrants had spent in the new culture, the more similar their emotional pattern became to the average mainstream pattern. Moreover, those immigrants who had frequent interactions with members of the new cultural context were emotionally more similar than immigrants who did not. As immigrants engage in relationships with members from their new culture, they seem to renegotiate their emotional interpretations and adjust their emotional patterns.

Recent research has shown just how quickly people adjust their meaning system when being exposed to (culturally) novel situations. In one experiment, Savani and colleagues (2011, Study 5) asked Indian and European American students to indicate the extent to which they would adjust to or influence interpersonal situations that were sampled from both India and the United States. In line with the American tendency to influence (e.g., Boiger, Mesquita, Tsai, & Markus, 2012; Morling et al., 2002; Weisz et al., 1984) and the Indian tendency to adjust (e.g., Roseman et al., 1995), U.S. participants initially reported more influence and Indian participants more adjustment across the range of situations from both cultures. However, this pattern changed after the participants had been exposed to a sufficiently large number of situations from the other culture: After 100 trials, the degree of adjustment reported by European American and Indian participants converged. Although this study did not investigate emotions, it does make a strong case for the idea that meaning making is afforded by the situations that people commonly experience; it is conceivable that similar situational affordances affect appraisal processes and consequent emotions (cf. Roseman et al., 1995).

A major shortcoming of previous cross-cultural research on emotion, at least in terms of our sociodynamic perspective, is that most studies focused exclusively on culture-level differences of otherwise noncontextualized individual responses; very few studies explored how cultural values and practices define people's emotional responses during their interactions with relevant others. Research on the socialization of emotion in children is one such exception. For example, Trommsdorff and Kornadt (2003) report very different ways in which conflict situations unfold in German and Japanese mother–child dyads. While the former tend to engage in escalating interactions of reciprocal resistance during which mothers and children enforce their perspective, the latter tend to make mutual concessions in order to maintain harmony and a feeling of oneness (*ittaikan*). The different interaction patterns between German and Japanese mothers and children had long-term effects on children's emotional patterns: Escalation of interactions in early childhood predicted the level of empathy-based altruism and aggression 9 years later (Kornadt & Tachibana, 1999, as cited in Trommsdorff & Kornadt, 2003). These socialization practices can be understood from the different cultural ideals in Germany and Japan: The German children learn to assert themselves and have their needs met, while the Japanese children learn to accommodate other people's desires irrespective of their individual goals.

In summary, the prevalent cultural values and practices afford different emotions and emotional patterns across cultures; some of these differences seem to occur because cultural contexts constrain the range of likely appraisals *in situ*, whereas others operate by promoting certain (culturally desirable) social interactions over others. Moreover, as people move between cultures, they adjust to the emotional patterns afforded by their new cultural contexts. Finally, even though most cross-cultural studies explored mean differences in individuals' emotions, a few studies convincingly showed how cultural values and practices "trickle down" through the culturally preferred relational arrangements to afford culturally functional emotional constructions in the moment.

Two Sides of the Same Coin:
Psychological and Sociodynamic Construction

Emotions emerge dynamically from interactions with others, they are grounded in relational patterns and meanings, and they are defined by the values and practices of the larger cultural context. Although we have emphasized how emotional experience, expression, and perception are situated in the social world, this does not mean sociodynamic construction replaces psychological construction; rather, sociodynamic and psychological construction are two sides of the same coin. Emotions occur in social contexts, and as we have shown, it is hard to imagine an emotional episode that is not in one way or another played out in the context of ongoing interactions, relationships, or one's culture. At the same time, emotions are also individual experiences that rely on individual minds. The point is not to emphasize sociodynamic construction at the expense of psychological construction, but rather to underline that the mind always operates in context.

In our sociodynamic view of emotion construction, an individual's emotions are strategic moves *given* the ongoing interaction with the social environment (Frijda, 2007; Solomon, 2003). Emotions are online responses that can be understood when taking into consideration the combined emotions of all people involved in the dynamically evolving interaction or relationship, which themselves are afforded and constrained by cultural values and practices. Given this contextualized view of emotions, it may be more appropriate to speak of people *doing emotions* (with others) than of having emotions (alone). What unites our sociodynamic and a psychological constructionist perspective (Barrett, 2009a, 2009b; Gendron & Barrett, 2009; Gross & Barrett, 2011; Russell, 2003) is that both emphasize the role of meaning making in emotional episodes.

In fact, we believe that sociodynamic and psychological perspectives on emotion construction are complementary—and a promising direction for future research would combine the predictions that both perspectives make. Combining both perspectives is possible because the "under-the-hood" predictions that psychological construction makes can complement our predictions about the dynamic role of social contexts. For example, the *conceptual act theory* (Barrett, 2006; Lindquist & Barrett, 2008) states that people continuously apply conceptual knowledge to their perception of the world, and that emotions emerge when emotional knowledge is applied to internal and external sensory information. A sociodynamic perspective would emphasize that activation of the relevant conceptual knowledge is contingent on the current context; that is, meaning making is continuously afforded by interactional, relational or cultural affordances. To give an example, conceptual knowledge of anger (e.g., "Someone has just blocked my goals; I feel hot and under pressure to retaliate") is more likely to be activated during an escalating interaction in a strained relationship between two individuals who have been socialized and currently engage in an autonomy-promoting cultural context. Investigating the interplay of sociodynamic and psychological construction means to see emotions for what they are: powerful connections between inner psyches and outer worlds.

REFERENCES

Algoe, S. B., Gable, S. L., & Maisel, N. C. (2010). It's the little things: Everyday gratitude as a booster shot for romantic relationships. *Personal Relationships, 17*(2), 217–233.

Algoe, S. B., Haidt, J., & Gable, S. L. (2008). Beyond reciprocity: Gratitude and relationships in everyday life. *Emotion, 8*(3), 425–429.

Anderson, C., Keltner, D., & John, O. P. (2003). Emotional convergence between people over time. *Journal of Personality and Social Psychology, 84*(5), 1054–1068.

Averill, J. R. (1982). *Anger and aggression: An essay on emotion.* New York: Springer.

Azuma, H. (1984). Secondary control as a heterogeneous category. *American Psychologist, 39*(9), 970–971.

Barrett, L. F. (2006). Solving the emotion paradox: Categorization and the experience of emotion. *Personality and Social Psychology Review, 10*(1), 20–46.

Barrett, L. F. (2009a). The future of psychology: Connecting mind to brain. *Psychological Science, 4*(4), 326–339.

Barrett, L. F. (2009b). Variety is the spice of life: A psychological construction approach to understanding variability in emotion. *Cognition and Emotion, 23*(7), 1284–1306.

Blascovich, J., & Mendes, W. B. (2000). Challenge and threat appraisals: The role of affective cues. In J. Forgas (Ed.), *Feeling and thinking: The role of affect in social cognition* (pp. 59–82). New York: Cambridge University Press.

Boiger, M., & Mesquita, B. (2012). The construction of emotion in interactions, relationships, and cultures. *Emotion Review, 4,* 221–229.

Boiger, M., Mesquita, B., Tsai, A. Y., & Markus, H. R. (2012). Influencing and adjusting in daily emotional situations: A comparison of European and Asian American action styles. *Cognition and Emotion, 26*(2), 332–340.

Boiger, M., Mesquita, B., Uchida, Y., & Barrett, L. F. (2013). Condoned or condemned: The situational affordance of anger and shame in the US and Japan. *Personality and Social Psychology Bulletin, 39*(4), 540–553.

Briggs, J. L. (1970). *Never in anger: Portrait of an Eskimo family.* Cambridge, MA: Harvard University Press.

Bruder, M., Dosmukhambetova, D., Nerb, J., & Manstead, A. S. R. (2012). Emotional signals in nonverbal interaction: Dyadic facilitation and convergence in expressions, appraisals, and feelings. *Cognition and Emotion, 26*(3), 480–502.

Butler, E. A. (2011). Temporal interpersonal emotion systems: The "TIES" that form relationships. *Personality and Social Psychology Review, 15*(4), 367–393.

Butner, J., Diamond, L. M., & Hicks, A. M. (2007). Attachment style and two forms of affect coregulation between romantic partners. *Personal Relationships, 14,* 431–455.

Chekhov, M. (1953). *To the actor: On the technique of acting.* New York: Harper & Row.

Coan, J. A., Schaefer, H. S., & Davidson, R. J. (2006). Lending a hand: Social regulation of the neural response to threat. *Psychological Science, 17*(12), 1032–1039.

De Leersnyder, J., Mesquita, B., & Kim, H. S. (2011). Where do my emotions belong?: A study of immigrants' emotional acculturation. *Personality and Social Psychology Bulletin, 37*(4), 451–463.

Fredrickson, B. L. (2001). The role of positive emotions in positive psychology: The broaden-and-build theory of positive emotions. *American Psychologist, 56*(3), 218–226.

Frijda, N. H. (2007). *The laws of emotion.* Hillsdale, NJ: Erlbaum.

Frijda, N. H., Kuipers, P., & Ter Schure, E. (1989). Relations among emotion, appraisal, and emotional action readiness. *Journal of Personality and Social Psychology, 57*(2), 212–228.

Gendron, M., & Barrett, L. F. (2009). Reconstructing the past: A century of ideas about emotion in psychology. *Emotion Review, 1*(4), 316–339.

Gibson, J. J. (1979). *The ecological approach to visual perception.* Hillsdale, NJ: Erlbaum.

Gottman, J. M., & Levenson, R. W. (2000). The timing of divorce: Predicting when a couple will divorce over a 14-year period. *Journal of Marriage and Family, 62*(3), 737–745.

Gross, J. J., & Barrett, L. F. (2011). Emotion generation and emotion regulation: One or two depends on your point of view. *Emotion Review, 3*(1), 8–16.

Hatfield, E., Cacioppo, J. T., & Rapson, R. L. (1994). *Emotional contagion.* New York: Cambridge University Press.

Heerey, E. A., & Kring, A. M. (2007). Interpersonal consequences of social anxiety. *Journal of Abnormal Psychology, 116*(1), 125–134.

Hofer, M. A. (1984). Relationships as regulators: A psychobiologic perspective on bereavement. *Psychosomatic Medicine, 46*(3), 183–197.

Kitayama, S., Markus, H. R., & Kurokawa, M. (2000). Culture, emotion, and well-being: Good feelings in Japan and the United States. *Cognition and Emotion, 14*(1), 93–124.

Kitayama, S., Markus, H. R., Matsumoto, H., & Norasakkunkit, V. (1997). Individual and collective processes in the construction of the self: Self-enhancement in the United States and self-criticism in Japan. *Journal of Personality and Social Psychology, 72*(6), 1245–1267.

Kitayama, S., Mesquita, B., & Karasawa, M. (2006). Cultural affordances and emotional experience: Socially engaging and disengaging emotions in Japan and the United States. *Journal of Personality and Social Psychology, 91*(5), 890–903.

Kubacka, K. E., Finkenauer, C., Rusbult, C. E., & Keijsers, L. (2011). Maintaining close relationships: Gratitude as a motivator and a detector of maintenance behavior. *Personality and Social Psychology Bulletin, 37*(10), 1362–1375.

Kuppens, P., Van Mechelen, I., Smits, D. J. M., & De Boeck, P. (2003). The appraisal basis of anger: Specificity, necessity and sufficiency of components. *Emotion, 3*(3), 254–269.

Lambert, N. M., Clark, M. S., Durtschi, J., Fincham, F. D., & Graham, S. M. (2010). Benefits of expressing gratitude: Expressing gratitude to a partner changes one's view of the relationship. *Psychological Science, 21*(4), 574–580.

Larson, R., & Almeida, D. (1999). Emotional transmission in the daily lives of families: A new paradigm for studying family process. *Journal of Marriage and the Family, 61,* 5–20.

Lazarus, R. S. (1991). *Emotion and adaptation.* New York: Oxford University Press.

Leary, M. R., Landel, J., & Patton, K. (1996). The motivated expression of embarrassment following a self-presentational predicament. *Journal of Personality, 64,* 619–363.

Leary, M. R., & Leder, S. (2009). The nature of hurt feelings: Emotional experience and cognitive appraisals. In A. Vangelisti (Ed.), *Feeling hurt in close relationships* (pp. 15–33). New York: Cambridge University Press.

Levenson, R. W., & Gottman, J. M. (1983). Marital interaction: Physiological linkage and affective exchange. *Journal of Personality and Social Psychology, 45*(3), 587–597.

Levy, R. I. (1978). Tahitian gentleness and redundant controls. In A. Montagu (Ed.), *Learning non-aggression: The experience of non-literate societies* (pp. 222–235). New York: Oxford University Press.

Lewis, C. C. (1995). *Educating hearts and minds.* New York: Cambridge University Press.

Lindquist, K. A., & Barrett, L. F. (2008). Constructing emotion: The experience of fear as a conceptual act. *Psychological Science, 19*(9), 898–903.

Markus, H. R., & Kitayama, S. (1991). Culture and the self: Implications for cognition, emotion, and motivation. *Psychological Review, 98*(2), 224–253.

Meisner, S., & Longwell, D. (1987). *Sanford Meisner on acting.* New York: Random House.

Mesquita, B., & Ellsworth, P. C. (2001). The role of culture in appraisal. In K. R. Scherer & A. Schorr (Eds.), *Appraisal processes in emotion: Theory, methods, research* (pp. 233–248). New York: Oxford University Press.

Miller, J. G., Bersoff, D. M., & Harwood, R. L. (1990). Perceptions of social responsibilities in India and in the United States: Moral imperatives or personal decisions? *Journal of Personality and Social Psychology, 58*, 33–47.

Morling, B., Kitayama, S., & Miyamoto, Y. (2002). Cultural practices emphasize influence in the United States and adjustment in Japan. *Personality and Social Psychology Bulletin, 28*(3), 311–323.

Parkinson, B., & Simons, G. (2009). Affecting others: Social appraisal and emotion contagion in everyday decision making. *Personality and Social Psychology Bulletin, 35*(8), 1071–1084.

Roseman, I. J., Dhawan, N., Rettek, S. I., Naidu, R. K., & Thapa, K. (1995). Cultural differences and cross-cultural similarities in appraisals and emotional responses. *Journal of Cross-Cultural Psychology, 26*(1), 23–48.

Russell, J. A. (2003). Core affect and the psychological construction of emotion. *Psychological Review, 110*(1), 145–172.

Savani, K., Morris, M. W., Naidu, N. V. R., Kumar, S., & Berlia, N. V. (2011). Cultural conditioning: Understanding interpersonal accommodation in India and the United States in terms of the modal characteristics of interpersonal influence situations. *Journal of Personality and Social Psychology, 100*(1), 84–102.

Saxbe, D., & Repetti, R. L. (2010). For better or worse?: Coregulation of couples' cortisol levels and mood states. *Journal of Personality and Social Psychology, 98*(1), 92–103.

Sbarra, D. A., & Hazan, C. (2008). Coregulation, dysregulation, self-regulation: An integrative analysis and empirical agenda for understanding adult attachment, separation, loss, and recovery. *Personality and Social Psychology Review, 12*(2), 141–167.

Smith, C. A., & Ellsworth, P. C. (1985). Patterns of cognitive appraisal in emotion. *Journal of Personality and Social Psychology, 48*(4), 813–838.

Solomon, R. C. (2003). *Not passion's slave: Emotions and choice.* New York: Oxford University Press.

Specht, M. (2010). Women in Korea (I). *The Korea Times.* Retrieved from *www.koreatimes.co.kr/www/news/opinon/2010/03/137_61602.html.*

Stein, N. L., Trabasso, T., & Liwag, M. (1993). The representation and organization of emotional experience: Unfolding the emotion episode. In M. Lewis & J. M. Haviland (Eds.), *Handbook of emotions* (pp. 279–300). New York: Guilford Press.

Trommsdorff, G., & Kornadt, H. (2003). Parent–child relations in cross-cultural perspective. In L. Kuczynski (Ed.), *Handbook of dynamics in parent–child relations* (pp. 271–305). Thousand Oaks, CA: Sage.

Tsai, J. L. (2007). Ideal affect: Cultural causes and behavioral consequences. *Perspectives on Psychological Science, 2*(3), 242–259.

Valdesolo, P., & DeSteno, D. (2011). Synchrony and the social tuning of compassion. *Emotion, 11*(2), 262–266.

Wang, Q. (2001). "Did you have fun?": American and Chinese mother–child conversations about shared emotional experiences. *Cognitive Development, 16,* 693–715.

Weisz, J. R., Rothbaum, F. M., & Blackburn, T. C. (1984). Standing out and standing in: The psychology of control in America and Japan. *American Psychologist, 39*(9), 955–969.

White, M. I., & LeVine, R. A. (1986). What is an *ii ko* (good child). In H. Stevenson, H. Azuma, & K. Hakuta (Eds.), *Child development and education in Japan* (pp. 55–67). New York: Freeman.

Wilson-Mendenhall, C. D., Barrett, L. F., Simmons, W. K., & Barsalou, L. W. (2011). Grounding emotion in situated conceptualization. *Neuropsychologia, 49*(5), 1105–1127.

CHAPTER 16

Evolutionary Constraints and Cognitive Mechanisms in the Construction of an Emotion

Insights from Human and Nonhuman Primates

JENNIFER M. B. FUGATE

Do nonhuman primates have emotion? Is a chimp that bares its teeth afraid? Is it possible to answer these questions? As with most things psychological, the answer is: "It depends." According to some emotion traditions asking such questions makes sense because such traditions treat emotions as *natural kinds*, existing in nature and independent of the mind of a perceiver (see Barrett, 2006a, 2006b, 2009, 2011a, 2011b, 2012; Barrett, Wilson-Mendenhall, & Barsalou, Chapter 4, this volume). For example, in "basic" theories, emotions are treated as triggered events (e.g., Allport, 1924; Ekman, Friesen, & Ellsworth, 1972; Izard, 1971; McDougall, 1908/1921; Panksepp, 1998; Tomkins, 1962), in which each emotion is elicited by a dedicated, evolutionary conserved mechanism in the brain. In fact, such an approach has long been the backbone of evolutionary and comparative psychology (e.g., Tooby & Cosmides, 1990; Pinker, 1997) and stems back to the work of Darwin (1872) who noted the similarities in facial displays across the Animal kingdom.[1] Contemporary theories of this approach recognize somewhere between five and seven "basic" emotions in humans (e.g., fear, anger, sadness, happiness, disgust, surprise) (Ekman et al., 1972; Izard, 1971; Tomkins, 1962), yet a somewhat mismatching list in nonhuman animals (e.g., seeking, rage, fear, lust, care, panic, and play,

1. *If emotions are psychological events constructed from more basic ingredients, then what are the key ingredients from which emotions are constructed? Are they specific to emotion or are they general ingredients of the mind? Which, if any, are specific to humans?*

A psychological primitive requires that it not be capable of being broken down into psychologically meaningful components. Yet, as I have shown here, language and categorization (two "psychological primitives" formerly described; Barrett 2006a, 2006b, 2011a, 2011b, 2012) share a bidirectional and complex relationship, in which language is a powerful means by which humans categorize, and which allows for ontologically subjective categories (albeit not the only way). I would suggest that we explore the more basic ingredients that underlie inferred causation and collective agreements, the basis of ontologically subjective categories. I have proposed several in this chapter, including analogical reasoning, mental state sharing, and the ability to understand causal forces. I do not believe that any of these are specific to language, although they are necessary for language.

2. *What brings these ingredients together in the construction of an emotion? Which combinations are emotions and which are not (and how do we know)?*

Part of psychological constructionism states that the primitives can be used interchangeably to construct multiple emergent states that alone were once considered mental faculties. Instrumental to this system of interchange is that a perceiver's attention can direct categorization. When attention is placed on an organism's bodily sensations and this information is prioritized and categorized—along whatever category lines the organism has—it has the potential to be an "emotion." As I have suggested in this chapter, however, the categorization abilities among nonhuman primates (mainly great apes) and humans show some fundamental differences that are reflected in structural and connectivity changes in the brain since a great ape–human common ancestor. This is not to say that organisms that do not possess these primitives do not have bodily sensations nor does it mean that they are automatically unable to categorize these sensations in biologically adaptive ways.

3. *How important is variability (across instances within an emotion category, and in the categories that exist across cultures)? Is this variance epiphenomenal or a thing to be explained? To the extent that it makes sense, it would be desirable to address issues such as universality and evolution.*

Psychological constructionists have also been criticized for being "antievolutionary." I would disagree. This approach to emotion suggests that core affect is shared among all organisms. I would add that the framework provided in this chapter shows that the conceptual system necessary for some of the

(continued)

building blocks of emotion exists on an evolutionary continuum. As a result, we may start to answer a set of questions that includes an evolutionary emphasis. In this sense, variability is also represented along evolutionary lines.

4. What constitutes strong evidence to support a psychological construction to emotion? Point to or summarize empirical evidence that supports your model or outline what a key experiment would look like. What would falsify your model?

The approach taken in this chapter builds on the idea that some categories, including emotion, are ontologically subjective and their creation and maintenance depend on certain advanced cognitive abilities that evolved in response to growing environmental complexities and increased social living. The evidence, then, is in the range of cognitive complexities that individual species exhibit. Thus, categories such as "emotion" will be different among species whose cognitive architecture and abilities differ. The approach taken in this chapter suggests that emotion and other ontologically subjective categories exist on a continuum across species. In recognizing this, a new list of scientific questions can be generated that might help to draw some consilience among basic, appraisal, social, and psychological constructionist accounts of emotion. For example, we might push for scientists to distinguish consistently between "emotion" and "core affect," in which the latter is shared among most (at least vertebrate) organisms and is one necessary component in the construction of emotion.

Testing the bidirectional evolutionary relationship between the brain's architecture and its resulting abilities is impossible. Yet, if we agree that language requires the psychological primitives I've outlined in this chapter (although there are likely other ways), then we might be able to look at studies which have taught a formalized language system (e.g., American Sign Language [ASL]) to a great ape species to gain some insight. Although there have been several efforts to teach ASL to chimpanzees (and other great apes) with varying success, emotion perception tasks have not been administered to see how the individual's performance changes with the acquisition of language. Some of the best evidence that we have comes piecemeal from studies with captive chimpanzees performing categorical perception tasks. Although categorical perception tasks of emotion may not be the only indicator of discrete emotion perception, they are widely used (for a review, see Fugate, 2013). For example, my dissertation (Fugate, 2008) showed that chimpanzees—who had not been language trained but who had extensive practice with sorting chimpanzee facial depictions—did not show universal categorical perception for conspecific facial expressions. In further research, I showed that adult humans do not show categorical perception for these same faces unless they are first taught a word-like anchor for the category (Fugate, Gouzoules, & Barrett, 2010). Additionally, a study by Martin-Malivel and Okada (2007) showed that only

(continued)

chimpanzees who have been taught a formalized language system showed categorical perception for conspecific identity, whereas those who had not been taught a language did not show the ability. Although this study was done with identity (and not emotion), it does provide support that teaching a formalized language system allows for a change in which information is organized and used to make meangingful categories. Specifically it allows for information and comparisons to be made at a higher-order level, which is the basis of analogical reasoning, and, as I argue, is necessary in the construction of an emotion. Based on this work, my colleagues and I have suggested that the reason humans show categorical perception for human facial expressions is because they have language (specifically emotion words) that they have learned throughout their development and readily apply when looking at faces. That is, emotion words serve as relational anchors.

This is a good start to answer some of the questions laid out, yet categorical perception tasks don't tell us how these anchors are used as relational devices nor do they address the other cognitive skills that I've argued are necessary in the construction of an emotion.

based mainly on detailed neuroanatomical work in the rat brain) (Panksepp, 1998, 2000, 2007). In other natural kinds views, such as "appraisal" theories, emotions are treated as the products of some kind of meaning analysis (e.g., Arnold, 1960a, 1960b; Ellsworth & Scherer, 2003; Fridja, 1986; Lazarus, 1991; Roseman, 1991; but see Ortony & Clore, Chapter 13, this volume). Like all faculty models of psychology, however, these models of emotion all assume that there are objective indicators of a person's mental (or emotional) state. From the view that emotions are the things of explanation, it makes sense to question whether a chimpanzee baring its teeth is angry.

For other traditions, emotions are not *natural kinds;* rather, they are psychological constructs—the product of minds that share a similar system for categorizing information and a collective agreement. Said another way, they are ontologically subjective categories (see Searle, 1995; Barrett, 2006a, 2006b, 2009, 2011a, 2011b, 2012; Barrett et al., Chapter 4, this volume). In this view, emotions are constructed in the minds of a group of perceivers who agree that they exist because they are important as explanatory constructs (i.e., they provide utility) that fit our folk psychology of how things work (Barrett, 2006a, 2006b, 2009, 2011a, 2011b, 2012; Barrett et al., Chapter 4, this volume). According to this approach, emotions (like all mental states) arise from a set of more basic psychological ingredients that are not themselves specific to any discrete emotion category, or to the category "emotion" more broadly (Barrett, 2006a, 2006b, 2009, 2011a, 2011b, 2012; Barrett et al., Chapter 4, this volume; Russell, 2003a; Russell, Chapter 17, this volume).

In the conceptual act theory of psychological constructionism, language is one such ingredient (Barrett, 2006a, 2006b, 2009, 2011a, 2011b, 2012; Barrett et al., Chapter 4, this volume; Barrett, Lindquist, & Gendron, 2007; Lindquist & Barrett, 2012; Lindquist et al., 2012; Oosterwijk, Touroutoglou, & Lindquist, Chapter 5, this volume). Emotion words, such as *anger*, introduce a kind of statistical regularity that allow various instances of bodily sensations, behaviors, and subjective feelings to be grouped together into a single category (Lindquist, Barrett, Bliss-Moreau, & Russell, 2006; Barrett et al., 2007; Fugate et al., 2010; Gendron, Lindquist, Barsalou, & Barrett, 2012). For example, you might experience yourself as angry or see another person's face as angry (or experience a dog's behavior as angry), but anger does not exist independently of your perception of it.

From this perspective, Cartesian questions that tend to guide a natural kinds approach do not apply. This is not to say that emotions are not real or not worth studying: They are, but measuring facial muscle movements, vocal acoustics, cardiovascular responses, hormones, or neurotransmitters alone cannot reveal them (cf. Barrett, 2012).[2] Therefore, this approach leads us to ask a different set of questions. Rather than asking whether an animal (or person) has an emotion, we should first ask: What are the elemental building blocks of emotion, and how do they come together in different ways depending on the cognitive architecture and environmental conditions of the organism? Only once we have identified what is necessary for the creation of a psychological construct that is ontologically subjective might we begin to ask whether other species have these abilities and whether the end product, an emotion, is the same as it is for humans. This is the approach I take in this chapter. Of course, many other evolutionary accounts exist, some that treat emotions as natural kinds, and others that do not. Even among those evolutionary accounts that treat emotions as constructed, none emphasize the cognitive architecture and functioning that is needed to understand emotion as an ontologically subjective category.[3]

In the first section of this chapter, I look at how language both supports and creates ontologically subjective categories, such as emotion. As part of this section, I question whether language is necessary for emotion and outline what I think are some more primitive "building blocks" of the mental life that includes emotion: (1) analogical reasoning, (2) shared mental states, and (3) causal inference. In the second section, I summarize the extent to which these "building blocks" for mental life exist in other species (mainly nonhuman primates). In the third section, I look briefly at some neural and structural changes during the evolution of the primate brain that may subserve these skills. Finally, I suggest what the end product of these building blocks, "emotion," may look like in other species.

Language Helps to Create and Support Emotion Categories

> Concepts that take on the garb of language seem to acquire a life of their own; thus we talk about ideas, we talk about concepts. . . . But we often forget that these things are "talk." We forget that it is we who have labeled some behaviors memory, learning, and other perception. We perceive some patterns of behavior that we can characterize as having common elements, and we give those patterns a name. . . . We come to believe then that because these patterns have a name, they are more than behaviors.
>
> —SAVAGE-RUMBAUGH, SHANKER, AND TAYLOR (1998, p. 226)

The Role of Language in Ontologically Subjective Categories

The idea that language plays a role in the development and instantiation of ontologically subjective categories, such as emotion, comes from two major sources. The first is the role that words play in how children acquire abstract categories more broadly. Words help highlight commonalities between objects that share few perceptual or structural features (Balaban & Waxman, 1997; Ferry, Hespos, & Waxman, 2010; Fulkerson & Waxman, 2007; Waxman & Booth, 2003). Along these lines, words have also been called "invitations" to form new categories (Waxman & Markow, 1995) and "essence placeholders" to categorize new objects as a certain kind (Dewar & Xu, 2009; Xu, 2000; Xu, Cote, & Baker, 2005).

Emotion words likely act similarly to how object names anchor abstract categories: Every time an emotion word is applied or made explicit, diverse patterns of behavior, physiology, and brain activity are made into meaningful categories. That is, emotion words serve as a "conceptual glue," creating a kind of statistical regularity (Barrett, 2006a, 2006b; Barrett et al., Chapter 4, this volume; for reviews of how words anchor emotion categories, see Barrett et al., 2007; Fugate, 2013; Lindquist & Gendron, 2013). Several lines of research are consistent with the role language plays in the perception of emotion categories. For example, limiting or restricting access to emotion words reduces people's agreement about whether two faces match in emotion, and their ability to characterize the faces into discrete categories (Gendron et al., 2012; Lindquist et al., 2006; Roberson & Davidoff, 2000; Roberson, Damjanovic, & Pilling, 2007). Giving people emotion words or using emotion words as primes facilitates both types of judgments (Fugate et al., 2010; Fugate & Barrett, 2014). For additional references and ways in which words ground emotion categories, I direct the reader to the chapter by Barrett and colleagues (Chapter 4, this volume).

The second source supporting the idea that language plays a role in the development and instantiation of ontologically subjective categories comes from its role in developing a *theory of mind*, which is broadly defined as the ability to attribute mental states (Premack & Woodruff, 1978). Several related capacities have been identified as parts of a theory of mind, including gaze monitoring, joint attention, mirror self-recognition, goal-based behavior (intentionality), knowledge states, and manipulation of knowledge (false beliefs). The false-belief task is one such theory of mind test typically given to children (Wimmer & Perner, 1983). In this test, children are often asked what someone else believes based on whether or not that person was present for some new source of information. In one such study, deaf children, who had not learned a signed language, were delayed in performing this task (Peterson & Siegal, 2000). In another study, children given linguistic training performed the task earlier than children who were not given such training (Lohmann & Tomasello, 2003). Nicaraguan deaf individuals who had learned a nascent version of sign language (deplete of mental state verbs) did not pass the false-belief task, whereas deaf signers in subsequent generations (in which such terms were included) were able to pass the test (Pyers & Senghas, 2009). The role of language in the development of cognition, specifically on the ability to construct and use a theory of mind, is due in part to a resurgence of the Whorfian hypothesis, which states that the language a person speaks creates (or at least shapes) a person's thinking about the world (Whorf, 1956). A thorough review of how language affects thought outside of its role in creating emotion is beyond the scope of this chapter, but I refer the interested reader to books by Gentner (Gentner & Goldin-Meadow, 2003) and Levinson and colleagues (Gumperz & Levinson, 1996; Levinson, 2003).

Is Language Necessary for Emotion?: Breaking Down Language into Primitive Cognitive Abilities

Analogical Reasoning

For humans who communicate via language, words serve as symbols that anchor perceptually ill-defined categories. In fact, it is the way in which these symbols are arranged (i.e., syntax) that allows for the type of relational thinking required to speak and understand a language.

Whereas the data suggest that language is important for humans to create and maintain ontologically subjective categories, from an evolutionary perspective, we might question whether language is necessary. Perhaps the cognitive skills necessary for language are sufficient by themselves. In the absence of words, an organism would need some other way to anchor categories whose members lack structural regularities or defining perceptual features.[4] An organism must not only have a way to ground these categories, but also this way must serve as a relational device from which information can be organized at a higher level. Having and using such relational devices is the key to forming and using analogies, a skill called *analogical reasoning*. I believe that analogical reasoning is a necessary building block of language. From an evolutionary perspective, then, we might ask do other species engage in analogical reasoning?

Mental State Sharing

In order for an ontologically subjective category to exist, people must collectively agree and make a declaration about its existence (Searle, 1995). I believe that a key part of making such a collective declaration is that those involved in its inception must be able to share and understand their own and others' mental states. From an evolutionary perspective, then, we might ask do other species have an understanding of others' minds, and to what extent do they engage in mental state sharing? Most of the comparative empirical and theoretical research on mental state sharing has been conducted under the larger heading of "social intelligence" (Byrne & Whiten, 1988) and has drawn its empirical claims from tasks requiring a "mind-reading system" (see Baron-Cohen, 1995), which fall under the construct of a theory of mind. For the purposes of this chapter, I focus on two such abilities for mental state sharing: joint attention and false beliefs.

Causal Inference

Finally, ontologically subjective categories exist as explanatory mechanisms that fit a group's folk psychology of how things should function (Searle, 1995). These categories have the capacity to impose functions on objects and people that are not based solely on the nature of their physical properties. For example, a dollar bill does not derive its function (as money) from its molecular structure; rather, a dollar bill acquires value when individuals agree that it can be traded for material goods. Once an ontologically subjective category is agreed upon, its "essence" is established and it becomes very real. The category, by virtue of its newly recognized essence, becomes a "stand in" for the process and commitment. The result is that the category itself takes on the process and a causal mechanism is either revealed or inferred by those engaged in the use of the category. It is the very reason why to us, as humans, emotions seem like *natural kinds* with essences and predictable relationships (see Barrett, 2006a, 2006b, 2009, 2012). From an evolutionary perspective we might ask what is the evidence that other species recognize and use hypothetical or hidden forces as the basis of categorization? Addressing these questions will begin to provide us the answer about the perception and experience of emotion in other species.

The Cognitive System on a Continuum: Evidence for Three Primitive Cognitive Abilities across Species

Analogical Reasoning

Analogical reasoning is most often tested with either relational or same-different tasks.[5] Many nonhuman species (including bees, pigeons, parrots, and several species of monkeys and apes) have been shown to perform relational and same–different tasks (for detailed reviews, see Penn, Holyoak, & Povinelli, 2008; Thompson & Oden, 2000). Many questions, however, have been raised about whether these tests actually require that the individual understands *sameness* and *difference* as abstract concepts that are (1) independent of a particular stimulus and (2) available to serve as a basis for higher-order inferences in a systematic fashion (see Penn et al., 2008; Thompson & Oden, 2000). That is, do individuals who perform these tests understand these concepts symbolically and, furthermore, do they engage in relational use of these symbols? Many researchers have been quick to point out that the success of an organism to pass these tests can be explained more parsimoniously by *chunking* or *segmentation* (Halford, Wilson, & Phillips, 1998), such that an animal can evaluate the variability within a pair and apply a straightforward rule to select the appropriate choice (Cook & Wasserman, 2006; Young & Wasserman, 1997; Fagot, Wasserman, & Young, 2001; see discussion in Penn et al., 2008; but also see Premack, 2010). Such a rule may look like this: If the variability within the pair is *low*, then select the choice with the *low* variability. For example, let's assume that a Fruit Loop and a Cheerio serve as the basis for the category *same*. An individual is then asked to identify whether a broom and a stick have a similar relationship. This only requires an individual to select an answer based on whether or not the two objects for comparison are as physically similar as the Fruit Loop and Cheerio (in the case of a *same* answer). An answer does not require that the individual understand that the individual items or the relationship can be based on a more abstract level of categorization (e.g., food vs. tool).

True analogical reasoning would require that an individual is able to *extract a general rule* that can be applied to not only novel instances but also instances in which there is asymmetry among the variability (Premack, 1976, 1983a, 1983b). Thompson and Oden (2000) describe such a rule in the following way: Given *AA* as the anchor, an individual would have to compare *A* to *A* and encode as "identity (*I*)." Then it would have to compare the individual members in two choices (*BB* and *EF*). In doing so, the individual would need to encode *BB* as "identity (*I*)" and *EF* as "nonidentity (*NI*)." Last, the individual would have to compare the two choices with the anchor: *I* & *I* = *same*; *I* & *NI* = *different* and *NI* & *NI*

= *same*. As a result, the individual would have learned a relationship that involved a symbolic understanding of the relationship between items. This is in fact what humans do when they use their language to compare items on abstract, or perceptually ill-defined, criteria (Genter, 1983; Genter & Markman, 1997; Holyoak & Thagard, 1997; Premack, 1983a, 1983b).

The evidence for this type of more formal analogical reasoning is sparse among other species. In fact, the only compelling demonstration comes from Sarah, a language-trained chimpanzee. Once Sarah had acquired the symbols for "same" and "different," she was able to judge the functional relationship between padlock/keys and can/cap opener (Gillan, Premack, & Woodruff, 1981; Oden, Thompson, & Premack, 2001; Premack, 1988). Although learning a symbol seemed to have a surprising effect on Sarah's ability to use analogical reasoning, similar results have also been achieved by extensively training chimpanzees on like and unlike relationships (300+ trials; Premack, 1988). The key difference is that chimpanzees do not show analogical reasoning in the absence of symbolic learning or extensive training. Human children, on the other hand, show the ability as young as age 10 months (Chen, Sanchez, & Campbell, 1997).

What seems to be the case is that many species are able to discriminate among a variety of items whose perceptual features vary. Many species are able to solve similar problems with new exemplars (i.e., learn a rule). In fact, the ability to discriminate accurately among items and respond appropriately to changes is the basis of successful learning and survival. Some species may even be able to extend knowledge from one domain to another or show more flexible rule use. There is limited empirical evidence, however, that, in the absence of language (or symbolic training) or extensive training, an individual is capable of encoding relationships at a higher level at which the rule transcends perceptual features and can be used flexibly.

Other researchers have similarly noted that analogical reasoning may be a watershed in the evolution of cognition. Penn and colleagues (2008, p. 127) proposed the *relational reinterpretation hypothesis*, in which they say that human and nonhuman minds differ in their ability to reinterpret relationships into rule-governed relationships.[6] Consistent with this view, it seems that learning a language or a symbolic token system removes the bias that animals inherently have to match perceptually and instead allows them to respond using an abstract code (see also Premack, 1983b). Deacon (1997) suggests that symbolic learning allows for a "freeing" or "unlinking" of relationships between otherwise obvious relationships.

Mental State Sharing

Another key ability in the creation and use of an ontologically subjective category is that an individual can engage with others in this process. Although some beliefs are individual and personal, other beliefs are shared despite individual differences. A key part of this sharing is based on an understanding of how minds work. A large amount of research has examined whether nonhuman species are capable of "mind sharing" and possess the skills needed for a theory of mind. Two of these are joint attention and false belief (for a more thorough review, see Penn et al., 2008). The evidence suggests that many species, not just nonhuman primates, are capable of gaze monitoring and joint attention (e.g., Povinelli & Eddy, 1996; Call, Hare, & Tomasello, 1998; Miklosi, Polgardi, Topal, & Csanyi, 1998; Hare & Tomasello, 1999). For example, not only chimpanzees but also capuchin monkeys show differential requesting behavior that varies with respect to a human's attentional state (e.g., Hattori, Kuroshima, & Fujita, 2007; Hattori, Tomonaga, & Fujita, 2011; Hostetter, Russell, Freeman, & Hopkins, 2007; Kaminski, Call, & Tomasello, 2008; Povinelli & Eddy, 1996). Some nonhuman primate species, such as chimpanzees, are also fairly good at understanding what another knows and does not know (knowledge–ignorance), but they do not appear to understand that others' beliefs can differ from their own (false-beliefs).[7] For example, chimpanzees will avoid pursuing a piece of food that they believe can be seen by another (more dominant) individual in preference for a piece of food outside the other's view (Hare, Call, Agnetta, & Tomasello, 2000; Hare, Call, & Tomasello, 2001). They do not, however, change their strategy when they witness that the more dominant individual has not seen the food being moved elsewhere; that is, the chimpanzees do not appear to take advantage of the competitor's likely false belief (cf. Kaminski et al., 2008). Human children have been shown to perform the false-belief task as early as age 2.5 years (He, Bolz, & Baillargeon, 2011). As a result, a fully developed theory of mind does not seem to be present even in our closest ancestors. Interestingly, but beyond the focus of this chapter, is that other large-brained, socially living animals may have more complex knowledge of others' false beliefs than do nonhuman primates (e.g., bootlenose dolphins, Tomonaga, Uwano, Ogura, & Saito, 2010; Xitco, Gory, & Kuczaj, 2004).

Inferring Causation

Most individuals of other species are apt problem solvers and show a great ability to learn from trial and error and from experiential learning, especially when motivated by a biological drive such as food. In these instances, individuals discover contingencies about their behavior and the likelihood of obtaining an outcome. Such contingencies are at the heart of understanding cause and effect. There is well-documented evidence that several species of monkeys, chimpanzees, and corvids can learn simple cause-and-effect contingencies, such as into which end of a tube a stick should be inserted to bypass a trap in order to obtain food (Visalberghi & Limongelli, 1994;

Mulcahy & Call, 2006; Povinelli, 2000; Seed, Tebbich, Emery, & Clayton, 2006). Yet when experimenters turn the tube upside down, making the trap nonfunctional, individuals do not show flexibility in their responding. That is, they continue to engage in the more effortful, learned behavior. They do not show evidence that they understand the forces of gravity, and that gravity does not apply when the tube is rotated so that the trap is irrelevant (Visalberghi & Limongelli, 1994; see also Cacchione & Call, 2010). On the other hand, even human infants are not surprised when a moving object goes behind a barrier and comes out the other side (Aguiar & Baillargeon, 1999).

A special type of cause-and-effect understanding involves ascribing hypothetical forces, such as causal mechanisms, in the absence of any. This is known as inferred causation. Many of the folk categories we have as humans involve inferred causation and explain why ontologically subjective categories (e.g., emotion) seem as if they must be real. Humans appear to be unique in that we also prioritize causal information over perceptual content or physical forces in forming categories (e.g., Lien & Cheng, 2000; Waldmann & Holyoak, 1992). There is no compelling demonstration that other nonhuman species do this regularly. People also reason about unseen forces, invent their own theories about how the world works, distinguish between real and spurious causes, reason diagnostically, and intuit theories (Hagmayer & Waldmann, 2004; Lien & Cheng, 2000; Saxe, Tannebaum, & Carey, 2005; Waldmann & Holyoak, 1992). They are the basis for our superstitions and religion and scientific thinking (see Bloom, 2012; Gelman & Legare, 2011). Although many species show a great ability to learn and navigate their environments, learn contingencies, and perhaps even possess a rudimentary understanding of cause and effect, there is little evidence that other species besides our own make such elaborate inferences about causation or hypothetical forces.

Summary

In summary, many species (not just nonhuman primates) are capable of relational matching based on first- and second-order instances (see Thompson & Oden, 2000; Penn et al., 2008). Yet there is very little evidence to suggest that other species (except apes trained to use symbols) extract more general rules from second-order relationships so that the items/instances can be appreciated at a higher level. I have argued that analogical reasoning of this sort is necessary to create emotion categories for which there exist no diagnostic or predictive features (or for which features do not share any perceptual similarity). Analogical reasoning by itself, however, is not sufficient for such categories. I have argued that ontologically subjective categories also involve sharing mental states (e.g., for the concept of *anger* to be useful it should allow an organism to perceive *anger* in a conspecific or individual from another species). Although many species engage in joint attention, it seems as if not even our closest living ancestors are able to engage in the most complex abilities underlying a theory of mind, including understanding another's false beliefs. Finally, emotion categories also require an attribution of an underlying cause (since emotions are not the elicitors or consequence of behavior). Although some nonhuman species understand simple cause-and-effect contingencies, there is no evidence that they understand hypothetical or unseen forces, or use them to infer causation.

Language as Product and Instigator of Change in the Brain

The relationship between thought and language is highly debated and contentious from both an evolutionary and a theoretical view (for a review of different theories, see Christensen, 2001). Perhaps most plausible is a view that is bidirectional, in which language required certain cognitive changes in order to develop, but once in place also altered the cognitive system. Deacon (1997) calls the relationship between language and cognition a "coevolution," in which symbol acquisition resulted in a back-and-forth escalation for greater development of the prefrontal cortex (PFC), more efficient articulatory and auditory capacities, and probably a suite of other ancillary capacities that in turn eased the acquisition and use of language. That is, language (and the abilities that underlie it) likely amplified a difference in the cognitive system that already existed in a shared common ancestor between great apes and humans (Premack, 1988). In the next paragraphs, I review some of the key changes in the evolution of brain structure, connectivity, and function that support this idea. Many of these changes are in brain regions that have been identified as part of the "neural reference space" that underlies the mental activity necessary for emotion experience and perception (see Barrett et al., Chapter 4, and Oosterwijk et al., Chapter 5, this volume; Barrett & Satpute, 2013; Kober et al., 2008; Lindquist et al., 2012).

Changes in Structure

Primates have many cortical areas that have no obvious counterparts in small-brain mammals, including those species that are evolutionary related to primates (e.g., shrews and bats). These regions include the higher-order sensory areas and higher-order association areas (dorsolateral PFC [dlPFC] and posterior parietal and inferotemporal cortex; Allman, 1977; Kaas, 1987; Preuss, 1995, 2007; Preuss & Kaas, 1999). Within the Primate order, the dlPFC is less developed in nonhumans than in humans (Preuss, 1995; Wise, 2008). The dlPFC is important in alternative interpretations and alternative scenario constructions and flexible behavioral responding (Passingham, Toni, & Rushworth, 2000; for a review, see Bunge et al., 2005). All of these tasks require using information "against itself" in ways that require shifting attention and directing action to alternative responding. These skills are instrumental to analogical reasoning because they all involve the "freeing" of constraints associated with obvious responding/associations (for a more thorough evolutionary discussion, see Deacon, 1997). The dlPFC is part of the executive attention network in the neural workspace of brain activity, which is important for deciding whether to attend to sensations in the body or to those from external factors (see Kober et al., 2008; Lindquist et al., 2012; Lindquist & Barrett, 2012; Oosterwijk et al., Chapter 5, this volume; Oosterwijk et al., 2012).

Portions of the PFC, but not the entire frontal lobe, became disproportionally large as hominins evolved. The lateral PFC accounts for approximately 29% of neocortex in humans, but only 17% in chimpanzees (Preuss, 1993). In addition, parts of the orbitofrontal cortex (OFC; (specifically, Brodmann area [BA] 13) are slightly smaller than expected in humans, whereas the ventral and dorsomedial PFC (specifically, BA 10) and the medial anterior cingulate cortex (ACC) are slightly larger in humans than would be expected based on body size (Schenker, Desgouttes, & Semendeferi, 2005; Semendeferi, Armstrong, Schleicher, Ziles, & van Hoesen, 2001). The OFC is a heteromodal association area that integrates sensory inputs from the body and the external world to help create a multimodal representation of the present (Mesulam, 2000). It also plays a role in the detection of threat and reward and hedonic evaluation, including contribution (along with other brain areas) to the experience of pleasure (e.g., Kringelbach & Rolls, 2004; Kringelbach & Berridge, Chapter 10, this volume). The medial and lateral parts of the OFC have been identified as part of the visceromotor network in the neural reference space, which is important for the generation of core affect (see Barrett & Bliss-Moreau, 2009; Lindquist et al., 2012; Kober et al., 2008).

Changes in Connectivity and Function

Most subdivisions of the lateral PFC have strong connections with higher-order parietal and temporal regions (including posterior parietal [PP], inferior temporal [IT], and superior temporal sulcus [STS]). That is, as brains enlarged throughout evolution, they did not minimize the length of all connections (i.e., they did not necessarily become more modular). Rather they retained some very long connections that serve as "shortcuts" to distant regions (Streidter, 2005). As the neocortex became more interconnected, it became more capable of influencing the activity of other regions (Streidter, 2005). As a result, instead of parallel distributed processing, brains evolved more serial circuits arranged hierarchically (Streidter, 2005). For example, in primates, portions of the ventromedial PFC (including parts of BA 10 and portions of the ACC) project directly to the hypothalamus and brainstem (Barbas, Saha, Rempel-Clower, & Ghashghaei, 2003; Ongur & Price, 2000), whereas other parts of the orbital sector have direct connections to these regions through the amygdala and striatum (Amaral, Price, Pitkanen, & Carmichael, 1992; Ghashghaei & Barbas, 2002). In both cases, these connections are not present in other nonprimate mammalian species, such as rats, and suggest a reorganization of connectivity. A likely result is that such connections allowed for a richer conceptualization of internal bodily and external sensory information leading to a more flexible arrangement of behavioral outcomes (see Barrett et al., 2007).

The arcuate fasciculus also shows notable changes in its projections among human and nonhuman primates (Rilling et al., 2007). Humans have more and stronger terminations extending from the arcuate posteriorly in the medial and inferior temporal gyrus, as well as anteriorly in the pars orbitalis (BA 47). This suggests that the frontal cortex of the left hemisphere is more strongly connected with the medial and inferior temporal lobe and includes more connections ventral and anterior to Wernicke's area in humans. In macaques, this area is mainly extrastriate cortex, whereas in humans it is known for processing word meaning (Rilling & Seligman, 2002).

Although areas BA 44 and 45 (including Broca's area) are structurally homologous among primate species, they most likely have undergone a function change to become associated with speech production in humans (Preuss, 2007). In addition, humans show a lateralized asymmetry in Broca's area that is not present in the chimpanzee brain (Preuss, 2011). Interestingly, however, humans and chimpanzees have a similar structural asymmetry in the planum temporale (which includes Wernicke's area and shows significant activation when listening to speech; Gannon, Holloway, Broadfield, & Braun, 1998). Microstructure differences between chimpanzees and humans, such as the lateralization of the minicolumns in the planum temporale, however, have been noted (Buxhoeveden, Switala, Litaker, Roy, & Casanova, 2001).

Finally, there are notable changes in the activity of what has been called the "default network" of the brain (Raichle et al., 2001) among human and nonhuman primates. The "default network" comprises a large network of areas and shows ample activity when an individual is at rest (Rilling et al., 2007; see Yeo et al., 2011 for a recent review). It has been implicated in a variety of tasks ranging from theory of mind to autobiographical memory, to moral reasoning, to representations of the self, and to mental projection.

The default network has been described as part of the neural workspace important for categorization, which is important for making meaning of sensory and bodily information and for the situated conceptualizations that underlie the category learning (Barrett et al., Chapter 4, and Ooster-wijk et al., Chapter 5, this volume; Lindquist & Barrett, 2012; Lindquist et al., 2012). A comparison of the underlying activity of this network showed that chimpanzees at rest, like humans, have high levels of activity in the network especially in the rostrolateral and dlPFC (Rilling et al., 2007). Humans, however, show more activity in dorsal areas of the medial PFC (BAs 9 and 32), whereas chimpanzees show more distributed activity (in the homologue of BA 10). Moreover, humans have strongly left-lateralized activity throughout the network, whereas chimpanzees do not show a high degree of lateralization. Given that monkeys also show a fair degree of activity of the default network at rest (Vincent et al., 2007) it is likely that these areas in the human brain may have undergone a change in function.

Summary

This limited look at some of the connective and anatomical changes that occurred in the brain during hominid evolution suggest that the brain underwent not only major enlargement but also major reorganization and massive changes in connectivity during the last 6 million or so years since chimpanzees and modern day humans shared a common ancestor. I direct the interested reader to Preuss (2011) for a more detailed review of brain evolution.

What Do "Emotions" in Other Species Look Like?

> "Many animals hide but don't know they are hiding.
> Many animals flock but don't think they are flocking."
> —DENNETT (1996, p. 119)

All organisms (at least those with a centralized nervous system) experience an ongoing array of bodily sensations and sensory input. These moment-to-moment bodily sensations, often called "core affect," can generally be described along two dimensions: valence (i.e., what is pleasant vs. unpleasant) and arousal (i.e., what is highly vs. lowly arousing) (Barrett & Russell, 1999; Russell, 2003, this volume).[8] Core affect is considered to be evolutionary conserved and likely biologically hardwired, and is a key force in deciding whether and how fast an organism will approach or avoid a stimulus (see Barrett & Bliss-Moreau, 2009). Most organisms derive action immediately from core affect through innate or learned behavioral contingencies from past associations (in which categorization is not necessary). Some species might situate the same changes in core affect into categories that provide an added layer of meaning and behavioral flexibility. For many of these species, such categories exist solely along perceptual lines (i.e., they are defined by structural regularities). For others, categories are more complex, blurring perceptual lines, and are defined by more abstract behavioral contingencies. And some species situate changes in core affect (along with incoming sensory information) into categories that exist only at a level of abstraction that is truly symbolic and reflects an underlying societal need to figure out how things work.

In this chapter I have argued that the category of emotion is this last type of category. These categories require a conceptual system capable of analogical reasoning, mental state sharing, and inferred causation. Most organisms, however, do not possess the cognitive capabilities to place and flexibly assign their core affect (in the case of emotion experience) or another's core affect (in the case of emotion perception) into different mental categories that allow for relationships among category members. Most organisms do not postulate causal mechanisms or understand that another can possess false beliefs. If we require these cognitive capabilities in order to construct an emotion, then we should conclude that animals without such capabilities do not have emotion in the way defined herein.

This is not to say, however, that nonhuman animals do not feel pain or that they are incapable of using sensory information in biological and adaptive ways. It also does not preclude an individual from using past experiences in its behavioral choices. For most species, there is little need to intuit a causal mechanism or infer causation because the relationship between features is a good predictor given certain circumstances. Relationships, in this case, are based on contingency and/or correlation (see Deacon, 1997). As long as an animal has no obligation or opportunity to communicate about its behaviors (or mental states), then there is no direct selective pressure for the cognitive abilities underlying ontologically subject categories to evolve (see also Dennett, 1996). Said another way, each species evolved in its own ümwelt and is a sui generis for its niche (von Uexküll, 1926; see also Lorenz, 1981; Tinbergen, 1951).

Other researchers have suggested views similar to the one I am advancing here. For example, LeDoux (2012) suggests to the extent that the mechanisms of consciousness and cognition exist, *feelings* (by which I infer him to mean *emotion*) will differ between animals that possess those brain structures and capabilities and those that do not. He goes on to say that different levels of consciousness may be present among different animals, but that without language, an animal would not be able to experience or perceive specific emotions (fear, anger, sadness, etc.). Russell (Chapter 17, this volume) outlines a similar position when he says some organisms can direct their core affect *at* something, meaning they can link a change in core affect to a cause. But whether an animal is capable of such will depend on the cognitive abilities of the species. Furthermore, Russell states that emotion (at least the meta-experience) is a psychologically constructed state that might require language and therefore be limited to humans (Russell, Chapter 17, this volume).

Conclusion

In this chapter I have argued that viewing emotions as ontologically subjective categories, rather than as *natural kinds*, sets a new scientific agenda for discovery. From this perspective, it makes better sense to ask questions about process rather than existence. If we can identify the cognitive abilities which are necessary for the creation of a psychological construct that is ontologically subjective, then we might begin to investigate their existence in other animals, and whether the end product, an emotion, is the same as it is for humans.[9]

In this chapter, I have indentified three such abilities: analogical reasoning, mental state sharing, and inferring causation. I have argued that these abilities are likely unique among symbolically trained or linguistic animals. This is not to say that animals without symbolic abilities or language training do not have categories. Rather it is to say that they have different categories than those which do. In the former case, these categories are likely based on stable relationships, predictability, or structural similarities among category members. This does not make them any less interesting or less successful; it just makes them different than those we as humans use so readily—those categories on which we build societies, teach our young, and cause theoretical debates which we struggle to objectively study.

I have also laid the groundwork to show that although most nonhuman animals do not have the necessary cognitive capabilities for the skills that are required for an emotion, there may be a small subset that do (e.g., great apes and possibly other large-brained, socially living animals, such as dolphins and elephants—admittedly neglected in this chapter). Furthermore, we can use my framework to emphasize the cognitive capabilities an organism possesses as a way to understand how different end products (e.g., emotion) are created from similar underlying and shared processes (e.g., core affect).

ACKNOWLEDGMENTS

I would like to thank Lisa Feldman Barrett and members of the Interdisciplinary Affective Science Laboratory for insightful discussion and feedback on these ideas, including comments on an early version of this chapter. I would also like to thank Jim Russell for his comments and editorial feedback.

NOTES

1. Darwin's systematic analysis of similarities in facial displays was intended to provide evidence for his theory of evolution rather than to explain the emotional experience of animals. For example, Darwin noted that similarities in the appearance of expressions suggest a similar ancestor. Such similarities say nothing, however, about their function or utility in humans. The idea that these similarities in appearance underlie a universal set of emotions (in which each emotion is represented by a dedicated circuit in the brain) was set forth and written about by later theorists in the late 1800s and early 1900s and more recently by Tomkins, Ekman, Izard, and Panksepp (for a historical review, see Gendron & Barrett, 2009). Despite this, most "basic" theorists cite Darwin as the academic father of this view.

2. According to this view, the "emotional circuits" that have been well-detailed in the animal research literature represent the basis for a few, very specific survival behaviors (e.g., *freezing* or *unconditioned threat*). They do not, however, represent the neuroanatomical basis that is inclusive of all instances of the category of emotion (or any specific emotion) or the experiential feeling of emotion (or any specific emotion) (see Barrett, 2006a, 2006b; 2009, 2011a, 2011b, 2012; Barrett et al., 2007; Barrett et al., Chapter 4, this volume; Lindquist & Barrett, 2012; Lindquist et al., 2012; Oosterwijk et al., Chapter 5, this volume). The circuits might also be better thought of as representing fixed action patterns, more specific and biologically inflexible responses, than as *behaviors* per se. A growing number of researchers who previously argued hard for emotional circuits in animals (e.g., see LeDoux, 2012) now accept this distinction.

3. Although many members of the Interdisciplinary Affective Science Laboratory were helpful to me in forming this evolutionary view, I would like to thank Lisa Feldman Barrett for pushing me to articulate the cognitive abilities necessary to create and use an ontologically subjective category like emotion.

4. A word anchors an ontologically subjective category with its phonological form.

5. In a typical same–different paradigm, subjects are asked to respond one way if two stimuli are the same and another way if they are different. In a relational matching paradigm, subjects are typically required to select a choice in which perceptual similarity among elements is the same as that within the sample; this is sometimes referred to as the ability to make relational comparisons (see Thompson & Oden, 2000).

6. According to their "relational reinterpretation hypothesis" (Penn et al., 2008), many species have perceptually grounded categories of the world and are able to use these categories in flexible decision making. Only humans, however, possess the additional capability of reinterpreting these perceptually grounded categories in terms of "higher-order, role-governed, inferentially systematic, explicitly structured relations" (p. 127).

7. Povinelli and Vonk (2003, 2004) have suggested that the current paradigms we have for testing theory of mind do not provide evidence that uniquely supports mental states (but see Tomasello, Call, & Hare, 2003a, 2003b). Specifically, Povinelli and Vonk suggest that theory of mind tests must meet two conditions to entertain mental states in addition to behavior: the cue on which the inferences to a mental state are based must be arbitrary, and there can be no exposure to the others' behaviors in association with that cue.

8. Many researchers use "core affect" or "affects" to refer to more basic and less differentiated states of *feelings* (Panksepp, 1998, 2005; Damasio, 1994, 1999).

9. Identifying these abilities, however, is only part of the picture. How these abilities scaffold one another, and how the brain implements them in both space and time, is another issue (see Cunningham, Dunfield, & Stillman, Chapter 7, this volume). Even elemental theories, in which the final product contains the individual components, must first identify the underlying abilities. Emergent theories (i.e., in which individual components can no longer be identified) propose an additional challenge and additional level of complexity that is beyond the scope of this chapter.

REFERENCES

Aguiar, A., & Baillargeon, R. (1999). 2.5-month-old infants' reasoning about when objects should and should not be occluded. *Cognitive Psychology, 39*, 116–157.

Allman, J. M. (1977). Evolution of the visual system in early primates. In J. M. Sprague & A. N. Epstein (Eds.), *Progress in psychology and physiological psychology* (pp. 1–53). New York: Academic Press.

Allport, F. H. (1924). *Social psychology*. New York: Houghton Mifflin.

Amaral, D. G., Price, J. L., Pitkanen, A., & Carmichael, S. T. (1992). Anatomical organization of the primate amygdaloid complex. In J. P. Aggleton (Ed.), *The amygdala* (pp. 1–67). New York: Wiley-Liss.

Arnold, M. B. (1960a). *Emotion and personality: Vol. 1. Psychological aspects*. New York: Columbia University Press.

Arnold, M. B. (1960b). *Emotion and personality: Vol. 2. Physiological aspects*. New York: Columbia University Press.

Balaban, M. T., & Waxman, S. R. (1997). Do words facilitate object recognition in 9 month olds? *Journal of Experimental Child Psychology, 64*, 3–26.

Barbas, H., Saha, S., Rempel-Clower, N., & Ghashghaei, T. (2003). Serial pathways for primate prefrontal cortex to autonomic areas may influence emotional expressions. *BMC Neuroscience, 10*, 4–25.

Barrett, L. F. (2006a). Emotions as natural kinds? *Perspectives on Psychological Science, 1,* 28–58.

Barrett, L. F. (2006b). Solving the emotion paradox: Categorization and the experience of emotion. *Personality and Social Psychology Review, 10,* 20–46.

Barrett, L. F. (2009). The future of psychology: Connecting mind to brain. *Perspectives on Psychological Science, 4,* 326–339.

Barrett, L. F. (2011a). Constructing emotion. *Psychological Topics, 3,* 359–380.

Barrett, L. F. (2011b). Was Darwin wrong about emotional expressions? *Current Directions in Psychological Science, 20,* 400–406.

Barrett, L. F. (2012). Emotions are real. *Emotion, 12,* 413–429.

Barrett, L. F., & Bliss-Moreau, E. (2009). Affect as a psychological primitive. *Advances in Experimental Social Psychology, 41,* 167–218.

Barrett, L. F., Lindquist, K., & Gendron, M. (2007). Language as context for the perception of emotion. *Trends in Cognitive Science, 11,* 327–332.

Barrett, L. F., & Russell, J. A. (1999). Structure of current affect. *Current Directions in Psychological Science, 8,* 10–14.

Barrett, L. F., & Satpute, A. (2013). Large-scale brain networks in affective and social neuroscience: Towards an integrative architecture of the human brain. *Current Opinion in Neurobiology, 23,* 361–372.

Baron-Cohen, S. (1995). *Mindblindness.* Cambridge, MA: MIT Press.

Bloom, P. (2012). Religion, morality, evolution. *Annual Review of Psychology, 63,* 179–199.

Bunge, S. A., Wallis, J. D., Parker, A., Brass, M., Crone, E. A., Hoshi, E., et al. (2005). Neural circuitry underlying rule use in humans and nonhuman primates. *Journal of Neuroscience, 25,* 10347–10350.

Buxhoeveden, D. P., Switala, A. E., Litaker, M., Roy, E., & Casanova, M. F. (2001). Lateralization of minicolumns in human planum temporale is absent in nonhuman primate cortex. *Brain and Behaviorial Evolution, 57,* 349–358.

Byrne, R. W., & Whiten, A. (1988). *Machiavellian intelligence: Social expertise and the evolution of intellect in monkeys, apes, and humans.* Oxford, UK: Oxford University Press.

Cacchione, T., & Call, J. (2010). Intuitions about gravity and solidity in great apes: The tubes task. *Developmental Science, 13,* 320–330.

Call, J., Hare, B., & Tomasello, M. (1998). Chimpanzee gaze following in an object choice task. *Animal Cognition, 1,* 89–100.

Chen, Z., Sanchez, R. P., & Campbell, T. (1997). Analogical transfer of problem-solving abilities in children. *Trends in Cognitive Science, 12,* 187–192.

Christensen, K. R. (2001). The co-evolution of language and the brain: A review of two contrastive views (Pinker & Deacon). *Grazer Linguistische Studien, 55,* 1–20.

Cook, R. G., & Wasserman, E. A. (2006). Relational discrimination learning in pigeons. In E. A. Wasserman & T. R. Zentall (Eds.), *Comparative cognition: Experimental explorations in animal intelligence* (pp. 307–324). New York: Oxford University Press.

Damasio, A. R. (1994). *Descartes' error: Emotion, reason, and the human brain.* New York: Gosset/Putnam.

Damasio, A. R. (1999). *The feeling of what happens: Body and emotion in the making of consciousness*. New York: Harcourt Brace.

Darwin, C. (1872). *The expression of the emotions in man and animals*. London: Fontana Press.

Deacon, T. W. (1997). *The symbolic species: The co-evolution of language and the brain*. New York: Norton.

Dennett, D. (1996). *Kinds of minds: Toward an understanding of consciousness*. New York: Basic Books.

Dewar, K., & Xu, F. (2009). Do early nouns refer to kinds or distinct shapes?: Evidence from 10-month-old infants. *Psychological Science, 20*, 252–257.

Ekman, P., Friesen, W. V., & Ellsworth, P. (1972). *Emotion in the human face*. New York: Pergamon Press.

Ellsworth, P. C., & Scherer, K. R. (2003). Appraisal processes in emotion. In R. J. Davidson, K. R. Scherer, & H. H. Goldsmith (Eds.), *The handbook of affective science* (pp. 572–595). New York: Oxford University Press.

Fagot, J., Wasserman, E. A., & Young, M. E. (2001). Discriminating the relation between relations: The role of entropy in abstract conceptualization by baboons (*Papio papio*) and humans (*Homo sapiens*). *Journal of Experimental Psychology: Animal Behavior Processes, 27*, 316–328.

Ferry, A. L., Hespos, S. J., & Waxman, S. R. (2010). Categorization in 3- and 4-month-old infants: An advantage of words over tones. *Child Development, 81*, 472–479.

Frijda, N. H. (1986). *The emotions*. New York: Cambridge University Press.

Fugate, J. M. B. (2008). *Perception and classification of chimpanzee (pan troglodytes) facial expressions and vocalizations*. Unpublished dissertation, Emory University, Atlanta, GA.

Fugate, J. M. B. (2013). Categorical perception for emotional faces. *Emotion Review, 5*(1), 84–89.

Fugate, J. M. B., & Barrett, L. F. (2014). *Emotion words: Adding face value*. Manuscript in preparation.

Fugate, J. M. B., Gouzoules, H., & Barrett, L. F. (2010). Reading chimpanzee faces: A test of the structural and conceptual hypotheses. *Emotion, 10*, 544–554.

Fulkerson, A. L., & Waxman, S. R. (2007). Words (but not tones) facilitate object categorization: Evidence from 6- and 12-month olds. *Cognition, 105*, 218–228.

Gannon, P. J., Halloway, R. L., Broadfield, D. C., & Braun, A. R. (1998). Asymmetry of chimpanzees planum temporale: humanlike pattern of Wernicke's brain language area homolog. *Science, 279*, 220–222.

Gelman, S., & Legare, C. H. (2011). Concepts and folk theories. *Annual Review of Anthropology, 40*, 379–398.

Gendron, M., & Barrett, L. F. (2009). Reconstructing the past: A century of ideas about emotion in psychology. *Emotion Review, 1*, 1–24.

Gendron, M., Lindquist, K. L., Barsalou, L., & Barrett, L. F. (2012). Language helps construct emotional percepts. *Emotion, 12*, 314–325.

Gentner, D. (1983). Structure-mapping: A theoretical framework for analogy. *Cognitive Science, 7*, 155–170.

Gentner, D., & Goldin-Meadow, S. (2003). *Language in mind: Advances in the study of language and thought.* Cambridge, MA: MIT Press.

Gentner, D., & Markman, A. B. (1997). Structure mapping in analogy and similarity. *American Psychologist, 52,* 45–56.

Ghashghaei, H. T., & Barbas, H. (2002). Pathways for emotion: Interactions of prefrontal and temporal pathways in the amygdala of the rhesus monkey. *Neuroscience, 115,* 1261–1279.

Gillan, D. J., Premack, D., & Woodruff, G. (1981). Reasoning in the chimpanzee: I. Analogical reasoning. *Journal of Experimental Psychology: Animal Behavior Processes, 7,* 1–17.

Gumperz, J. J., & Levinson, S. J. (1996). *Rethinking linguistic relativity.* Cambridge, UK: Cambridge University Press.

Hagmayer, Y., & Waldmann, M. R. (2004). Seeing the unobservable: Inferring the probability and impact of hidden causes. In *Proceedings of the 26th annual conference of Cognitive Science Society* (pp. 523–528). Mahwah, NJ: Erlbaum.

Halford, G. S., Wilson, W. H., & Phillips, S. (1998). Processing capacity defined by relational complexity: Implications for comparative, developmental, and cognitive psychology. *Behavioral and Brain Sciences, 21,* 803–831.

Hare, B., Call, J., Agnetta, B., & Tomasello, M. (2000). Chimpanzees know what conspecifics do and do not see. *Animal Behaviour, 59,* 771–785.

Hare, B., Call, J., & Tomasello, M. (2001). Do chimpanzees know what conspecifics know? *Animal Behaviour, 61,* 771–785.

Hare, B., & Tomasello, M. (1999). Domestic dogs (*Canis familiaris*) use human and conspecific social cues to locate hidden food. *Journal of Comparative Psychology, 113,*173–177.

Hattori, Y., Kuroshima, H., & Fujita, K. (2007). I know you are not looking at me: Capuchin monkeys' (*Cebus apella*) sensitivity to human attentional states. *Animal Cognition, 10,* 141–148.

Hattori, Y., Tomonaga, M. & Fujita, K. (2011). Chimpanzees (*Pan troglodytes*) show more understanding of human attentional states when requesting food held by a human. *Animal Cognition, 12,* 418–429.

He, Z., Bolz, M., & Baillargeon, R. (2011). False-belief understanding in 2.5-year-olds: Evidence from violation-of-expectation change-of-location and unexpected-contents tasks. *Developmental Science, 14*(2), 292–305.

Holyoak, K. J., & Thagard, P. (1997). The analogical mind. *American Psychologist, 52,* 35–44.

Hostetter, A. B., Russell, J. L., Freeman, H., & Hopkins, W. D. (2007). Now you see me, now you don't: Evidence that chimpanzees understand the role of the eyes in attention. *Animal Cognition, 10,* 55–62.

Izard, C. E. (1971). *The face of emotion.* New York: Appleton-Century-Crofts.

Kaas, J. H. (1987). The organization and evolution of neocortex. In S. P. Wise (Ed.), *Higher brain function: Recent explorations of the brain's emergent properties* (pp. 347–378). New York: Wiley.

Kaminski, J., Call, J., & Tomasello, M. (2008). Chimpanzees know what others know, but not what they believe. *Cognition, 109,* 224–234.

Karnath, H.-O. (2001). New insights into the functions of the superior temporal cortex. *Nature Reviews Neuroscience, 2,* 568–576.

Kober, H., Barrett, L. F., Joseph, J., Bliss-Moreau, E., Lindquist, K. A., & Wager, T. D. (2008). Functional networks and cortical–subcortical interactions in emotion: A meta-analysis of neuroimaging studies. *NeuroImage, 42,* 998–1031.

Kringelbach, M. L., & Rolls, E. T. (2004). The functional neuroanatomy of the human orbitofrontal cortex: Evidence from neuroimaging and neuropsychology. *Progress in Neurobiology, 72,* 341–372.

Lazarus, R. S. (1991). *Emotion and adaptation.* New York: Oxford University Press.

LeDoux, J. (2012). Rethinking the emotional brain. *Neuron, 73,* 653–676.

Levinson, S. C. (2003). *Space in language and cognition: Explorations in cultural diversity.* Cambridge, UK: Cambridge University Press.

Lindquist, K. A., & Barrett, L. F. (2012). A functional architecture of the human brain: Emerging insights from the science of emotion. *Trends in Cognitive Sciences, 16,* 533–540.

Lindquist, K. A., Barrett, L. F., Bliss-Moreau, E., & Russell, J. (2006). Language and the perception of emotion. *Emotion, 6,* 125–138.

Lindquist, K. A., & Gendron, M. (2013). What's in a word?: Language constructs emotion perception. *Emotion Review, 5*(1), 66–71.

Lindquist, K. A., Wager, T. D., Kober, H., Bliss-Moreau, E., & Barrett, L. F. (2012). The brain basis of emotion: A meta-analytic review. *Behavioral and Brain Sciences, 35,* 121–143.

Lien, Y., & Cheng, P. W. (2000). Distinguishing genuine from spurious causes: A coherence hypothesis. *Cognitive Psychology, 40,* 87–137.

Lohmann, H., & Tomasello, M. (2003). The role of language in the development of false belief understanding: A training study. *Child Development, 74,* 1130–1144.

Lorenz, K. (1981). *The foundations of ethology: The principle ideas and discoveries in animal behavior.* New York: Simon & Schuster.

Martin-Malivel, J., & Okada, K. (2007). Human and chimpanzee face recognition in chimpanzees (*Pan troglodytes*): Role of exposure and impact on categorical perception. *Behavioral Neuroscience, 121,* 1145–1155.

McDougall, W. (1921). *An introduction to social psychology.* Boston: John W. Luce. (Original work published 1908)

Mesulam, M. M. (2000). *Principles of behavioral and cognitive neurology* (2nd ed.). New York: Oxford University Press.

Miklosi, A., Polgardi, R., Topal, J., & Csanyi, V. (1998). Use of experimenter-given cues in dogs. *Animal Cognition, 1,* 113–121.

Mulcahy, N. J., & Call, J. (2006). How great apes perform on a modified trap-tube task. *Animal Cognition, 9,* 193–199.

Oden, D. L., Thompson, R. K. R., & Premack, D. (2001). Can an ape reason analogically?: Comprehension and production of analogical problems by Sarah, a chimpanzee (*Pan troglodytes*). In D. Gentner, K. J. Holyoak, & B. N. Kokinov (Eds.), *The analogical mind* (pp. 471–498). Cambridge, MA: MIT Press.

Ongur, D., & Price, J. L. (2000). The organization of networks within the orbital and medial prefrontal cortex of rats, monkeys and humans. *Cerebral Cortex, 10*(3), 206–219.

Oosterwijk, S., Lindquist, K. A., Anderson, E., Dautoff, R., Moriguchi, Y., & Barrett, L. F. (2012). Emotions, body feelings, and thoughts share distributed neural networks. *NeuroImage, 62*, 2110–2128.

Panksepp, J. (1998). *Affective neuroscience: The foundations of human and animal emotions.* New York: Oxford University Press.

Panksepp, J. (2000). Emotions as natural kinds within the mammalian brain. In M. Lewis & J. Haviland (Eds.), *Handbook of emotions* (2nd ed., pp. 87–107). New York: Guilford Press.

Panksepp, J. (2005). Affective consciousness: Core emotional feelings in animals and humans. *Consciousness and Cognition, 14*, 81–88.

Panksepp, J. (2007). Neurologizing the psychology of affects: How appraisal-based construction and basic emotion theory can coexist. *Perspective in Psychological Science, 2*, 281–296.

Passingham, R. E., Toni, I., & Rushworth, M. F. (2000). Specialization within the prefrontal cortex: The ventral prefrontal cortex and associative learning. *Experimental Brain Research, 111*, 103–113.

Penn, D. C., Holyoak, K. J., & Povinelli, D. J. (2008). Darwin's mistake: Explaining the discontinuity between human and nonhuman minds. *Behavioral and Brain Sciences, 31*, 109–178.

Peterson, C., & Siegal, M. (2000). Insights into theory of mind from deadness and autism. *Mind and Language, 15*, 123–145.

Pinker, S. (1997). *How the mind works.* New York: Norton.

Povinelli, D. J. (2000). *Folk physics for apes: The chimpanzee's theory of how the world works.* New York: Oxford University Press.

Povinelli, D. J., & Eddy, T. J. (1996). What young chimpanzees know about seeing. *Monograph of the Society for Research in Child Development 61*, 1–152.

Povinelli, D. J., & Vonk, J. (2003). Chimpanzees' minds: Suspiciously human? *Trends in Cognitive Neuroscience, 7*, 157–160.

Povinelli, D. J., & Vonk, J. (2004). We don't need a microscope to explore the chimpanzee's mind. *Mind and Language, 19*, 1–28.

Premack, D. (1976). Language and intelligence in ape and man. *American Scientist, 64*, 674–683.

Premack, D. (1983a). Animal cognition. *Annual Review of Psychology, 34*, 351–362.

Premack, D. (1983b). The codes of man and beast. *Behavioral and Brain Sciences, 6*(1), 125–137.

Premack, D. (1988). Minds with and without language. In L. Weiskrantz (Ed.), *Thought without language* (pp. 46–65). New York: Oxford University Press.

Premack, D. (2010). Why humans are unique: Three theories. *Perspectives on Psychological Science, 5*, 22–32.

Premack, D., & Woodruff, G. (1978). Does the chimpanzee have a theory of mind? *Behavioral and Brain Sciences, 4*, 515–526.

Preuss, T. M. (1993). The role of the neurosciences in primate evolutionary biology: Historical commentary and prospectus. In R. D. E. MacPhee (Ed.), *Primates and their relatives in phylogenetic perspective* (pp. 333–362). New York: Plenum Press.

Preuss, T. M. (1995). The argument from animals to humans in cognitive neuroscience. In M. S. Gazzaniga (Ed.), *The cognitive neurosciences* (pp. 1227–1241). Cambridge, MA: MIT Press.

Preuss, T. M. (2007). Evolutionary specializations of primate brain systems. In M. J. Ravosa & M. Dagosto (Eds.), *Primate origins, adaptations and evolution* (pp. 625–675). New York: Springer.

Preuss, T. M. (2011). The human brain: Rewired and running hot. *Annals of the New York Academy of Sciences, 1225*, E182–E191.

Preuss, T. M., & Kaas, J. H. (1999). Human brain evolution. In F. E. Bloom, S. C. Landis, J. L. Robert, L. R. Squire, & M. J. Zigmond (Eds.), *Fundamental neurosciences* (pp. 1283–1311). San Diego, CA: Academic Press.

Pyers, J. E., & Senghas, A. (2009). Language promotes false belief understanding: Evidence from learners of a new signed language. *Psychological Science, 20*, 805–812.

Raichle, M. E., MacLeod, A. M., Snyder, A. Z., Powers, W. J., Gusnard, D. A., & Shulman, G. L. (2001). A default mode of brain function. *Proceedings of the National Academy of Sciences, 98*, 676–682.

Rilling, J. K., Barks, S. K., Parr, L. A., Preuss, T. M., Faber, T. L., Pagnoni, G., et al. (2007). A comparison of resting-state brain activity in humans and chimpanzees. *Proceedings of the National Academy of Sciences, 104*, 17146–17151.

Rilling, J. K., & Seligman, R. A., (2002). A quantitative morphometric comparative analysis of the primate temporal lobe. *Journal of Human Evolution, 42*, 505–533.

Roberson, D., Damjanovic, L., & Pilling, M. (2007). Categorical perception of facial expressions: Evidence for a "category adjustment" model. *Memory and Cognition, 35*, 1814–1829.

Roberson, D., & Davidoff, J. (2000). The categorical perception of color and facial expressions: The effect of verbal interference. *Memory and Cognition, 28*, 977–986.

Roseman, I. J. (1991). Appraisal determinants of discrete emotions. *Cognition and Emotion, 5*, 161–200.

Russell, J. A. (2003). Core affect and the psychological construction of emotion. *Psychological Review, 110*, 145–172.

Savage-Rumbaugh, S., Shanker, S. G., & Taylor, T. J. (1998). *Apes, language and the human mind*. New York: Oxford University Press.

Saxe, R., Tenenbaum, J. B., & Carey, S. (2005). Secret agents: Inferences about hidden causes by 10- and 12-month old infants. *Psychological Science, 16*, 235–239.

Schenker, N. M., Desgouttes, A. M., & Semendeferi, K. (2005). Neural connectivity and cortical substrates of cognition in hominoids. *Journal of Human Evolution, 49*, 547–569.

Searle, J. R. (1995). *The construction of social reality*. New York: Free Press.

Seed, A. M., Tebbich, S., Emery, N. J., & Clayton, N. S. (2006). Investigating physical cognition in rooks (*Corvus frugilegus*). *Current Biology, 16*, 697–701.

Semendeferi, K., Armstrong, E., Schleicher, A., Zilles, K., & Van Hoesen, G. W. (2001). Prefrontal cortex in humans and apes: A comparative study of Area 10. *American Journal of Physical Anthropology, 114*, 224–241.

Streidter, G. F. (2005). *Principles of brain evolution.* Sunderland, MA: Sinauer Associates.

Thompson, R. K. R., & Oden, D. L. (2000). Categorical perception and conceptual judgments by nonhuman primates: The paleological monkey and the analogical ape. *Cognitive Science, 24*, 363–396.

Tinbergen, N. (1951). *The study of instinct.* New York: Oxford University Press.

Tomasello, M., Call, J., & Hare, B. (2003a). Chimpanzees understand psychological states—the question is which ones and to what extent. *Trends in Cognitive Sciences, 7*(4), 153–156.

Tomasello, M., Call, J., & Hare, B. (2003b). Chimpanzees vs. humans: It's not that simple. *Trends in Cognitive Sciences, 7*, 239–240.

Tomkins, S. S. (1962). *Affect, imagery, and consciousness: Vol. 1. The positive affects.* New York: Springer.

Tomonaga, M., Uwano, Y., & Ogura, S. (2010). Bottlenose dolphins' (*Tursiops truncatus*) theory of mind as demonstrated by responses to their trainers' attentional states. *International Journal of Comparative Psychology, 23*, 386–400.

Tooby, J., & Cosmides, L. (1990). The past explains the present: Emotional adaptations and the structure of ancestral environments. *Ethological Sociobiology, 11*, 375–424.

Vincent, J. L., Patel, G. H., Fox, M. D., Synder, A. Z., Baker, J. T., Van Essen, D. C., et al. (2007). Intrinsic functional architecture in the anaesthetized monkey brain. *Nature, 447*, 83–86.

Visalberghi, E., & Limongelli, L. (1994). Lack of comprehension of cause–effect relations in tool-using capuchin monkeys (*Cebus paella*). *Journal of Comparative Psychology, 108*, 15–22.

von Uexküll, J. (1926). *Theoretical biology.* New York: Harcourt Brace.

Waldmann, M. R., & Holyoak, K. J. (1992). Predictive and diagnostic learning within causal model: Asymmetries in cue competition. *Journal of Experimental Psychology: General, 121*, 222–236.

Waxman, S. R., & Booth, A. E. (2003). The origins and evolution of links between word learning and conceptual organization: New evidence from 11-month-olds. *Developmental Science, 6*, 128–135.

Waxman, S. R., & Markow, D. B. (1995). Words as invitations to form categories: Evidence from 12 to 13 month old infants. *Cognitive Psychology, 29*, 257–302.

Whorf, B. L. (1956). *Language, thought, and reality.* Cambridge, MA: Technology Press of MIT.

Wimmer, H., & Perner, J. (1983). Beliefs about beliefs—representation and constraining function of wrong beliefs in young children's understanding of deception. *Cognition, 13*, 103–128.

Wise, S. P. (2008). Forward frontal fields: Phylogeny and fundamental function. *Trends in Neuroscience, 31,* 599–608.

Xu, F. (2002). The role of language in acquiring object kind concepts in infancy. *Cognition, 85,* 223–250.

Xu, F., Cote, M., & Baker, A. (2005). Labeling guides object individuation in 12-month old infants. *Psychological Science, 16,* 372–377.

Yeo, B. T. T., Krienen, F. M., Sepulcre, J., Sabuncu, M. R., Lashkari, D., Hollinshead, M., et al. (2011). The organization of the human cerebral cortex estimated by intrinsic functional connectivity. *Journal of Neurophysiology, 106,* 1125–1165.

Young, M. E., & Wasserman, E. A. (1997). Entropy detection by pigeons: Response to mixed visual displays after same–different discrimination training. *Journal of Experimental Psychology: Animal Behavior Processes, 23,* 157–170.

PART V

INTEGRATION AND REFLECTION

CHAPTER 17

The Greater Constructionist Project for Emotion

JAMES A. RUSSELL

Ortony, Clore, and Collins (1988, p. 2) characterized the study of emotion as a "very confused and confusing field of study." With the emergence of psychological construction, an end of the confusion is in sight. It is perhaps natural in the early stages of scientific progress to view different research programs as competing with one another. In this chapter, I propose that the emergence of psychological construction and the evidence it inspired opens the door to integrating those programs at least to some extent.

The concepts of emotion, fear, anger, disgust, and so on are folk concepts that predate psychology. The set of events called *emotions*, or all those called *fear* or *anger* or some other type of emotion, are heterogeneous. This heterogeneity has long been recognized but, all the same, underappreciated. The category of fear indeed includes what Panksepp (2012) took to be the paradigm case of fear: the unconditioned reflex of a rat freezing when shocked—with no appraisal, attribution, labeling, goal setting, or categorizing. But the category of fear also includes the prolonged view of the future of a man who just lost his job and sees no prospect for another or of avoiding financial ruin—this case includes appraisal, attribution, labeling, goal setting, and categorizing, but no freezing. Theorists seem puzzled that the category of disgust is equally heterogeneous. It includes not only the revulsion of biting into rotten food but also the moral abhorrence of hypocritical politicians. Psychologists ask whether some of the cases are metaphorical, but no clear line separates the literal from the metaphorical use of the word *disgust*. Failure to take into account the heterogeneity of emotion and types of emotion may be one reason emotion is a "very confused and confusing field of study" (Ortony et al., 1988, p. 2).

The heterogeneity of other categories named in folk psychology is recognized in other areas of psychology. The types of processes assumed in folk psychology are therefore not necessarily the most basic processes of the human mind but are instead constructed from more basic ones. The folk psychological concept of memory is challenged by research showing that memory is not one process. That is, memory, as understood in folk psychology, has moved to the status of chapter heading and been replaced in working models with a series of more specific processes, each beginning with different input and operating by different rules. Rather than assume that folk psychologists knows the basic processes of the mind, we must use scientific methods to discover them (Bickle, 2012).

The proposal that an emotional episode must be constructed anew on each occurrence out of more basic processes creates a new research program for emotion, which I call the Greater (meaning bigger, not better) Constructionist Project, and of which psychological construction is but one part. The project includes levels of analysis from evolutionary to sociocultural and timescales from seconds to a lifetime. Among emotion researchers, the word *construction* is sometimes used synonymously with extreme cultural relativism. Here, however, I use *construction* in a way that is agnostic relative to the nature–nurture issue—except to say that genes, epigenetic processes, and experiences are all essential to emotion (Nesse, 1990).

The chapters of this book represent the beginning of the Greater Constructionist Project, including under one umbrella accounts that previously would have been considered competing: basic emotion, appraisal, and social construction, as well as, of course, psychological construction. A near neighbor in exploring the broadly constructionist account is a recent analysis by Faucher (2013). For biological, psychological, and sociocultural accounts, he distinguished between what he called strong and weak versions. Strong versions assume that emotion is, at some level, defined by a common core, whereas weak versions do not. He argued that although strong versions compete with one another, weak versions are compatible with one another. I prefer the term *traditional* over *strong*, and *modern* over *weak*, but, in any case, the Greater Constructionist Project starts with the premise that emotions have no common core. Thus, biological, psychological, and sociocultural accounts do not compete, and they can be integrated.

At a minimum, the Greater Constructionist Project questions preconceptions found in both lay and scientific understanding of emotion. And it offers a new and useful way to understand emotion. Psychological construction was already an attempt to integrate categorical and dimensional perspectives on emotion, and the Greater Constructionist Project continues the expansion. Here, I argue that the assumptions just outlined allow us to integrate seemingly incompatible accounts of emotion. What divided the various accounts—basic emotion theories, psychological constructionist theories, appraisal theories, and social constructionist theories—are incompatible assumptions about the common core to emotions. With those assumptions of a common core gone, the various theories can be at least partly integrated. This is the topic of this chapter. This is the Greater Constructionist Project.

Background Assumptions

For centuries, emotion has defied explanation, despite efforts by humanists, natural philosophers, and scientists. Part of the reason is an unwarranted preconception, namely, the assumption that every emotional episode is a a recurrent pattern of predetermined components caused by an unseen entity called the *emotion*, in turn, triggered by an eliciting event. (One alternative is that each emotional episode must be actively constructed at the time of its occurrence.) Challenging this preconception has resulted in a family of theories, celebrated in this book. The proposals seen in this book will be criticized for being negative and vague. They are indeed sometimes negative, in that a major premise is a denial of this very preconception. They are indeed sometimes vague, in that together they form a research project, with the specifics to be determined by the data. Data have been gathered from different conceptual frameworks, and the proposed Greater Constructionist Project opens the door to integrating that evidence. Still, the main purpose of this project is to inspire the gathering of new data.

The preconception that emotions have a common core is rarely defended—or even stated—explicitly. Rather, having a common core is often a background, intuitive, implicit, underlying preconception of emotions. In everyday talk, we English-speakers treat emotion as qualitatively different from other psychological processes, as in the distinction between heart and mind, passion and reason, or feeling and thought. Lakoff (1987) and Kövecses (2003) offered evidence and analyses of everyday talk about emotion. We speak of emotions in a way very different from the way we speak about reasoning. (Scientists then proceed as if emotion is distinct from reasoning, perception, cognition, memory, etc.) We speak of an emotion as if it were a force that we encounter and battle from time to time. We speak of ourselves as victims of that force when we talk of struggling with our emotions, being overwhelmed by grief, or overcoming our fear. (Scientists once described emotions as disruptive forces and currently study emotion regulation.) We speak of an emotion as separate from its components when we speak of the facial expression *of* the emotion or the feeling *of* the emotion. (Scientists then write of various events as emotion's indicators, as if emotion were an entity separate from those indicators.) We speak of an emotion as if it were an entity inside the person: Tom was unaware of how much he loved her. (Scientists write of emotions as entities within the person much as psychoanalysts write of id, ego, and superego as entities within the person.) We speak of those internal entities as having certain powers, such as the power to cause their own components: Jill's fear made her heart beat fast and her hands sweat. Jack's jealousy drove him to make wild accusations. (Scientists then describe their research as showing, for example, the effects of fear on the autonomic nervous system or on facial expressions.) We speak of an emotion as if it were an entity with the power to influence other psychological processes. (Thus, correlational studies are routinely interpreted as showing that emotions *influence* changes in other processes; for example, disgust is said to influence moral judgments. In their textbook for college students, Gilovich, Keltner, and Nisbett [2011] aroused their students' interest by asking questions such as "How do emotions influence reasoning?")

These folk notions about emotions are not merely ways of speaking. Rather, our way of speaking reveals assumptions that underlie perceptions and expectations about emotion. We directly see anger in others and directly feel anger in ourselves—or so it seems. Folk assumptions about emotion therefore appear not just in affective science. When researchers who study music, morality, memory, or any other psychological topic ask how emotion bears on that topic, they often begin by taking for granted the background folk assumptions about emotion. Philosophers search for definitions of emotion, anger, fear, and the rest, on the assumption that there are necessary and sufficient features to be found. Still, folklore is a topic for a scientific account rather than a substitute for it. Science has a way of turning folk theories upside down. Maraun (1998) argued that everyday folk concepts (his term: "garden-variety concepts") cannot be measured. If so, difficulties in establishing a science of emotion are not surprising.

To think of emotions as heterogeneous is hard. As a consequence, constructionist accounts are easily misunderstood. Indeed, challenges to the idea that emotions are natural kinds, for example, seems to imply, absurdly, that emotions are unnatural. Thus, challenges to the idea that emotions are prepackaged modules are often met with incredulity. Some even seem to think that anyone denying the predetermined nature of emotion must believe some obviously absurd notion: that emotions do not exist, that emotions are not real, or that people (or nonhuman animals) do not actually ever undergo emotional episodes. And if emotions are not real, then they do not need to be explained. This *reductio ad absurdum* would refute the constructionist perspective, except that constructionists do not believe these particular absurd notions. Emotional episodes exist, are natural, and are real. Emotional episodes are caused and must be explained.

A human being is a complex system with many coordinated parts. As we go about our business, we benefit from understanding, predicting, and influencing each other. Folklore provides a set of concepts that help us do so—albeit not perfectly. Folk concepts are primitive tools, molded by cognitive economy, much as the theory of the four elements (earth, air, fire, and water) and the related theory of the four humours (blood, black bile, yellow bile, and phlegm) were primitive tools in early physical science and medicine. Folk concepts are not automatically invalid, but they do need to be tested and, historically, tend not to stand up to scientific scrutiny. They are first approximations that will eventually be replaced with scientifically honed concepts. (One complication exists in psychology because folk concepts are part of psychology's subject matter in a way that folk concepts of plants are not the subject matter of botany. More important, folk concepts of emotion are influences on other psychological processes, including those involved in emotional episodes.)

The word *emotion* has been a recurring source of difficulty when used to name a scientific concept. Scientists have used the English term *emotion* to express different concepts at different times (Dixon, 2012). *Emotion* is an English word that lacks an exact counterpart in various other languages (Russell, 1991) and that has changed through history: "even the very concept of 'emotion' hardly existed in the 16th century" (Tissari, 2010, p. 322). *Emotion* today includes a variety of types of events: occurrent events and dispositions, response syndromes and the inferred cause of those syndromes, automatic and controlled events, intentional and nonintentional mental states, mental states and bodily states, temporary and chronic states, fixed action patterns and complex epistemic states, and so on. *Emotion* is so heterogeneous that it is often unclear what a writer means by the term; misunderstanding between emotion scholars is widespread. This heterogeneity is especially damaging to interdisciplinary work or even dialogue, because a folk emotion term can be implicitly defined differently in different disciplines. Explicit definitions of emotion are often so broad it is hard to imagine what is not an emotion so defined. Verbal reports, overt emotional behaviors, nonverbal expressive gestures, and physiological indices have not proven to be interchangeable measures or indicators of the same event.

Folk concepts for types of emotions present a similar recurring problem in affective science. Although *fear, anger, sadness, love,* and the rest have been the terms with which we ask questions and formulate answers, these terms defy definition. In medieval English, *fear* referred to a property of the external world rather than to an inner experience (Barfield, 1954). Emotion concepts in different languages cannot always be translated one-to-one (Russell, 1991; Russell & Sato, 1995; Wierzbicka, 1999). Fear and other types of emotional episodes lack a common core; instances of fear bear a family resemblance to one another, each drawing from a "shifting menu of components" (Zachar, 2012, p. 9).

Some emotion researchers now acknowledge this heterogeneity within *emotion, fear,* and the rest, but the question is what to do about it. We want scientifically valid and well-defined concepts, but at the same time, many require that scientific formulations of emotion agree with ordinary language. Yet any concept with well-defined boundaries cannot coincide with a concept with blurry boundaries, even if given the same name. Neologisms are stillborn, leaving everyday terms seeming to be the only option. Science is a social enterprise, and we need to work toward consensus on a solution. Part of the solution, I suggest, is to replace *emotion* and the rest with a series of more narrowly and stipulatively defined terms. When, as in the Greater Constructionist Project, folk theories are not confused with scientific theories, affective science faces the formidable challenge of replacing folk concepts with stipulatively defined concepts that must then be validated.

Because the category named *emotion* is heterogeneous, examples can be found that fit different theories of emotion: A basic emotion theorist can point to (or at least imagine) an emotional episode in which a bear in the woods triggers a coordinated syndrome of predicted physiological, nonverbal, subjective, and instrumental responses that corresponds to their account of fear. Panksepp (2012) pointed to unconditioned reflexes as primary emotions and conditioned reflexes as secondary; anything more complex was tertiary. An appraisal theorist can point to an emotional episode of severe fear that is an appraisal of distant prospects as potential danger, that drives important decisions, but that lacks the assumed physiological and nonverbal signature of fear (and, on a more theoretical level, can point out that emotion and cognition are both examples of information processing). A social constructionist can point to an emotional syndrome common in a foreign land but unnamed in English; *amae, song, fago,* and *liget* are some well-known examples.

Affective science studies a broad range of phenomena, including emotional episodes, feelings, moods, sentiments, stress, evaluations, emotional dispositions, preferences, and many more events that are difficult to categorize. In the remainder of this chapter, I leave most of these phenomena for another day and focus on the emotional episode, each token of which is an occurrent event that takes place in a specific time and place. I argue that basic emotion theory, appraisal theory, social construction theory, and psychological construction theory, at least in part, can be integrated into a single account of emotional episodes.

Basic Emotion Theory

The dominant research program in the study of emotion, basic emotion theory (a.k.a. discrete emotion theory, differential emotion theory, affect program theory), presupposes that emotions divide into natural kinds, and that each kind has a common core. For example, in one version, all episodes of fear have in common the fear affect program, which automatically triggers a specific set of responses. The basic emotion research program raised valuable questions about the evolutionary history of emotion and led to valuable research on causal antecedents, functional and adaptive consequences, psychophysiological correlates, neural circuitry, nonverbal expressions, and subjective experiences of emotion. In the Greater Constructionist Project, each of these topics, including the evolutionary history of emotions, is seen as an empirical question. Basic emotion theory led to the development of useful tools, such as the Facial Action Coding System (Ekman & Friesen, 1978). More importantly, this research program made explicit many assumptions that previously were implicit, leading to their empirical scrutiny.

Basic emotion theory is already constructionist in two senses. First, the basic emotions involve multiple components: peripheral physiological changes, expressive changes, instrumental action, and so on. On one version, the affect program constructs the emotional episode from these components. (Unlike my psychological constructionist account, however, basic emotion theory has all cases of the same basic emotion stemming from the same origin, such as an affect program.) Second, all emotional episodes other than the occurrence of the basic ones are constructed: They are mixtures of the basic emotions. Izard (1991) defined love as a combination of interest and joy (p. 394); anxiety as the combination of fear, sadness, shame, and guilt (p. 312). Indeed, the occurrence of pure basic emotions is nowadays said to be rare (Izard, 2011), and, if so, most emotional episodes are constructed out of the basic ones. (In psychological construction, they are constructed not out of basic emotions but out of processes that are not themselves emotions.)

Basic emotion theory is also evolving. Parts of the theory have been reformulated in a way that is consistent with the Greater Constructionist Project. For example, some basic emotion theorists have abandoned the assumption that a basic emotion must have all the components in place; instead, they view emotion as multicomponential, with no single defining component. (The common core is then presumably the affect program or emotion-specific generating mechanism.) Some have abandoned the assumption that emotions are fixed action patterns triggered by predetermined elicitors; instead, they view the emotion's components as probabilistic or as tendencies. Some have abandoned the assumption that types of emotion can be defined with clear boundaries; instead, they use the metaphor of emotion families. Ellsworth and Scherer (2003, p. 574) noted this change:

> As originally proposed by Tomkins (1962, 1963, 1984), Ekman 1972), and Izard (1977), these theories suggested that each of these basic emotions is produced by an innate hardwired neuromotor program with

characteristic neurophysiological, expressive, and subjective components. More recent versions have loosened up the model somewhat, to
better capture the variety and subtlety of human emotional life, and now
speak of "families" of emotions (Ekman, 1992).

Specific components have also been reconceptualized. Although Levenson, Soto, and Pole (2007) defined emotion within the basic emotion
perspective (as "a hardwired organized set of response tendencies"), they
abandoned the idea that the subjective conscious experience of the emotion is simply a hardwired sensation. Rather, according to their account,
the subjective conscious experience of the emotion (what I call *emotional
meta-experience* and is often called *feeling*) is an end product based on the
perception of other processes, such as feedback from facial movements and
from changes in the autonomic nervous system, and—here is the important part—the experience is not fixed by that feedback but varies with cultural understanding. Thus, there is no fixed number of qualitatively different types of subjectively experienced emotions. Levenson et al.'s (2007)
constructionist account of subjective emotional experience was based on
empirical results that undoubtedly were surprising to a basic emotion theorist. Levenson et al. (2007) found that members of two different cultures
with the same facial expression and the same autonomic nervous system
activity nonetheless reported very different subjective emotional states.

I see no distance between Levenson et al.'s (2007) account of subjective
emotional states and four other accounts that do not share the assumptions
of basic emotion theory—although each theorist used a different term for
the subjective emotional state. James (1884) used the word *emotion*. He
argued that emotion so defined emerges from nonemotional ingredients:
It is a form of perception and is based on feedback from bodily changes,
including instrumental behavior, and from an interpretation of the "exciting fact." (See Ellsworth, 2014, for a discussion of James's theory that
brings out the implicit appraisal of the external situation in his account.)
LeDoux (2012) used the term *emotional feelings*. He presented a detailed
neuroscience account in which emotional feelings emerge from nonemotional ingredients: behavioral and physiological responses in the body,
brain arousal, memory, and cognitive evaluation, to name a few. Scherer
(2001) used the phrase *feeling component*. He hypothesized that the feeling
component is an integration of all the other components in an emotional
episode. And I (Russell, 2003) used the term *emotional meta-experience* in
an explicitly constructionist account that mirrors Levenson (2011), James
(1884), LeDoux (2012), and Scherer (2001). So it is possible to conceptualize at least one component of an emotional episode in a way that reconciles
basic emotion theory with the Greater Constructionist Project.

Another candidate would be instrumental behavior. Change from theorizing that emotion triggers a specific set of actions (e.g., fight or flight)

to theorizing that emotion entails "action tendencies" is a change from a predetermined view of emotion to a more open-ended one. After all, if emotion entails only a tendency, then another process must be invoked to account for the actual specific behavior that occurs. Other theorists go further. Scherer (2001) argued that human emotion is decoupled from instrumental behavior, which must therefore be formed through other means. There are recent proposals in which emotional behavior is accounted for not as an effect of emotion at all but through a separate process (Baumeister, Vohs, DeWall, & Zhang, 2007; Strack & Deutsch, 2004).

Tamir (2009) offered hypotheses and evidence that an emotion is not always a passive automatic process triggered by an external stimulus, but that individuals seek and regulate emotion.

Even "facial expressions of emotion" can be reconceptualized. Camras (2011) described the genesis of a facial expression not as stemming from a central, top-down affect program, but as the result of a bottom-up dynamical system. Fridlund (1994) described a facial expression not as a signal broadcasting an emotion to any and all who happen to see it, but as a signal of a specific behavioral intention aimed at a specific audience. Buss (in press) argued from an evolutionary perspective that facial expressions need not be a sign of a basic emotion.

In a recent statement, Izard (2011) distinguished basic emotions (his preferred term: *first-order emotions*) from emotion schemas. Whereas first-order emotions lack higher-order cognitive processes, emotion schemas are close to the prototypical emotional episodes described in psychological construction. "Except for the period of early development and relatively rare occasions of emergencies, highly threatening or challenging situations, emotion schemas (not first-order emotions) are typical of everyday life" (p. 372). Moreover, Izard (2010) also expressed doubts about the very concept of emotion: "I agree that the term *emotion* may have a fate in psychological science similar to the term *constellation* in the science of astronomy" (p. 383).

Izard (2011) did, however, express confidence that the concepts of first-order emotions, such a fear and anger, would remain viable scientific concepts. In his defense of basic emotion theory, Scarantino (Chapter 14, this volume) has abandoned even that claim. He acknowledged problems with traditional basic emotion theory and suggested abandoning the categories at the heart of that theory (fear, anger, etc.). He proposed a basic emotion theory in which those categories are replaced by "basic fear," "basic anger," and so on. Elsewhere, Scarantino (2012) proposed multiple categories for each of the basic emotions: so, "basic fear1," "basic fear2" and so on. Furthermore, even within the new categories, exemplars are not guided by the same neural circuitry, and the resulting components need not be the same from one exemplar to the next. I can find little in Scarantino's new basic emotion theory that is inconsistent with the Greater Constructionist Project.

Each such abandonment of a prior assumption and each reconceptualization of a component is a step toward integration of basic emotion theory into the Greater Constructionist Project. Especially encouraging is Levenson et al.'s (2007) observation that "one of the failings of most theories of emotion . . . is that they have treated emotion as a monolith" (p. 788).

Appraisal Theory

I use the term *appraisal theory* to capture a family of accounts in which a person's emotional episode depends on his or her subjective interpretation of an event rather than on the event itself. Appraisal theory so defined therefore includes accounts that focus on not only appraisals but also cognitive interpretations (Reisenzein & Schoenpflug, 1992), judgments (Solomon, 1976), attributions (Weiner, 1985), goals (Mandler, 1975; Stein & Levine, 1987, 1990), and communications (Oatley & Johnson-Laird, 2011).

Clore and Ortony (2008) offered an appraisal theory of emotion explicitly compatible with a constructionist perspective. Still, many emotion researchers likely think appraisal theories and constructionist theories are incompatible because of the historical evolution of the two. Most early appraisal theorists worked within the tradition of basic emotions (e.g., Roseman, 2011; Lazarus, 1991), whereas constructionists sat on the opposition bench. To make the case for compatibility, I distinguish between two types of appraisal theories—which for convenience I call *early* and *modern*. I group early ones with the basic emotion approach, but I see modern ones as compatible with a broad constructionist approach.

In an *early appraisal theory*, appraisal is added to a hardwired emotion process. Ekman's (1992) addition of an appraisal step to his account of emotion illustrates this type of theory. For emotion-eliciting stimuli other than innate elicitors, an appraisal process is needed to code the stimulus on a set of appraisal variables (goal relevance, agency, evaluation, etc.). Early appraisal theories posited a limited number of patterns among the appraisal variables. Each pattern, in turn, triggers a different discrete emotion. Thus, appraisal and emotion are sharply distinguished, they are said to occur in a fixed order, and there remains a fixed number of discrete categories of emotion. The immediate cause of an emotion is one or more appraisal outcomes, and appraisals are a necessary condition for an emotion. Different individuals can appraise the same stimulus differently; therefore, the same stimulus can result in different emotions. The emotion (or affect program) triggers a predetermined package of components, such as observable behaviors and physiological changes. Thus, a causal chain is envisioned: stimulus, appraisal, emotion/program, and behavioral and physiological changes. Because appraisal is necessary, any feedback mechanism that alters the emotion must operate via reappraisal. To say that all emotions follow this causal chain is to say that emotions have a common core.

In contrast, emergent *modern appraisal theories* change key assumptions of the basic emotion approach. Not all modern appraisal theorists agree with all the changes, but a version of appraisal theory can be articulated that abandons any assumption that emotions have a common core. Appraisal outcomes (the eliciting event being coded on evaluation, goal relevance, etc.) are distinguished from the processes that lead to those outcomes. Scherer (2001) found his appraisal theory to be compatible with dimensions of emotion: valence, activation, and power; although some episodes qualify as anger, fear, and so on, many other patterns of components do not. Frijda (2009) found no discrepancy between modern appraisal theories and my psychological construction on two major points: the multicomponential nature of an emotional episode and a rejection of the idea that emotions are hardwired packages. Perhaps the two most significant modern ideas are assuming (1) that appraisals are *typical* rather than necessary for emotion—Moors (2012) listed Frijda (2007), Scherer (1984), and Roseman and Smith (2001) as seeing appraisals as typical—and (2) that there is a near infinite number of types of emotional episodes rather than a fixed number of discrete emotions—Scherer (1984) and Ellsworth (2013) endorsed this idea. Ellsworth (2013, p. 125) wrote that "like dimensional theories dating back to Wundt (1902), [modern appraisal theorists] see emotional experience as continuous, with infinite variations in a multidimensional space, rather than as separate, independent categories or programs." Moors, Ellsworth, Scherer, and Frijda (2013) and Ellsworth (2013) articulated further commitments of their modern appraisal theories that resonate with a broad constructionist approach: (1) An "emotion" is taken to mean an emotional episode (see also Moors, 2009) and (2) the relations among antecedents, components, and consequences are not strict, but probabilistic. An amalgamated version of modern appraisal theory can therefore be made compatible with a broad constructionist approach at a deep level. Of course, specific formulations by specific theorists differ, but such differences can best be thought of as empirically testable details within a common framework.

Indeed, I believe that when examined more closely, apparent differences between modern appraisal theories and even my specific psychological construction shrink. Both accounts start with the premise that emotional episodes typically result from a subjective interpretation of an event rather than from the event itself. Because my account left the appraisal part of that interpretation as a promissory note (presumably to be fulfilled by appraisal theorists), appraisal theories are, to their credit, much more detailed than my psychological construction in their treatment of appraisal. The question is whether there are deep conceptual differences.

One apparent difference is the role of appraisal. Modern appraisal theories continue to view appraisal as the driving force of the other components of the emotional episode. In contrast, in psychological construction, the emotional episode can be influenced by all manner of factors, including purely physical processes and all sensory–perceptual–conceptual information processing. Yet this apparent difference is likely smaller than it first appears. First, because appraisal theorists have not agreed upon a definitive list of appraisal outcome variables, some differences may concern just what counts as an appraisal outcome. Second, drawing on advances in several appraisal theories, Moors (2012) took a broad view of what can influence the appraisal outcome. Put differently, unlike early appraisal theories, appraisal *processes* need bear no one-to-one correspondence to appraisal *outcomes*. Moors described how appraisal outcomes are influenced by three kinds of processes (rule-based, associative, and sensorimotor), and she agreed that these processes can be controlled or automatic, conscious or nonconscious. Thus, all manner of sensory–perceptual–conceptual information processing plays a role in emotional episodes, but according to the modern appraisal account, they do so by influencing appraisal outcomes. Moors thus found one assumption in modern appraisal theories that is not in my specific account: The appraisal outcome mediates the effects of all information processing on all other components of the emotional episode.

In psychological construction, in contrast, there is no fixed sequence of events; rather, components are ongoing processes continuously interacting with one another. Appraisal outcome is but one component of the emotional episode, and any component can influence any other. Core affect, for example, might directly influence emotional behavior and emotional meta-experience, and in turn be influenced. In short, modern appraisal theories and psychological construction share enough common ground to point to a specific testable hypothesis. Furthermore, a contrast between the two may raise questions. For example, as did early appraisal theories, modern appraisal theories often treat the emotional episode as a single event; the theorist might ask about, for example, the appraisal outcome profile for anger or fear. Psychological construction, in contrast, emphasizes dissociations among components. The question that then arises is how a given appraisal outcome is related to each component separately. The mediation hypothesis can then be seen as a family of hypotheses: Appraisal outcomes mediate peripheral autonomic nervous system changes, behavioral changes, and so on.

Another apparent difference is that in psychological construction, appraisal is not the only cause of the other components of an emotional episode, which, for example, may be influenced by purely physical processes (e.g., hormones, drugs, and bodily changes), some of which are mediated by core affect. Moors (2012) explicitly addressed claims that some causes of emotion are not appraisals, but found such claims consistent with modern appraisal theory. She considered purely physical processes, mental processes of minimal complexity, social appraisal (an estimation of audience reactions to future emotional behavior), activation of an emotion network in memory, beliefs and desires, and categorization. Moors acknowledged that some of these possible causes are not appraisals, and that their existence challenges early appraisal theories (which claim appraisals are necessary causes), but they do not challenge modern ones (which claim that appraisals are typical but not necessary causes). Second, regarding the remaining possible causes, she found it unclear whether and how the alternative processes put forward by the critics differ from appraisal. Thus, again, on Moors's account, all the processes mentioned in psychological construction occur and influence other components of the emotional episode, but, she adds, they do so by influencing appraisal outcomes. In short, on these matters, Moors's appraisal theory and my psychological construction again differ only on a specific empirically testable hypothesis: the mediation hypothesis. Either account could easily be modified to accommodate empirical evidence on this matter.

Of course, there are differences between the particular hypotheses I proposed and those proposed by appraisal theorists—just as there are differences among appraisal theorists. Still, I see fundamental similarities. Agreement seems to have been hidden by the way we name ourselves and the groups with which we historically identify. Having separate camps, each with its own name, is becoming more costly than helpful. I therefore offer the Greater Construction Project as a broad enough banner for both. Moving in this direction may free us from unanswerable questions. To illustrate, consider a question debated by appraisal theorists. The theory of fixed emotions presupposed that the antecedent is one thing and the emotional reaction another. This presupposition led to disputes: Is appraisal a part of the antecedent or a part of the emotional reaction? In the Greater Constructionist Project, the attempt to define the borders of the emotion itself is abandoned. Emotional episodes involve many components, each continuously unfolding over time while interacting with each other, with other psychological processes, and with the external world. Pointing to the beginning or the end, or pointing to which one of these components is or is not the emotion has not proved useful. Moving beyond unanswerable questions would allow us to focus our efforts on devising empirical means to examine specific testable hypotheses—such as modern appraisal theory's mediation hypothesis.

Social Construction

Social construction focuses on sociocultural processes in assembling an emotional episode. A version of social construction could be defined as if an emotional episode were predetermined, by assuming, for example, that cultural or social practices constitute emotion, that the essence of emotion is to be found in a social institution, or that all emotions are roles or another socially fixed process. Such assumptions are incompatible with the Greater Construction Project. But assuming that the emotion is located at the sociocultural level, then relegating other levels to secondary status has not proved useful. If those assumptions are abandoned, then social-cultural, psychological, and biological levels can all be seen as legitimate, compatible, and far from independent of one another. Integration of the various levels is possible and highly desirable. Averill (2012), Boiger and Mesquita (Chapter 15, this volume), and Rogers, Schroeder, and von Scheve (2014) presented versions of social construction consistent with a Greater Constructionist Project. Faucher's (2013) analysis similarly distinguished strong from weak versions of social construction. Here I continue this work of integration by arguing that the Greater Construction Project can be expanded to take into account a sociocultural level. I begin with a focus on the individual, then touch on larger aggregates.

It is difficult to name any aspect of the emotional life of the individual that is not influenced by immediate social context and society's longer term impact. In the first place, most (but not all) emotional episodes are principally reactions to external events, and different societies present different external events to the individual. In some societies in some places, especially in the Pleistocene, dangerous animals, disease, lack of food, and extreme weather were common; in other societies, places, and times, such confrontations occur rarely. Emotion theorists have written an inordinate amount about the bear in the woods or the snake in the path, but bears and snakes (and epidemics, starvation, and extreme cold) are more frequent in some societies than in others. Instead, most events with emotional impact, especially nowadays, involve the actions of another person or a collection of other persons. The frequency of such social events varies from one society to another.

Furthermore, the meaning of the event encountered is often (although not always) defined by social means. Events that involve other persons are obvious examples. Emotional episodes are rarely single events that can be understood through the traditional stimulus–response scheme; instead, they typically unfold moment to moment during an interaction between persons, each trying to understand the other, and each having a socially defined relationship to the other. Even a reaction to a single physical event, however, involves the social meaning of that event: Consider the seemingly most basic of basic emotions, disgust. Herz (2012) detailed examples of the same physical event being disgusting in one society but valued in another. Disgust depends on beliefs about what is disgusting, and the beliefs are socially determined. In an experimental demonstration of this point, disgust was elicited by a smell labeled "vomit" but not by the same smell labeled "Parmesan cheese" (Herz & von Clef, 2001).

Whereas psychological construction and appraisal theory emphasize that the emotional episode typically results from the person's interpretation of the eliciting event rather than from the event itself, social construction expands the account by examining the origin of the interpretation. Humans live in social reality. Part of culture is a set of ideas, assumptions, and beliefs that underlie the individual's expectations about and appraisal of a given situation. Much of our knowledge about the world is acquired by social means rather than directly. Properties and even the existence of events and situations are often known, not directly, but through information provided by others. Part of that knowledge concerns the affective qualities of objects and events. Another part concerns the status of the object or event on the dimensions of appraisal. Features of situations can be highlighted in some cultures but ignored in others. Indeed, what the individual takes to be the reality of the situation is this culturally permeated perception. Thus, much of the interpretation of an eliciting event can be traced to its cultural meaning.

Finally and most importantly, much of human reality is socially constituted. Laws, money, borders, and universities exist, but only because a group of people agree they exist. Thus, their defining properties are socially constituted. Emotional episodes that are reactions to events involving socially constituted reality occur highly frequently in modern life. Thus, an account of differences between different societies and groups within those societies in the socially constituted reality is needed if we are to understand the situations that initiate many emotional episodes. The socially constituted moral order is an especially potent source of emotion. We feel good when upholding the moral order (and label that feeling *pride*), and we feel bad when violating the moral order (and label that feeling *guilt* or *shame*). We admire others who uphold the moral order, especially at their personal sacrifice, and we feel anger toward those who violate it.

Just as there is a social origin to most eliciting situations, certain components of the emotional episode are directed at social outcomes. Changes in the peripheral nervous system are preparations for action, and action is often directed at other persons. Fridlund (1994) showed that so-called emotional facial expressions depend on the audience a person confronts or even imagines.

Part of culture that is absorbed by the individual is a set of roles, norms, feeling rules, ideals, values, and practices that play their part in emotional episodes. For example, enacting one's role is typically a positive experience; failing at that role is a negative one. Role is part of one's self-identity, which then helps one plan actions in response to the eliciting event. Similarly, these aspects of culture play a clear part in what at a psychological level is called *emotion regulation*.

Linguistic relativity, sometimes dismissed within much of psychology, is underscored by social construction. Language provides a system of concepts/categories (*fear, shame, liget, fago*) that underlies the individual's emotional meta-experience and perception of emotion in others. Thus, the language community must be studied for the words it provides to the child and the assumptions inherent in those words. Earlier, I pointed to an account of emotional meta-experience emerging from theorists at different levels of analysis and different research traditions (Levenson et al., (2007), James (1884), LeDoux (2012), and Scherer (2001), in addition to my own account) according to which the perception of one's own emotion (the conscious subjective experience of having a specific emotion) involves the culture-specific concepts named by the society's language.

Emotion is also not restricted to the individual level. The behavior of the shortstop in a baseball game cannot be understood outside the context of the whole game. Similarly, many emotional episodes cannot be understood outside their social context. They occur in face-to-face dyad or larger group. Mimicry, convergence, imitation, contagion, and escalation are best understood by examining not the individual but the dyad, the group, or the society, as the case may be. Abandoning the preconception that an emotion is an entity within a person that causes its components opens the door to thinking of some emotional episodes as being best understood to be more like a baseball game, a series of interactions that unfold over time in a way that is dependent on the context (Parkinson, 2012).

REFERENCES

Averill, J. R. (2012). What should theories of emotion be about? In P. Zachar & R. D. Ellis (Eds.), *Categorical versus dimensional models of affect: A seminar on the theories of Panksepp and Russell* (pp. 203–224). Amsterdam: Benjamins.

Barfield, O. (1954). *History in English words.* London: Methuen.

Baumeister, R. F., Vohs, K. D., DeWall, C. N., & Zhang, L. (2007). How emotion shapes behavior: Feedback, anticipation, and reflection rather than direct causation. *Personality and Social Psychology Review, 11,* 167–203.

Bickle, J. (2012). Lessons for affective science from a metascience of "molecular and cellular cognition." In P. Zachar & R. D. Ellis (Eds.), *Categorical versus dimensional models of affect: A seminar on the theories of Panksepp and Russell* (pp. 175–188). Amsterdam: Benjamins.

Buss, D. M. (in press). Evolutionary criteria for considering an emotion "basic": Jealousy as an illustration. *Emotion Review.*

Camras, L. A. (2011). Differentiation, dynamical integration, and functional emotional development. *Emotion Review, 3*(2), 138–146.

Clore, G. L., & Ortony, A. (2008). Appraisal theories: How cognition shapes affect into emotion. In M. Lewis, J. M. Haviland-Jones, & L. F. Barrett (Eds), *Handbook of emotions* (3rd ed., pp. 628–642). New York: Guilford Press.

Coan, J. A. (2010). Emergent ghosts of the emotion machine. *Emotion Review, 2,* 274–285.

Dixon, T. (2012). "Emotion": The history of a keyword in crisis. *Emotion Review, 4*, 338–344.

Ekman, P. (1992). An argument for basic emotions. *Cognition and Emotion, 6*, 169–200.

Ekman, P., & Friesen, W. V. (1978). *Manual of the Facial Action Coding System (FACS)*. Palo Alto, CA: Consulting Psychologists Press.

Ellsworth, P. C. (2013). Appraisal theory: Old and new questions. *Emotion Review, 5*(2), 125–131.

Ellsworth, P. C. (2014). Basic emotions and the rocks of New Hampshire. *Emotion Review, 6*(1), 21–26.

Ellsworth, P. C., & Scherer, K. R. (2003). Appraisal process in emotion. In R. J. Davidson, K. R. Scherer, & H. H. Goldsmith (Eds.), *Handbook of affective sciences* (pp. 572–595). Oxford, UK: Oxford University Press.

Faucher, L. (2013). Comment: Constructionism? *Emotion Review, 5*(4), 374–378.

Fridlund, A. J. (1994). *Human facial expressions: An evolutionary view*. San Diego, CA: Academic Press.

Frijda, N. H. (2007). *The laws of emotion*. Mahwah, NJ: Erlbaum.

Frijda, N. H. (2009). Emotions, individual differences and time course: Reflections. *Cognition and Emotion, 23*(7), 1444–1461.

Gilovich, T., Kletner, D., & Nisbett. R. E. (2011). *Social psychology* (2nd ed.). New York: Norton.

Herz, R. S. (2012). *That's disgusting: Unraveling the mysteries of repulsion*. New York: Norton.

Herz, R. S., & von Clef, J. (2001). The influence of verbal labeling on the perception of odors: Evidence for olfactory illusions. *Perception, 30*, 381–391.

Izard, C. E. (1991). *The psychology of emotions*. New York: Plenum.

Izard, C. E. (2010). More meanings and more questions for the term "emotion." *Emotion Review, 2*(4), 383–385.

Izard, C. E. (2011). Forms and functions of emotions: Matters of emotion-cognition interactions. *Emotion Review, 3*(4), 371–378.

James, W. (1884). What is an emotion? *Mind, 34*, 188–205.

Kövecses, Z. (2003). *Metaphor and emotion: Language, culture, and body in human feeling*. Cambridge, UK: Cambridge University Press.

Lakoff, G. (1987). *Women, fire, and dangerous things: What categories reveal about the mind*. Cambridge, UK: Cambridge University Press.

Lazarus, R. S. (1991). *Emotion and adaptation*. New York: Oxford University Press.

Levenson, R. W. (2011). Basic emotion questions. *Emotion Review, 3*, 379–388.

Levenson, R. W., Soto, J., & Pole, N. (2007). Emotion, biology, and culture. In *Handbook of cultural psychology* (pp. 780–796). New York: Guilford Press.

Mandler, G. (1975). *Mind and emotion*. New York: Wiley.

Maraun, M. D. (1998). Measurement as a normative practice: Implications of Wittgenstein's philosophy for measurement in psychology. *Theory and Psychology, 8*, 435–461.

Moors, A. (2009). Theories of emotion causation: A review. *Cognition and Emotion, 23*, 625–662.

Moors, A. (2012). Comparison of affect program theories, appraisal theories, and psychological construction theories. In P. Zachar & R. Ellis (Eds.), *Categorical versus dimensional model of affect* (pp. 257–278). Amsterdam: Benjamins.

Moors, A., Ellsworth, P. C., Scherer, K. R., & Frijda, N. H. (2013). Appraisal theories of emotion: State of the art and future development. *Emotion Review, 5*(2), 119–124.

Nesse, R. (1990). Evolutionary explanations of emotions. *Human Nature, 1,* 261–289.

Oatley, K., & Johnson-Laird, P. N. (2011). Basic emotions in social relationships, reasoning, and psychological illnesses. *Emotion Review, 3*(4), 424–433.

Ortony, A., Clore, G. L., & Collins, A. (1988). *The cognitive structure of emotions.* Cambridge, MA: Cambridge University Press.

Panksepp, J. (2012). In defense of multiple core affects. In P. Zachar & R. Ellis (Eds.), *Categorical versus dimensional model of affect* (pp. 31–78). Amsterdam: Benjamins.

Parkinson, B. (2012). Piecing together emotion: Sites and time-scales for social construction. *Emotion Review, 4,* 291–298.

Reisenzein, R., & Schoenpflug, W. (1992). Stumpf's cognitive-evaluative theory of emotion. *American Psychologist, 47,* 34–45.

Rogers, K., Schroeder, T., & von Scheve, C. (2014). Dissecting the sociality of emotion: A multi-level approach. *Emotion Review, 6,* 124–133.

Roseman, I. J. (2011). Emotional behaviors, emotivational goals, emotion strategies: Multiple levels of organization integrate variable and consistent responses. *Emotion Review, 3*(4), 434–443.

Roseman, I. J., & Smith, C. A. (2001). Appraisal theory: Overview, assumptions, varieties, controversies. In K. R. Scherer, A. Schorr, & T. Johnstone (Eds.), *Appraisal processes in emotion* (pp. 3–34). New York: Oxford University Press.

Russell, J. A. (1991). Culture and the categorization of emotion. *Psychological Bulletin, 110,* 426–450.

Russell, J. A. (2003). Core affect and the psychological construction of emotion. *Psychological Review, 110,* 145–172.

Russell, J. A., & Sato, K. (1995). Comparing emotion words between languages. *Journal of Cross-Cultural Psychology, 26,* 384–391.

Scarantino, A. (2012). Discrete emotions: From folk psychology to causal mechanisms. In P. Zachar & R. D. Ellis (Eds.), *Categorical versus dimensional models of affect: A seminar on the theories of Panksepp and Russell* (pp. 135–154). Amsterdam: Benjamins.

Scherer, K. R. (1984). On the nature and function of emotions: A component process approach. In K. R. Scherer & P. Ekman (Eds.), *Approaches to emotion* (pp. 293–317). Hillsdale, NJ: Erlbaum.

Scherer, K. R. (2001). Appraisal considered as a process of multi-level sequential checking. In K. R. Scherer, A. Schorr, & T. Johnstone (Eds.), *Appraisal processes in emotion* (pp. 92–120). New York: Oxford University Press.

Solomon, R. C. (1976). *The passions: The myth and nature of human emotion.* Garden City, NY: Anchor.

Stein, N. L., & Levine, L. J. (1987). Thinking about feelings: The development and organization of emotional knowledge. In R. E. Snow & M. Farr (Eds.), *Aptitude, learning, and instruction* (Vol. 3, pp. 165–198). Hillsdale, NJ: Erlbaum.

Stein, N. L., & Levine, L. J. (1990). Making sense out of emotion: The representation and use of goal-structured knowledge. In N. L. Stein, B. Leventhal, & T. Trabasso (Eds.), *Psychological and biological approaches to emotion* (pp. 45–73). Hillsdale, NJ: Erlbaum.

Strack, F., & Deutsch, R. (2004). Reflective and impulsive determinants of social behavior. *Personality and Social Psychology Review, 8,* 220–247.

Tamir, M. (2009). What do people want to feel and why?: Pleasure and utility in emotion regulation. *Current Directions in Psychological Science, 18*(2), 101–105.

Tissari, H. (2010). English words for emotions and their metaphors. In M. E. Winders, H. Tissari, & K. Allan (Eds.), *Historical cognitive linguistics* (pp. 298–332). Berlin: de Gruyter.

Weiner, B. (1985). An attributional theory of achievement motivation and emotion. *Psychological Review, 92*(4), 548.

Wierzbicka, A. (1999). *Emotions across languages and cultures.* New York: Cambridge University Press.

Zachar, P. (2012). Introduction: Categories, dimensions, and the problem of progress in affective science. In P. Zachar & R. Ellis (Eds.), *Categorical versus dimensional model of affect* (pp. 1–30). Amsterdam: Benjamins.

CHAPTER 18

Construction as an Integrative Framework for the Science of the Emotion

LISA FELDMAN BARRETT

The science of emotion is a messy business. Debates about the nature of emotion have yet to be resolved, despite over a century of empirical effort. For example, emotions were initially characterized as evolved faculties (see Spencer [1855], McDougall [1908/1921], and particularly Allport [1924], whose ideas were mistakenly attributed to Darwin [see Barrett, 2011a]). The idea of "emotion faculties" was tested and rejected in the mid-20th century (e.g., Hunt, 1941; Duffy, 1934a, 1934b; 1941; Dunlap, 1932; Harlow & Stagner, 1932, 1933), only to be resurrected (after a brief detour into behaviorism) five decades later as "basic emotion" theory (Ekman, 1972; Izard, 1977; Tomkins, 1962, 1963) and as "appraisal" theory (Arnold, 1960a, 1960b; Lazarus, 1966). After much experimentation in the latter part of the 20th century, the idea of emotions as faculties was again criticized, for exactly the same reason, because a growing number of empirical findings disputed the claim that emotion words referred to natural kind categories (e.g., Mandler, 1975; Barrett, 2006; Ortony & Turner, 1990). In particular, the newer evidence in human brain imaging (Lindquist, Wager, Kober, Bliss-Moreau, & Barrett, 2012) and in brain evolution (reviewed in Barrett et al., 2007) does not support the idea of emotions as faculties. Nonetheless, scientific articles, textbooks, and even newspaper articles, television documentaries, and science shows continue to claim that universal, "basic" emotions exist, as if this is an air-tight empirical fact.

Given these events, it is tempting to assume that the science of emotion is in a preparadigmatic state, characterized by the philosopher Thomas Kuhn (1962/1996) as a situation in which competing schools of thought possess different metaphysical assumptions, different theoretical positions, and even different methods and procedures, such that continued debate about fundamentals prevents collective progress. Indeed, this was Kuhn's view of the social sciences more generally.

Yet I am not so sure. When taking the long-term view, progress in science occurs when theories guided by human experience are eventually replaced with theories that bear little resemblance to that experience. Such replacement does not usually happen in an incremental, gradual fashion. More typically, one generation's theories are overturned by the next, only to then be resurrected by the next, and so on, we hope, with improvement at each new incarnation along the way. Eventually, when a scientific revolution does materialize, it rarely answers the questions posed by the deposed paradigm. Instead, it replaces those questions with new ones, prompting new concepts and empirical strategies that reshape the scientific landscape.

A Scientific Revolution

In my view, psychological construction (as a research program) offers the opportunity to guide the science of emotion as it abandons (for the third or fourth time, depending on how one counts) the idea of emotion faculties (or the idea of emotions as natural kind categories; Barrett, 2006). It is not enough to show how a paradigm is wanting: True progress requires another research program to take its place in accounting for the phenomena of interest (even as the phenomena, as stipulated by the new approach, might be revised or otherwise changes). The chapters in this volume (along with other works, e.g., Uddin, Kinnison, Pessoa, & Anderson, 2014; Lane & Schwartz, 1987; LeDoux, 2012, 2014; Menon, 2011; Olsson & Ochsner, 2008; Roy, Shohamy, & Wager, 2012; Seth, 2013; Seth, Suzuki, & Critchley, 2012) embody a major shift in the assumptions that drive inquiry within the science of emotion. Here are three examples:

Emergence Rather Than Essentialism

In psychological construction accounts, emotional episodes are events (not processes) that *emerge* from the interplay of more basic processes. This assumption is embodied in nearly every chapter in this volume (perhaps Chapter 14 by Scarantino is the notable exception). This stands in contrast to the current state of a field still dominated by a research program guided by *essentialism* (as I noted in Chapter 3, and in Barrett, 2011b, 2013). In the tradition of faculty psychology, each emotion category (*anger, sadness, fear*, etc.) is an internal force (or is triggered by an internal force) that produces behavior. The mind is understood as a conglomeration of these internal forces, many of which battle with each other for control of behavior. Essentialism is not a special problem in the science of emotion. It is embedded in the assumptions and methods of psychological science more generally. Standard psychometric procedures in psychology are largely essentialistic (e.g., see Chapter 9; also see Barrett, 2000, 2006, 2011b). Even the use of a Gaussian distribution in statistical analysis assumes essentialism (because variance is modeled as random error around a modal [essential] tendency).

The Mind as Spontaneously Active versus at Rest until Perturbed

In psychological construction accounts, emotional episodes are constructed via the top-down processes that are part and parcel of a normal functioning mind and brain. In this sense, the mind is active. Emotional episodes are not reactions to events as much as they are part of the everyday ebb and flow of how sensory input is made meaningful. This hypothesis is particularly evident in Chapters 4–8, 13, and 16. The view stands in contrast to one where the mind is primarily bottom-up and *reactive* (internal forces are inactive until triggered by a stimulus or the interpretation of a stimulus, but a stimulus is required). For example, appraisal theories hypothesize top-down processes in emotion generation, but these are usually thought to react to and modulate in coming, bottom-up stimulation. Compare these to the conceptual act theory, which uses a more predictive coding approach. In predictive coding, top-down conceptual influences from the past drive perception and experience as predictions. These predictions are modulated and constrained by incoming sensations. As a consequence, sensations modulate, but do not drive, perception and experience. Top-down, meaning making occurs on a continuous basis and is not a stimulus-yoked process. In real-world settings, it usually determines what is (and what is not) a "stimulus."

Constructive Analysis and Holism versus Reductionism

In most versions of psychological construction, reductionism is impossible because the emotional episodes have new properties that emerge via the interactions of more basic processes. The idea is that the composite whole has properties not evident in its individual parts. This is similar to the observation that phenotypes have properties that are not due to genes or environment alone but result from their interplay. Emergentism is not metaphysical magic, but it does require different methods and statistical analysis than a more reductionist account. In particular, it requires methods that allow us to observe multiple systems interacting with each other in real time (because the function of each is conditional on the state of the whole system, an assumption called *holism, contextualism,* or *compositionalism*). Usually, it also requires modeling representations across different dimensionalities (to map less abstract features at higher dimensionalities to the emergent, more abstract properties at lower dimensionalities). Again, the authors of most chapters in this volume, other than Chapters 8, 10, and 14, attempt to discuss something like constructive analysis in their discussion. By contrast, current methods and explanations favor *reductionism*, because the goal is to search for the specific neuron, brain region, or network that is responsible for each emotion faculty or type, and study each in isolation of all others. This reductionism can be observed, in that the same concepts (*anger, sadness, fear,* etc.) are used for the psychological phenomena and for the physical mechanisms that cause the phenomena. As a result, it is tempting to reduce emotions ontologically to their physical aspects (e.g., Damasio & Carvalho, 2013).

Horizontal Integration

A scientific revolution does not necessarily mean abandoning all aspects of the theories that have come before. In this sense, psychological construction offers the opportunity to integrate important insights from other psychological research programs for emotion (i.e., it creates a framework that is well suited to "horizontal" integration; see Russell, Chapter 17, this volume). The construction paradigm incorporates several important insights from the basic emotion research program: (1) Any theory of emotions must be an evolutionary account (even if it is not the specific evolutionary account embodied in the basic emotion view; Barrett, 2013); (2) survival circuits in nonhuman animals are often ingredients in emotional episodes (even if there is no necessary or sufficient relation between a behavioral adaptation, its circuit, and a given category of emotion; Barrett, 2012); and (3) it is important to consider points of continuity and disjunction between humans and nonhuman animals (even if the species-general ingredients are not themselves sufficient for human emotion, this does not mean that they are unimportant to a scientific account of emotion; Barrett, 2012; Barrett et al., 2007).

Psychological construction incorporates several important insights from the appraisal research program: (1) Emotional episodes involve creating meaning (even if appraisals are not the literal cognitive mechanisms that produce meaning; Barrett, 2012); (2) emotional episodes are functional (even if function is not viewed in a teleological sense and is rooted in collective intentionality about emotion concepts; Barrett, 2012); and (3) emotional episodes have component parts (even if the appraisals do not coordinate or cause these parts per se).

Psychological construction also incorporates several insights from the social construction research program: (1) Emotional episodes are functional (even if the functions are not solely relational and might be homeostatic or regulatory; Barrett, 2012); (2) emotional episodes are situated in context, such that the situation is important for creating opportunities for emotion (Barrett, 2012, 2013); and (3) emotions are relational (because they are not only "afforded" by certain situations but also they are illocutionary acts that depend on collective intentionality; Barrett, 2012).

Psychological construction not only has value in integrating different research programs for the study of emotion, but it also has the potential to unify the social, cognitive, affective, and perceptual neurosciences into one science of the mind, with a common, unified functional architecture of the brain for creating cognitions, emotions, perception, actions, and social functioning (Chapter 5; also see Barrett & Satpute, 2013; Lindquist & Barrett, 2012). This is consistent with the move away from misguided attempts to map emotions, social cognitions, and nonsocial cognitions and perceptions to distinct brain networks, and toward a systems neuroscience approach that treats cognitions, emotions, perception, actions and social functioning not as separate processes but as psychological events that can be understood as emerging from the interactions within and between brain networks that compute domain-general functions. By shifting the empirical emphasis from the search for mental faculties as unified neurobiological categories toward development of a more constructionist functional architecture of the human brain, the overlap in empirical findings across psychological domains is not a problem for reverse inference; rather, it becomes the engine that drives a more valid approach to reverse inference, leading to a domain-general understanding of how the brain creates the mind.

Vertical Integration

In addition to providing a framework of consilience for other theories of emotion at the psychological level (i.e., horizontal integration), psychological construction provides a framework for integrating a science of emotion across levels of analysis. This should not be surprising given psychology's history as a discipline that straddles the natural and the social sciences (Barrett, 2009); psychology became a full-fledged experimental science as scholars used the methods of neurology and physiology to search for the physical basis of socially inspired mental categories. As exemplified in this volume, constructionist theories are articulated at the neurobiological, psychological, and social levels of analysis, and several theories make an explicit attempt to integrate construction processes as they occur at biological, psychological, and social levels (particularly Chapters 4–7 and 10–12;

see also Barrett & Satpute, 2013; Lindquist & Barrett, 2012). The goal is to have a unified theory of emotion in which concepts from physical, psychological, and social levels of analysis can be understood from within the same framework (see Chapter 2). In this sense, it is possible to view emotions as natural phenomena without relying on nativist assumptions.

This vertical integration is an important contribution of psychological construction, because it reminds scientists that not all biological evidence for emotions as coherent categories is evidence for an emotion faculty/natural kind view of emotion (see Chapter 3). For many years, the basic emotion research program was the only set of theories that offered a biological account of emotions, and for this reason, researchers often treat any biological evidence as support for a basic emotion view (e.g., Kassam, Markey, Cherkassky, Loewenstein, & Just, 2013; Vytal & Hamann, 2010). In fact, the basic emotion program makes very specific hypotheses about the nature of the biological evidence that would be supportive, and psychological construction accounts make very different hypotheses. For example, the faculty psychology/natural kind approach to emotion would hypothesize that each instance of a given emotion category (e.g., *anger*) will emerge from a distinct anatomically prescribed (and therefore inheritable), dedicated, emotion-specific region or network that should be homologous in nonhuman animals (e.g., in a recent review of the basic emotion research program, Tracy & Randles [2011, p. 398] wrote that the "agreed-upon gold standard is the presence of neurons dedicated to an emotion's activation"). A psychological construction hypothesis, however, would characterize different instances of emotion as being constructed from the interactions across distributed brain networks that are not specific to emotion per se but that subserve other basic processes, including attention, memory, action, and perception, as well as autonomic, endocrine, and metabolic regulation of the body (Chapters, 4–7, 10, and 11). Careful consideration of these two competing views makes it possible to design biological experiments that directly compare the two, providing a stronger inferential test than comparing each to the null hypothesis (e.g., Touroutoglou, Lindquist, Hollenbeck, Dickerson, & Barrett, 2014; Wilson-Mendenhall, Barrett, Simmons, & Barsalou, 2011).

Psychological construction's integration across levels of analysis prescribes a very different program of research than is currently the norm in studies of emotion. For the past half a century, emotion-related research, guided by the faculty psychology/natural kind research program, has had the goal to produce a Linnaean-type classification of emotions by identifying the autonomic nervous system (ANS) pattern, brain circuit, and social function for phenomena corresponding to a small group of emotion words (e.g., "anger," "sadness," "fear," "disgust," and sometimes "shame" and "guilt") using a variety of methods in a variety of contexts. Experiments are typically designed to discover the ANS, the central nervous system (CNS), and social functions that are repeatable across instances of the same emotion category (e.g., all instances of *anger*), and those that are maximally different across emotions (e.g., distinguishing *anger* from *fear*). From this perspective, there is progress in creating more precise classifications (e.g., Chapter 14; Gross & Canteras, 2012; Silva et al., 2013). Psychological construction, by contrast, prescribes an empirical approach for the science of emotion that does not evoke an emotion such as anger or fear as a unitary phenomenon, but instead maps each category's population variation in a context-driven way (e.g., Wilson-Mendenhall et al., 2011; Wilson-Mendenhall, Barrett, & Barsalou, 2014). This can be done at the biological level of analysis, using concepts such as degeneracy, and at the social level of analysis, by examining the varying functions that instances of the same emotion category can play (rather than assuming that each emotion category reflects only one modal function, or that the function varies primarily by culture).

To date, most of the evidence for psychological construction comes from experiments inspired by faculty psychology/"natural kind" research that has failed to produce evidence of emotion types. Within an individual experiment, different ANS variables might distinguish one emotional experience from another, but these findings do not replicate across studies (in which either no discrimination is found, or a different set of variables is distinctive in each study; see Barrett, 2013). This same variation can also be observed in studies that use multivariate pattern classifications in ANS variables, even when the same methods and stimuli are being used (cf. Kragel & LaBar, 2013; Stephens, Christie, & Friedman, 2010; for a review, see Barrett, 2013). A similar pattern of observation can also be found in brain imaging studies of emotion; for example, Kassam et al. (2013) reported a multivoxel pattern classification that distinguished emotions by broadly distributed brain activation patterns, but these patterns do not replicate a pattern classification of our meta-analytic database, as reported in Wager et al., 2014). More importantly, distributed brain patterns that classify different categories of emotion are not necessarily biomarkers for those emotions per se. A brain pattern for a category can be understood as a disjunction of sufficient features. For example, imagine the brain pattern for *anger* consists of 10,000 voxels that are active more than baseline, and each voxel can be thought of as a feature. Each instance classified as *anger* will have some number of those features (during each instance of *anger*, some number of those voxels will be active over baseline). But instance 1 and instance 2 need not have overlapping features (different subsets of active voxels can be present in the two instances). This means that the overall pattern cannot be interpreted as the essence of the category. In principle, the pattern itself need not appear in *any* instance of the category to work well in classifying its instances. The overall pattern is neither necessary nor sufficient for the category, even though its features can be used to diagnose the category's instances. (This is reminiscent of certain issues in the cognitive psychology categorization literature.)

Moreover, meta-analyses of task-dependent brain imaging studies also fail to find brain regions or networks that consistently and uniquely respond during each emotion, and that are active across different emotion categories (Lindquist et al., 2012; Vytal & Hamann, 2010). In effect, the very experiments inspired by the natural kind approach to emotion, that were designed to reveal the ANS and CNS patterns for each emotion, have instead produced evidence of heterogeneity of instances within each emotion category, as well as similarities across categories (Barrett, 2006). While these "natural kind" inspired experiments are consistent with psychological construction, they do not provide strong scientific evidence for the validity of construction theories. Only experiments that are designed with psychological assumptions in mind (e.g., an emotion category is a not a physical type but population of instances) can do that.

The Future

When taking the long view of scientific progress, this volume, along with key articles (e.g., Gendron & Barrett, 2009; Barrett, 2009, 2011b) represent an attempt to articulate the history, philosophical assumptions, and theoretical ideas embodied in a psychological construction research program. Faculty psychology is simple. Psychological construction is complex. To be maximally successful, this program will have to stimulate new experimental methods and statistical procedures to test its hypotheses properly, as is typically the case in paradigm shifts. Only time will tell, of course, whether psychological construction will mature into a full-fledged scientific revolution in the science of emotion. But I hope you agree that the chapters in this volume demonstrate that we are off to an interesting, if not a generative, start.

ACKNOWLEDGMENTS

Preparation of this chapter was supported by a National Institutes of Health Director's Pioneer Award (No. DP1OD003312); by grants from the National Institute on Aging (No. R01AG030311), the National Institute of Mental Health (No. R21MH099605), and the National Science Foundation (No. BCS-1052790); and by contracts from the U.S. Army Research Institute for the Behavioral and Social Sciences (Contract Nos. W5J9CQ-11-C-0046 and W5J9CQ-12-C-0049) to Lisa Feldman Barrett. The views, opinions, and/or findings contained in this article are solely those of the author(s) and should not be construed as an official Department of the Army or Department of Defense position, policy, or decision.

REFERENCES

Allport, F. H. (1924). *Social psychology.* New York: Houghton Mifflin.

Arnold, M. B. (1960a). *Emotion and personality: Vol. 1. Psychological aspects.* New York: Columbia University Press.

Arnold, M. B. (1960b). *Emotion and personality: Vol. 2. Physiological aspects.* New York: Columbia University Press.

Barrett, L. F. (2000, February). *Modeling emotion as an emergent phenomenon: A causal indicator analysis.* Paper presented at the annual meeting of the Society for Personality and Social Psychology, Nashville, TN.

Barrett, L. F. (2006). Emotions as natural kinds? *Perspectives on Psychological Science, 1,* 28–58.

Barrett, L. F. (2009). The future of psychology: Connecting mind to brain. *Perspectives in Psychological Science, 4,* 326–339.

Barrett, L. F. (2011a). Was Darwin wrong about emotional expressions? *Current Directions in Psychological Science, 20,* 400–406.

Barrett, L. F. (2011b). Bridging token identity theory and supervenience theory through psychological construction. *Psychological Inquiry, 22,* 115–127.

Barrett, L. F. (2012). Emotions are real. *Emotion, 12,* 413–429.

Barrett, L. F. (2013). Psychological construction: A Darwinian approach to the science of emotion. *Emotion Review, 5,* 379–389.

Barrett, L. F., Lindquist, K., Bliss-Moreau, E., Duncan, S., Gendron, M., Mize, J., et al. (2007). Of mice and men: Natural kinds of emotion in the mammalian brain? *Perspectives on Psychological Science, 2,* 297–312.

Barrett, L. F., & Satpute, A. B. (2013). Large-scale brain networks in affective and social neuroscience: Towards an integrative architecture of the human brain. *Current Opinion in Neurobiology, 23,* 361–372.

Damasio, A., & Carvalho, G. B. (2013). The nature of feelings: Evolutionary and neurobiological origins. *Nature Reviews Neuroscience, 14,* 143–152.

Duffy, E. (1934a). Is emotion a mere term of convenience? *Psychological Review, 41,* 103–104.

Duffy, E. (1934b). Emotion: An example of the need for reorientation in psychology. *Psychological Review, 41,* 184–198.

Duffy, E. (1941). An explanation of "emotional" phenomena without use of the concept "emotion." *General Journal of Psychology, 25,* 283–293.

Dunlap, K. (1932). Are emotions teleological constructs? *American Journal of Psychology, 44,* 572–576.

Ekman, P. (1972). Universals and cultural differences in facial expressions of emotion. In J. Cole (Ed.), *Nebraska Symposium on Emotion and Motivation* (pp. 207–283). Lincoln: University of Nebraska Press.

Gendron, M., & Barrett, L. F. (2009). Reconstructing the past: A century of ideas about emotion in psychology. *Emotion Review, 1,* 316–339.

Gross, C. T., & Canteras, N. S. (2012). The many paths to fear. *Nature Reviews Neuroscience, 13,* 651–658.

Harlow, H. F., & Stagner, R. (1932). Psychology of feelings and emotions: I. Theory of feelings. *Psychological Review, 39,* 570–589.

Harlow, H. F., & Stagner, R. (1933). Psychology of feelings and emotions: II. Theory of emotions. *Psychological Review, 40,* 184–195.

Hunt, W. A. (1941). Recent developments in the field of emotion. *Psychological Bulletin, 38*, 249–276.

Izard, C. E. (1977). *Human emotions.* New York: Springer.

Kassam, K. S., Markey, A. R., Cherkassky, V. L., Loewenstein, G., & Just, M. A. (2013). Identifying emotions on the basis of neural activation. *PLos ONE, 8*(6), e66032.

Kragel, P. A., & LaBar, K. S. (2013). Multivariate pattern classification reveals autonomic and experiential representations of discrete emotions. *Emotion, 13*(4), 681–690.

Kuhn, S. (1996). *The structure of scientific revolutions.* Chicago: University of Chicago Press. (Original work published 1962)

Lane, R., & Schwartz, G. E. (1987). Levels of emotional awareness: A cognitive-developmental theory and its application to psychopathology. *American Journal of Psychiatry, 144*, 133–143.

Lazarus, R. S. (1966). *Psychological stress and the coping process.* New York: McGraw-Hill.

LeDoux, J. (2012). Rethinking the emotional brain. *Neuron, 73*, 653–676.

LeDoux, J. E. (2014). Coming to terms with fear. *Proceedings of the National Academy of Sciences.* Available online at *www.cns.nyu.edu/home/ledoux/pdf/PNAS-2014-LeDoux-1400335111.pdf.*

Lindquist, K. A., & Barrett, L. F. (2012). A functional architecture of the human brain: Insights from the science of emotion. *Trends in Cognitive Sciences, 16*, 533–540.

Lindquist, K. A., Wager, T. D., Kober, H., Bliss-Moreau, E., & Barrett, L. F. (2012). The brain basis of emotion: A meta-analytic review. *Behavioral and Brain Sciences, 35*, 121–143.

Mandler, G. (1975). *Mind and emotion.* New York: Wiley.

McDougall, W. (1921). *An introduction to social psychology.* Boston: John W. Luce. (Original work published 1908)

Menon, V. (2011). Large-scale brain networks and psychopathology: A unifying triple network model. *Trends in Cognitive Sciences, 15*, 483–506.

Olsson, A., & Ochsner, K. N. (2008). The role of social cognition in emotion. *Trends in Cognitive Sciences, 12*, 65–71.

Ortony, A., & Turner, T. J. (1990). What's basic about basic emotions? *Psychological Review, 97*, 315–331.

Roy, M., Shohamy, D., Wager, T. D. (2012). Ventromedial prefrontal–subcortical systems and the generation of affective meaning. *Trends in Cognitive Sciences, 16*(3), 147–156.

Seth, A. K. (2013). Interoceptive inference, emotion, and the embodied self. *Trends in Cognitive Sciences, 17*, 565–573.

Seth, A. K., Suzuki, K., & Critchley, H. D. (2012). An interoceptive predictive coding model of conscious presence. *Frontiers in Psychology, 2*, 395.

Silva, B., Mattucci, C., Krzywkowski, P., Muana, E., Illarionova, A., Grinevich, V., et al. (2013). Independent hypothalamic circuits for social and predator fear. *Nature Neuroscience, 16*, 1731–1733.

Spencer, H. (1855). *Principles of psychology.* London: Longman, Brown, Green & Longmans.

Stephens, C. L., Christie, I. C., & Friedman, B. H. (2010). Autonomic specificity of basic emotions: Evidence from pattern classification and cluster analysis. *Biological Psychology, 84*, 463–473.

Tomkins, S. S. (1962). *Affect, imagery, consciousness: Vol. 1. The positive affects.* New York: Springer.

Tomkins, S. S. (1963). *Affect, imagery, consciousness: Vol. 2. The negative affects.* New York: Springer.

Touroutoglou, A., Lindquist, K. A., Hollenbeck, M., Dickerson, B. C., & Barrett, L. F. (2014). *Intrinsic connectivity in the human brain does not reveal networks for "basic" emotions.* Manuscript under review.

Tracy, J. L., & Randles, D. (2011). Four models of basic emotions: A review Ekman & Cordaro, Izard, Levenson, and Panksepp & Watts. *Emotion Review, 3*, 397–405.

Uddin, L., Kinnison, J., Pessoa, L., & Anderson, M. (2014). Beyond the tripartite cognitive–emotion–interoception model of the human insular cortex. *Journal of Cognitive Neuroscience, 26*(1), 16–27.

Vytal, K., & Hamann, S. (2010). Neuroimaging support for discrete neural correlates of basic emotions: A voxel-based meta-analysis. *Journal of Cognitive Neuroscience, 22*, 2864–2885.

Wager, T. D., Kang, J., Johnson, T. D., Nichols, T. E., Satpute, A. B., & Barrett, L. F. (2014*). A Bayesian model of category-specific emotional brain responses.* Manuscript under review.

Wilson-Mendenhall, C. D., Barrett, L. F., Simmons, W. K., & Barsalou, L. W. (2011). Grounding emotion in situated conceptualization. *Neuropsychologia, 49*, 1105–1127.

Wilson-Mendenhall, C., Barrett, L. F., & Barsalou, L. W. (2014). Variety in emotional life: Within-category typicality of emotional experiences is associated with neural activity in large-scale brain networks. *Social Cognitive and Affective Neuroscience.* Epub ahead of print.

Afterword

Emotional Construction in the Brain

JOSEPH LeDOUX

During the early 20th century, while the young field of psychology was going through an identity crisis that stemmed from its emphasis on subjective experience, another fledgling enterprise that involved mind and behavior was also taking root. This, of course, is what we now call *neuroscience*. In psychology, the behaviorists had gotten rid of mental states, but they did not eliminate mental state terms. *Emotions*, for example, were no longer conscious feelings that had a causal role in behavior; they were dispositions to behave in a certain way, determined by reinforcement history. But unconstrained by the limits of behaviorism, brain researchers interested in emotion talked freely about consciously experienced feelings in the brain and often gave these a causal role in behavior. Animals were angry when aggressive, afraid when defending, and they felt pleasure when they pressed a bar for electrical stimulation. And the brain areas that controlled innate emotional behaviors were also said to generate feelings. By the 1960s, basic emotions theory had come along and solidified the view that emotions are innate programs in the brain, providing conception of emotions that linked Darwin and psychology in the brain.

I would like to take this opportunity to offer a different view of how the brain experiences emotions, one that is compatible with constructionist ideas. In spite of often being thought of as part of the basic emotions camp, I have long maintained that the brain mechanisms that give rise innate emotional expressions are distinct from those that give rise to conscious emotional experiences. I therefore agree with basic emotions theorists that some responses that occur when people feel emotions are hardwired, but I do not think that the emotion, the feeling, is hardwired. It is imputed, assembled, constructed, or otherwise cognitively created.

I have to share some of the blame for being viewed as a basic emotions kind of researcher. For the past three decades, I have studied the neural mechanism underlying what is called *Pavlovian fear conditioning* (see LeDoux, 1996, 2002; Johansen, Cain, Ostroff, & LeDoux, 2011). In this work, I focused on how the brain detects and responds to learned threats. But I called the brain system that does this the *fear system*. This was a mistake. The common meaning of *fear* is the feeling of being afraid. It was therefore natural to think that when I used the term *fear system* I was talking about a system that gives rise to conscious feelings of fear. I have recently written several articles to clarify this point of view (LeDoux, 2012, 2013, 2014).

My view of how the feeling of fear comes about has not changed much over the many years I have been involved in this field. It has its origins in my PhD research on split-brain patients with Michael Gazzaniga in the 1970s. During this time, I was steeped in the emerging field of cognitive science, especially from a social psychology point of view. Leon Festinger's (1957) theory of cognitive dissonance, and Stanley Schachter and Jerome Singer's cognitive theory of emotion (Schachter, 1975) were central to my dissertation. Gazzaniga and I summarized this and other split-brain work in our 1978 book, *The Integrated Mind*.

After graduate school, I turned to rats as subjects because I wanted to pursue the brain mechanisms of emotion in more detail than is possible studying the human brain. I focused on the mechanisms that detect and respond to threats, not the mechanisms that give rise to feelings of fear, since I did not think we could know what, if anything, rats feel. But when I wrote about feelings in humans, my ideas were very much in the cognitive vein (LeDoux, 1984, 1987, 1996, 2002, 2008). Specifically, I have argued that feeling occur when working memory, via executive attention, integrates information about the immediate stimulus and long-term semantic and episodic memories triggered by the stimulus with information from subcortical systems and body feedback into a unified representation. These are non-emotional factors or ingredients that, when blended in working memory, emerge as feelings. More recently I have elaborated on the latter of these ideas in the form of survival circuits and global organismic states (LeDoux, 2012, 2014), but the fundamental ideas are the same.

Much confusion results when we label factors that contribute to emotions with emotion terms. Arousal, body responses and feedback, cognitive appraisal, and so forth, are not fundamentally emotional mechanisms. They did not evolve to make feelings. Arousal, for example, exists to regulate sleep and wakefulness, and alertness when awake. This capacity is present in bees, flies, and worms, as well as rats and humans. It is useful in creating feelings but is not itself a feeling or emotion mechanism.

Obviously, aspects of this point of view fit nicely with the constructionist position. The idea that fear does not erupt as a full-blown, prepackaged mental state when there is a threat, but instead requires the integration of information via a general-purpose system (working memory) is a prime example. I have even used a similar metaphor (ingredients) used by some constructionists, notably Barrett (2009). I have also proposed that feelings can come about when they are imposed in bottom-up fashion or because they are assembled in top-down fashion, but in both cases, working memory and cognitive work is required. In this view, fears that arise with the help of subcortical survival circuits (fear of a snake at your feet) come about in much the same way as fears that do not depend on survival circuits (abstract fears, such fear of not leading a meaningful life, or of the eventuality of death). In other words, I do not think that conscious experience of fear is ever the result of an innately stored feeling that is unleashed from a subcortical site when a threat occurs. Fear is always an interpretation that *you* are in harm's way.

One tricky area is deciding how to apply the term *general-purpose*. This seems to be a bit in the eye of the beholder. Is arousal general-purpose, since it can be used in lots of different behavioral settings, or is it specific, since it performs a particular function? The same could be said of working memory. It is general-purpose from some perspectives (e.g., sensory processing) but specific from another (it is the only brain system that can integrate diverse kinds of information).

Another caution has to do with whether to apply a notion-like construction across the board in mind or brain science. I am a constructionist when it comes to conscious emotional experiences (feelings) but more of a faculty psychology kind of guy when talking about survival circuits. In other words, I do think there are innate systems that are relevant to emotion, even if they do not directly make feelings.

Finally, when I say that working memory is important in feelings, I do not mean to imply that we understand how feelings are actually experienced. As with cognitive theories of consciousness in general, we need to understand how such experiences are cognitively accessed as part of the explanation of how they are experienced. The constructionist point of view provides ways to understand access, which is something lacking in theories that assume fear or other feelings are innately stored experiences waiting to be unleashed.

It is interesting that brain stimulation data in the early 20th century were interpreted in two ways. As noted, some described the stimulation as eliciting psychological states that were causal to the behavioral responses—cats were angry and fearful, not just aggressive and defensive (Hess, 1954).

But prominent theorists, such as Walter Cannon (1929) and James Papez (1937), concluded that without the cortex and its ability to interpret the event, the elicited behaviors were stripped of their experiential component, the feeling—rage so elicited was considered "sham rage." One could say that these brain researchers were early constructionists.

I have glossed over many of the details of my views, which can be found in three articles over the past several years (LeDoux, 2008, 2012, 2014). To summarize, the basic point is that emotions are feelings, and feelings are cognitively created conscious experiences. The other factors that contribute to feelings, such as arousal, body feedback, and so forth, are non-emotional ingredients that are neither necessary nor sufficient for an emotional experience. We can be afraid of something independent of activation of a defensive survival circuit. But when we integrate consequences of survival circuit activity information about an immediately present stimulus, and memories triggered that stimulus, the character of the feeling changes. Instead of being a concern or worry, it becomes a feeling of fear, panic, horror, or terror, depending on the way the individual interprets the particular blend of ingredients.

REFERENCES

Barrett, L. F. (2009). The future of psychology: Connecting mind to brain. *Perspectives on Psychological Science, 4*, 326–339.

Cannon, W. B. (1929). *Bodily changes in pain, hunger, fear, and rage*. New York: Appleton.

Festinger, L. (1957). *A theory of cognitive dissonance*. Evanston, IL: Row, Peterson.

Gazzaniga, M. S., & LeDoux, J. E. (1978). *The integrated mind*. New York: Plenum.

Hess, W. R. (1954). *Functional organization of the diencephalon*. New York: Grune & Stratton.

Johansen, J. P., Cain, C. K., Ostroff, L. E., & LeDoux, J. E. (2011). Molecular mechanisms of fear learning and memory. *Cell, 147,* 509–524.

LeDoux, J. E. (1984). Cognition and emotion: Processing functions and brain systems. In M. S. Gazzaniga (Ed.), *Handbook of cognitive neuroscience* (pp. 357–368). New York: Plenum.

LeDoux, J. E. (1987). Emotion. In F. Plum (Ed.), *Handbook of physiology 1: The nervous system: Vol. V. Higher functions of the brain* (pp. 419–460). Bethesda, MD: American Physiological Society.

LeDoux, J. E. (1996). *The emotional brain*. New York: Simon & Schuster.

LeDoux, J. E. (2002). *Synaptic self: How our brains become who we are*. New York: Viking.

LeDoux, J. E. (2008). Emotional colouration of consciousness: How feelings come about. In L. Weiskrantz & M. Davies (Eds.), *Frontiers of consciousness: Chichele lectures* (pp. 69–130). Oxford, UK: Oxford University Press.

LeDoux, J. E. (2012). Rethinking the emotional brain. *Neuron, 73,* 653 –676.

LeDoux, J. E. (2013). The slippery slope of fear. *Trends in Cognitive Sciences, 17,* 155–156.

LeDoux, J. E. (2014). Coming to terms with fear. *Proceedings of the National Academy of Sciences USA,.111,* 2871–2877.

Papez, J. W. (1937). A proposed mechanism of emotion. *Archives of Neurology and Psychiatry, 79,* 217 –224.

Schachter, S. (1975). Cognition and centralist–peripheralist controversies in motivation and emotion. In M. S. Gazzaniga & C. B. Blakemore (Eds.), *Handbook of psychobiology* (pp. 529–564). New York: Academic Press.

Index

An *f* following a page number indicates a figure;
n following a page number indicates a note;
t following a page number indicates a table.